MR in the Emergency Room

Editors

JOHN CONKLIN
MICHAEL H. LEV

MAGNETIC RESONANCE IMAGING CLINICS OF NORTH AMERICA

www.mri.theclinics.com

Consulting Editors
SURESH K. MUKHERJI
LYNNE S. STEINBACH

August 2022 • Volume 30 • Number 3

ELSEVIER

1600 John F. Kennedy Boulevard ● Suite 1800 ● Philadelphia, Pennsylvania, 19103-2899

http://www.mri.theclinics.com

MAGNETIC RESONANCE IMAGING CLINICS OF NORTH AMERICA Volume 30, Number 3
August 2022 ISSN 1064-9689, ISBN 13: 978-0-323-84932-6

Editor: John Vassallo (j.vassallo@elsevier.com)
Developmental Editor: Arlene Campos

Magnetic Resonance Imaging Clinics of North America (ISSN 1064-9689) is published quarterly by Elsevier Inc., 360 Park Avenue South, New York, NY 10010-1710. Months of issue are February, May, August, and November. Business and Editorial Offices: 1600 John F. Kennedy Blvd., Ste. 1800, Philadelphia, PA 19103-2899. Customer Service Office: 3251 Riverport Lane, Maryland Heights, MO 63043. Periodicals postage paid at New York, NY and additional mailing offices. Subscription prices are $408.00 per year (domestic individuals), $1053.00 per year (domestic institutions), $100.00 per year (domestic students/residents), $455.00 per year (Canadian individuals), $1069.00 per year (Canadian institutions), $573.00 per year (international individuals), $1069.00 per year (international institutions), $100.00 per year (Canadian students/residents), and $275.00 per year (international students/residents). International air speed delivery is included in all *Clinics* subscription prices. All prices are subject to change without notice. **POSTMASTER:** Send address changes to *Magnetic Resonance Imaging Clinics*, Elsevier Health Sciences Division, Subscription Customer Service, 3251 Riverport Lane, Maryland Heights, MO 63043. Customer Service (orders, claims, online, change of address): Elsevier Health Sciences Division, Subscription **Customer Service, 3251 Riverport Lane, Maryland Heights, MO 63043. Tel:1-800-654-2452 (U.S. and Canada); 314-447-8871 (outside U.S. and Canada). Fax: 314-447-8029. E-mail: journalscustomerservice-usa@elsevier.com (for print support); journalsonlinesupport-usa@elsevier.com (for online support).**

Reprints. For copies of 100 or more of articles in this publication, please contact the Commercial Reprints Department, Elsevier Inc., 360 Park Avenue South, New York, NY 10010-1710. Tel.: 212-633-3874; Fax: 212-633-3820; E-mail: reprints@elsevier.com.

Magnetic Resonance Imaging Clinics of North America is covered in the *RSNA Index of Imaging Literature, MEDLINE/PubMed (Index Medicus),* and *EMBASE/Excerpta Medica.*

Contributors

CONSULTING EDITORS

SURESH K. MUKHERJI, MD, MBA, FACR
Clinical Professor of Radiology and Radiation
Oncology, University of Illinois, Peoria, Illinois;
Robert Wood Johnson Medical School,
Rutgers University, New Brunswick, New
Jersey; Faculty, Otolaryngology–Head Neck
Surgery, Michigan State University,
Farmington Hills, Michigan; National Director of

Head and Neck Radiology, ProScan Imaging,
Carmel, Indiana, USA

LYNNE S. STEINBACH, MD, FACR
Emeritus Professor of Radiology on Full Recall,
Department of Radiology and Biomedical
Imaging, University of California, San
Francisco, San Francisco, California, USA

EDITORS

JOHN CONKLIN, MD, MS
Assistant Professor of Radiology, Harvard
Medical School, Director of Emergency MRI
and Emergency Radiology QA, Department of
Radiology, Massachusetts General Hospital,
Boston, Massachusetts, USA

MICHAEL H. LEV, MD
Professor of Radiology, Harvard Medical
School, Director of Emergency Radiology and
Emergency Neuroradiology, Department of
Radiology, Massachusetts General Hospital,
Boston, Massachusetts, USA

AUTHORS

LAURA AVERY, MD
Department of Radiology, Massachusetts
General Hospital, Boston, Massachusetts,
USA

KAREN BUCH, MD
Department of Radiology, Massachusetts
General Hospital and Harvard Medical School,
Boston, Massachusetts, USA

DAVID D.B. BATES, MD
Department of Radiology, Assistant Professor,
Cornell University, Memorial Sloan Kettering
Cancer Center, New York, New York, USA

PAUL M. BUNCH, MD
Department of Radiology, Wake Forest School
of Medicine, Winston-Salem, North Carolina,
USA

SANJEEV BHALLA, MD
Mallinckrodt Institute of Radiology,
Washington University School of Medicine, St
Louis, Missouri, USA

GARIMA CHANDRA, MD
Research Assistant, Department of Radiology,
Massachusetts General Hospital, Boston,
Massachusetts, USA

KHYATI BIDANI, MD
Research Assistant, Department of Radiology,
Massachusetts General Hospital, Boston,
Massachusetts, USA

HAILEY CHANG, MD
Department of Radiology, Radiology Resident,
Boston Medical Center, Boston,
Massachusetts, USA

JOHN CONKLIN, MD, MS
Assistant Professor of Radiology, Harvard
Medical School, Director of Emergency MRI
and Emergency Radiology QA, Department of
Radiology, Massachusetts General Hospital,
Boston, Massachusetts, USA

JORGE DELGADO, MD
Division of MSK Radiology, Massachusetts
General Hospital, Harvard Medical School,
Boston, Massachusetts, USA

RUHANI DODA KHERA, MD, MBA
Department of Radiology, Massachusetts
General Hospital and Harvard Medical School,
Boston, Massachusetts, USA

MARIA GABRIELA FIGUEIRO LONGO, MD
Division of Pediatric Radiology, Massachusetts
General Hospital, Harvard Medical School,
Boston, Massachusetts, USA

DAMIEN GALANAUD, MD, PhD
Department of Neuroradiology, Pitié
Salpêtrière Hospital, Boulevard de l'Hôpital,
Paris, France

MICHAEL S. GEE, MD, PhD
Division of Pediatric Radiology, Massachusetts
General Hospital, Harvard Medical School,
Boston, Massachusetts, USA

**RAMON GILBERTO GONZÁLEZ, MD, PhD,
FACR**
Professor and Neuroradiology Chief, Emeritus,
Division of Neuroradiology, Department of
Radiology, Massachusetts General Hospital,
Boston, USA

AVNEESH GUPTA, MD
Department of Radiology, Clinical Associate
Professor, Boston Medical Center, Boston,
Massachusetts, USA

RAJIV GUPTA, MD, PhD
Department of Radiology, Massachusetts
General Hospital, Boston, Massachusetts,
USA

JOSHUA A. HIRSCH, MD
Department of Radiology, Massachusetts
General Hospital and Harvard Medical School,
Neuro-Interventional Radiology,
Massachusetts General Hospital, Boston,
Massachusetts, USA

SUSIE HUANG, MD, PhD
Associate Professor of Radiology, Harvard
Medical School, Department of Radiology,
Massachusetts General Hospital, Boston,
Massachusetts, USA; Athinoula A. Martinos
Center for Biomedical Imaging, Charleston,
Massachusetts, USA

CAMILO JAIMES, MD
Department of Radiology, Boston Children's
Hospital, Harvard Medical School, Boston,
Massachusetts, USA

DOUGLAS S. KATZ, MD
Department of Radiology, NYU Langone
Hospital, Mineola, New York, USA

HILLARY R. KELLY, MD
Department of Radiology, Massachusetts
General Hospital, Department of Radiology,
Massachusetts Eye and Ear, Harvard Medical
School, Boston, Massachusetts, USA

BHARTI KHURANA, MD
Staff Radiologist, Division of Emergency
Radiology, Brigham and Women's Hospital,
Founder and Director, Trauma Imaging
Research and Innovation Center, Associate
Professor, Harvard Medical School, Boston,
Massachusetts, USA

MIN LANG, MD
Clinical Fellow in Radiology, Harvard Medical
School, Department of Radiology,
Massachusetts General Hospital, Boston,
Massachusetts, USA

CHRISTINA A. LEBEDIS, MD
Associate Professor, Department of Radiology,
Boston Medical Center, Boston, Massachusetts
USA

MICHAEL H. LEV, MD
Professor of Radiology, Harvard Medical
School, Director of Emergency Radiology and
Emergency Neuroradiology, Department of
Radiology, Massachusetts General Hospital,
Boston, Massachusetts, USA

MEGAN E. LIPFORD, PhD
Department of Radiology, Wake Forest School of
Medicine, Winston-Salem, North Carolina, USA

DANIEL R. LUDWIG, MD
Mallinckrodt Institute of Radiology,
Washington University School of Medicine, St
Louis, Missouri, USA

FEDEL MACHADO, MD
Department of Radiology, Boston Children's
Hospital, Harvard Medical School, Boston,
Massachusetts, USA

JACOB C. MANDELL, MD
Fellowship Director, Musculoskeletal Imaging
and Intervention, Staff Radiologist, Division of
Musculoskeletal Radiology, Assistant
Professor, Harvard Medical School, Brigham
and Women's Hospital, Boston,
Massachusetts, USA

JEANNETTE MATHIEU, MD
Department of Radiology and Biomedical
Imaging, UCSF and Zuckerberg San Francisco
General Hospital, San Francisco, California,
USA

MARIAM MOSHIRI, MD
Department of Radiology, Vanderbilt University
Medical Center, Nashville, Tennessee, USA

MICHAEL N. PATLAS, MD, FRCPC
Department of Radiology, McMaster
University, Hamilton General Hospital,
Hamilton, Ontario, Canada

RUBAL RAI, MD
Research Assistant, Department of Radiology,
Massachusetts General Hospital, Boston,
Massachusetts, USA

OTTO RAPALINO, MD
Assistant Professor of Radiology, Harvard
Medical School, Department of Radiology,
Massachusetts General Hospital, Boston,
Massachusetts, USA

CONSTANTINE A. RAPTIS, MD
Mallinckrodt Institute of Radiology,
Washington University School of Medicine, St
Louis, Missouri, USA

MARGARITA V. REVZIN, MD, MS
Department of Radiology and Biomedical
Imaging, Yale University, New Haven,
Connecticut, USA

JEFFREY R. SACHS, MD
Department of Radiology, Wake Forest School
of Medicine, Winston-Salem, North Carolina,
USA

SANJAY SAINI, MD, MBA
Department of Radiology, Massachusetts
General Hospital and Harvard Medical School,
Boston, Massachusetts, USA

AJAY KUMAR SINGH, MD
Assistant Professor, Department of Emergency
Radiology, Massachusetts General Hospital,
Boston, Massachusetts, USA

RAMANDEEP SINGH, MD
Clinical Fellow, Department of Emergency
Radiology, Massachusetts General Hospital,
Boston, Massachusetts, USA

ABIGAIL D. STANLEY, BM
OMS III, NYIT College of Osteopathic
Medicine, Old Westbury, Glen Head, New
York, USA

JASON F. TALBOTT, MD, PhD
Associate Professor in Residence, Department
of Radiology and Biomedical Imaging,
UCSF and Zuckerberg San Francisco
General Hospital, Brain and Spinal Injury
Center, Zuckerberg San Francisco
General Hospital, San Francisco, California,
USA

MILTIADIS TEMBELIS, MD
Department of Radiology, NYU Langone
Hospital, Mineola, New York, USA

LAWRENCE L. WALD, PhD
Professor of Radiology, Harvard Medical
School, Department of Radiology,
Massachusetts General Hospital, Boston,
Massachusetts, USA; Athinoula A. Martinos
Center for Biomedical Imaging, Charleston,
Massachusetts, USA

BRIAN WELLS, MD, MS, MPH
Department of Radiology, Brigham and
Women's Hospital, Boston, Massachusetts,
USA

THOMAS G. WEST, MD
Department of Radiology, Wake Forest School
of Medicine, Winston-Salem, North Carolina,
USA

Contents

> The role of MR imaging in the evaluation and management of ischemic stroke pa-
> tients is large, and to cover it all is far beyond the scope of one article. Thus, the
> focus will be on the role of MR imaging in the great leap forward in stroke therapy:
> endovascular thrombectomy of large vessel occlusions (LVOs). Diffusion MR imag-
> ing has played a key role in the research leading to the current standard of care for
> LVO stroke because it is the most sensitive and reliable method for the early delin-
> eation of the ischemic core.

> Although evaluation of suspected stroke is a major driver of MRI use in the emer-
> gency department (ED), the exquisite contrast resolution and flexibility provided
> by MRI are valuable in the workup of a broad variety of acute neurologic complaints.
> This article provides an overview, focused primarily on "non-stroke" neurologic
> emergencies encountered in ED brain MRI that emergency radiologists should be
> familiar with.

> This article is devoted to the MR imaging evaluation of spine emergencies, defined
> as spinal pathologic conditions that pose an immediate risk of significant morbidity
> or mortality to the patient if not diagnosed and treated in a timely manner. MR imag-
> ing plays a central role in the timely diagnosis of spine emergencies. A summary of
> MR imaging indications and MR imaging protocols tailored for a variety of spinal
> emergencies will be presented followed by a review of key imaging findings for
> the most-encountered emergent spine pathologic conditions. Pathologic conditions
> will be broadly grouped into traumatic and atraumatic pathologic conditions. For
> traumatic injuries, a practical and algorithmic diagnostic approach based on the
> AO Spine injury classification system will be presented focused on subaxial spine
> trauma. Atraumatic spinal emergencies will be dichotomized into compressive
> and noncompressive subtypes. The location of external compressive disease with
> respect to the thecal sac is fundamental to establishing a differential diagnosis for
> compressive emergencies, whereas specific patterns of spinal cord involvement
> on MR imaging will guide the discussion of inflammatory and noninflammatory
> causes of noncompressive myelopathy.

Use of magnetic resonance (MR) imaging in the emergency department continues to increase. Although computed tomography is the first-line imaging modality for most head and neck emergencies, MR is superior in some situations and imparts no ionizing radiation. This article provides a symptom-based approach to nontraumatic head and neck pathologic conditions most relevant to emergency head and neck MR imaging, emphasizing relevant anatomy, "do not miss" findings affecting clinical management, and features that may aid differentiation from potential mimics. Essential MR sequences and strategies for obtaining high-quality images when faced with patient motion and other technical challenges are also discussed.

The use of magnetic resonance (MR) imaging in the emergency department continues to increase. Although computed tomography is the first-line imaging modality for most head and neck emergencies, MR is superior in some situations and imparts no ionizing radiation. This article provides a symptom-based approach to nontraumatic head and neck pathologic conditions most relevant to emergency head and neck MR imaging, emphasizing relevant anatomy, "do not miss" findings affecting clinical management, and features that may aid differentiation from potential mimics. Essential MR sequences and strategies for obtaining high-quality images when faced with patient motion and other technical challenges are also discussed.

MR is often the most definitive imaging for assessment of musculoskeletal trauma and infection. Although it is not possible to address all the intricacies of these complex topics in a single article, this review will attempt to provide a useful toolbox of skills by discussing several common clinical scenarios faced by emergency radiologists in interpretation of adult trauma and infection. These scenarios include MR assessment of hip and pelvic fracture, traumatic soft tissue injuries, septic arthritis, soft tissue infection, and osteomyelitis.

As a complement to computed tomography and ultrasound for the emergency evaluation of penile and scrotal trauma, MR imaging provides unique advantages and anatomic delineation in the acute care setting. Rapid recognition of traumatic injuries helps guide appropriate clinical and surgical care to prevent long-term comorbidities. It is important for the radiologist to understand and identify these findings to optimize patient care in the emergency setting.

Thoracoabdominal and peripheral vasculature pathologies include a variety of severe and life threatening conditions that may be encountered in the emergent setting. Computed tomography angiography (CTA) is the first-line modality for imaging of the vasculature in this context, but magnetic resonance angiography (MRA) also plays an important and emerging role in the evaluation of carefully selected patients. Intravenous (IV) iodinated contrast is necessary for CTA, although MRA is most useful in patients who cannot receive IV iodinated contrast for reasons including prior severe allergic-like reaction to iodinated contrast, poor IV access, or severe renal insufficiency. Gadolinium-based contrast agents are administered for MRA when possible, as they generally improve the diagnostic quality and shorten the duration of the exam. In most clinical situations, however, noncontrast MRA is sufficient to obtain a diagnostic evaluation. In this review, we discuss the key strengths and limitations of MRA performed in the emergent setting, highlighting the role of MRA in the diagnosis of acute aortic syndromes, aortitis, aortic aneurysm, pulmonary embolism, and peripheral vascular disease.

This article presents the MR protocols, imaging features, diagnostic criteria, and complications of commonly encountered emergencies in pancreaticobiliary imaging, which include pancreatic trauma, bile leak, acute cholecystitis, biliary obstruction, and pancreatitis. Various classifications and complications that can arise with these conditions, as well as artifacts that may mimic pathology, are also included. Finally, the emerging utility of abbreviated MR protocols is discussed.

While computed tomography (CT) offers faster cross-sectional imaging in the emergency department, owing to its concerns for higher radiation exposure, magnetic resonance imaging (MRI) applications in acute settings are increasingly validated. A significant proportion of patients present to the emergency department with abdominopelvic symptoms, most commonly acute abdominal pain. Early detection with imaging and timely intervention can significantly decrease morbidity and mortality in conditions such as acute pancreatitis or ovarian torsion. MRI encompasses better soft-tissue resolution, nonusage of ionizing radiation and iodinated contrast media, nonoperator dependency, and higher reproducibility. This review discusses the MRI protocols and applications in abdominopelvic emergencies.

Evaluation of a pregnant patient presenting with acute abdominal pain can be challenging to accurately diagnose for a variety of reasons, and particularly late in pregnancy. Noncontrast MR remains a safe and accurate diagnostic imaging modality for the pregnant patient presenting with acute abdominal pain, following often an initially inconclusive ultrasound examination, and can be used in most settings to avoid the ionizing radiation exposure of a computed tomography scan. Pathologic processes discussed in this article include some of the more common gastrointestinal, hepatobiliary, genitourinary, and gynecologic causes of abdominal pain occurring in pregnancy, as well as traumatic injuries.

MAGNETIC RESONANCE IMAGING CLINICS OF NORTH AMERICA

SERIES OF RELATED INTEREST

Advances in Clinical Radiology
Neurologic Clinics
PET Clinics
Radiologic Clinics

VISIT THE CLINICS ONLINE!
Access your subscription at:
www.theclinics.com

MAGNETIC RESONANCE IMAGING CLINICS OF NORTH AMERICA

FORTHCOMING ISSUES

November 2022
Postoperative Joint MR Imaging
Luis Beltran, Editor

February 2023
MR Imaging of the Ankle
Cora B. Stein and Kim L. Sheppard, Editors

May 2023
Musculoskeletal MRI-Ultrasound Correlation
Jan Fritz

RECENT ISSUES

May 2022
MR Imaging of the Knee
Mary K. Jesse

February 2022
MR Imaging of Head and Neck Cancer
Ahmed Abdel Khalek Abdel Razek, Editor

November 2021
Pediatric Neuroimaging, State-of-the-Art
Mai-Lan Ho, Editor

PROGRAM OBJECTIVE

The goal of *Magnetic Resonance Imaging Clinics of North America* is to keep practicing physicians up to date with current clinical practice by providing timely articles reviewing the state of the art in patient care.

TARGET AUDIENCE

All practicing physicians and healthcare professionals who provide patient care utilizing findings from Magnetic Resonance Imaging.

LEARNING OBJECTIVES

Upon completion of this activity, participants will be able to:
1. Review the role, indications, protocols, and diagnostic applications of MRI in the emergency room as a first-line modality for assessment and evaluation.
2. Discuss the appropriate use of MRI based on clinical presentation in the emergency room, taking into account strengths, limitations, safety, protocols, and consent.
3. Recognize the importance of using MRI and its features in the evaluation and diagnosis of emergencies to reduce the risk of morbidity and mortality in patients.

ACCREDITATION

The Elsevier Office of Continuing Medical Education (EOCME) is accredited by the Accreditation Council for Continuing Medical Education (ACCME) to provide continuing medical education for physicians.

The EOCME designates this journal-based CME activity enduring material for a maximum of 14 *AMA PRA Category 1 Credit*(s)™. Physicians should claim only the credit commensurate with the extent of their participation in the activity.

All other healthcare professionals requesting continuing education credit for this enduring material will be issued a certificate of participation.

DISCLOSURE OF CONFLICTS OF INTEREST

The EOCME assesses conflict of interest with its instructors, faculty, planners, and other individuals who are in a position to control the content of CME activities. All relevant conflicts of interest that are identified are thoroughly vetted by EOCME for fair balance, scientific objectivity, and patient care recommendations. EOCME is committed to providing its learners with CME activities that promote improvements or quality in healthcare and not a specific proprietary business or a commercial interest.

The planning committee, staff, authors, and editors listed below have identified no financial relationships or relationships to products or devices they or their spouse/life partner have with commercial interest related to the content of this CME activity:

Laura Avery, MD; David D.B. Bates, MD; Sanjeev Bhalla, MD; Khyati Bidani; Karen Buch, MD; Paul M. Bunch, MD; Garima Chandra; Hailey Chang, MD; Jorge Delgado, MD; Ruhani Doda Khera, MD, MBA; Maria Gabriela Figueiro Longo, MD; Damien Galanaud, MD, PhD; Michael S. Gee, MD, PhD; R. Gilberto González, MD, PhD, FACR; Avneesh Gupta, MD; Joshua A. Hirsch, MD; Susie Huang, MD, PhD; Camilo Jaimes, MD; Douglas S. Katz, MD; Bharti Khurana, MD; Pradeep Kuttysankaran; Min Lang, MD; Christina A. LeBedis, MD; Michael H. Lev, MD; Megan E. Lipford, PhD; Daniel R. Ludwig, MD; Fedel Machado Rivas; Jacob C. Mandell, MD; Jeannette Mathieu, MD; Mariam Moshiri, MD; Michael N. Patlas, MD, FRCPC; Rubal Rai, MD; Otto Rapalino, MD; Constantine A. Raptis, MD; Margarita V. Revzin, MD, MS; Jeffrey R. Sachs, MD; Sanjay Saini, MD, MBA; Ramandeep Singh, MD; Ajay Kumar Singh, MD; Abigail D. Stanley, OMS III; Jason F. Talbott, MD, PhD; Miltiadis Tembelis, MD; Doreen Thomas-Payne, MSN, BSN, RN, PMHNP-BC; Brian Wells, MD, MS, MPH; Thomas G. West, MD

The planning committee, staff, authors and editors listed below have identified financial relationships or relationships to products or devices they or their spouse/life partner have with commercial interest related to the content of this CME activity:

John Conklin, MD, MS: *Researcher*: Siemens Healthineers

Rajiv Gupta, MD, PhD: *Consultant/Advisor*: Braintale, Idorsia Pharmaceuticals US Inc., Stryker; *Speaker*: Siemens Medical Solutions USA Inc.; *Researcher*: Samsung

Hillary R. Kelly, MD: *Researcher*: Bayer AG

Lawrence L. Wald, PhD: *Researcher*: Siemens Healthineers; *Consultant and Ownership Interest*: Neuro42 Inc.

UNAPPROVED/OFF-LABEL USE DISCLOSURE

The EOCME requires CME faculty to disclose to the participants:
1. When products or procedures being discussed are off-label, unlabelled, experimental, and/or investigational (not US Food and Drug Administration [FDA] approved); and
2. Any limitations on the information presented, such as data that are preliminary or that represent ongoing research, interim analyses, and/or unsupported opinions. Faculty may discuss information about pharmaceutical agents that is outside of FDA-approved labelling. This information is intended solely for CME and is not intended to promote off-label use of these

medications. If you have any questions, contact the medical affairs department of the manufacturer for the most recent pre-scribing information.

TO ENROLL

To enroll in the *Magnetic Resonance Imaging Clinics of North America* Continuing Medical Education program, call customer service at 1-800-654-2452 or sign up online at http://www.theclinics.com/home/cme. The CME program is available to sub-scribers for an additional annual fee of USD 281.00.

METHOD OF PARTICIPATION

In order to claim credit, participants must complete the following:

1. Complete enrolment as indicated above.
2. Read the activity.
3. Complete the CME Test and Evaluation. Participants must achieve a score of 70% on the test. All CME Tests and Evalua-tions must be completed online.

CME INQUIRIES/SPECIAL NEEDS

For all CME inquiries or special needs, please contact elsevierCME@elsevier.com.

Foreword

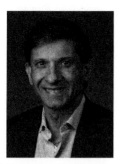

Suresh K. Mukherji, MD, MBA, FACR
Consulting Editor

"You want to order a what?... Why do you need an MRI performed on a patient from the emergency room?".... This was the common reply when I was a resident and junior faculty when a request was made for an emergent MRI from the ER, ...which was really not that long ago... ☺. Well, ...times have certainly changed, and the utilization of MR ordered from the emergency room has substantially increased with many institutions now installing MRI units in the ER.

There are numerous indications for performing MR in the emergency room setting, and this rapid expansion of utilization was the reason we decided to devote an issue to "MR in the ER." We are very fortunate to have Drs John Conklin and Michael Lev guest edit this important issue. The articles cover technique, indications, and common pathologic conditions that can be expected from emergent neuroradiology, musculoskeletal, thoracic, gastrointestinal, genitourinary, and pediatric imaging studies. The articles emphasize the key elements that should be included in the report and how this information will affect treatment and management.

I would also like to acknowledge the article authors for their wonderful contributions. All are recognized experts in their fields, and their content and image quality are superb. Finally, I again want to thank Drs Conklin and Lev. They have done a masterful job in creating this important issue, which will become an essential reference for many years to come!

Suresh K. Mukherji, MD, MBA, FACR
University of Illinois & ProScan Imaging
Carmel, IN 46074, USA

E-mail address:
sureshmukherji@hotmail.com

Magn Reson Imaging Clin N Am 30 (2022) xv
https://doi.org/10.1016/j.mric.2022.06.009
1064-9689/22/© 2022 Published by Elsevier Inc.

Preface

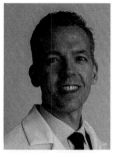 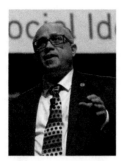

John Conklin, MD Michael H. Lev, MD

Editors

All significant medical advances ultimately depend on advances in technology, extending the sensitivity of the MD's eyes, ears, and fingers
—Robert H. Ackerman, MD, MPH, 2015

In a 2001 Medscape survey, physicians were asked to rank the 30 most important, impactful medical innovations of the prior 25 years; computed tomography (CT) and MR imaging were ranked number 1, at the top of this list. Indeed, since the invention of the stethoscope in 1816, technological developments have continued at an ever-increasing pace to enhance the ability of health care providers to diagnose, treat, and manage diverse diseases. The potential of imaging to noninvasively evaluate anatomy and physiology in living human patients was recognized from the outset, as underscored by the only 50 days between Wilhelm Conrad Röntgen's initial observation of X rays on November 8, 1895 and his provisional communication of this seminal discovery, "On a new kind of rays," in the *Proceedings of the Würzburg Physico-Medical Society* on December 28, 1895, for which he was awarded the first Nobel Prize in Physics 5 years later in 1901.[1]

It would be another 70 years until it became possible to reconstruct cross-sectional images from X rays using CT; the first CT scan was performed at Atkinson Morley Hospital, London, in 1971, for a patient with a brain tumor. By 1973, commercial head CT scanners manufactured by EMI (the record label for *The Beatles*) were being installed in Great Britain, as well as at the Mayo Clinic and Massachusetts General Hospital in the United States. Allan M. Cormack and Godfrey N. Hounsfield shared the Nobel Prize in Medicine for the development of CT in 1979.

The development of nuclear magnetic resonance scanning (NMR, soon renamed magnetic resonance imaging) quickly followed. Although the mathematical basis for MR imaging's use of magnetic field gradients to determine spatial localization and methods for fast gradient switching was introduced as early as 1973 by Paul Lauterbur and Peter Mansfield, respectively, it was not until 2003 that they shared the Nobel Prize in Medicine for the conception and development of MR imaging. Interestingly, one of Lauterbur's early Nobel Prize quality papers, "Image formation by induced local interactions: examples of employing nuclear magnetic resonance," was initially rejected by the journal *Science*.[2] Some of the first MR images of a human brain were obtained in 1978 at the Research Laboratories of Thorn EMI Ltd. Alfidi and colleagues suggested in 1982 that 3-dimensional images of blood vessels might be possible using MR imaging, and in 1985, Van Wedeen and colleagues published the first "modern" report of techniques for MR angiography (MRA) of the head and neck.[3]

In this issue of *Magnetic Resonance Imaging Clinics of North America*, we discuss emergency room applications of MR imaging. The authors, who run the spectrum from up and coming to established leaders in their respective areas of

Magn Reson Imaging Clin N Am 30 (2022) xvii–xix
https://doi.org/10.1016/j.mric.2022.05.001
1064-9689/22/© 2022 Published by Elsevier Inc.

mri.theclinics.com

expertise, have done a wonderful job. There is some overlap between authors as they review related topics from different perspectives, which benefit a field in this stage of its development. Certain recurrent themes emerge from the outset; foremost among these are the needs for (i) speed, (ii) accuracy, and (iii) safety.

Not only is speed important for issues of emergency department (ED) overcrowding and reducing acquisition/interpretation turn-around time (TAT), but also could be associated with improved patient access and hence greater patient satisfaction. Fast scanning is certainly fundamental to current efforts in minimizing TAT, and in the future, portable MR imaging scanning may play a role as well (see the chapter "Emerging Techniques and Future Directions: Ultrafast MRI and Portable MRI"). Speed, accuracy (eg, spatial and contrast resolution, artifact reduction), and safety (eg, metallic devices, sedation) all involve tradeoffs, including issues of cost for both patients and payors (eg, number of imaging slots per hour, number of sequences per imaging slot); efficient ED scanning has the potential to reduce the frequency of visits for follow-up imaging and primary care. Regarding safety, 1.5-T scanners might be preferable for embedded ED use compared with 3-T scanners, given the potential for more frequent patient exclusions owing to untested, conditional devices at higher field strengths (see the chapter "Safety, Consent, and Regulatory Considerations").

Specific indications for ED MR imaging scanning matter: when is an MR exam required in the ED, and when is it appropriate to wait for a nonemergent, outpatient scan? The top indications for ED MR imaging are well covered in the subsequent articles and include but are not limited to the following:

1. *Neurologic emergencies*: Vascular, infection, trauma; sequences such as diffusion-weighted imaging (for acute stroke detection), susceptibility-weighted imaging (for microbleed detection), and MRA (for occlusion, critical stenosis detection), are typically important for urgent assessments, whereas perfusion, spectroscopy, and functional MR imaging sequences are less relevant.
   Stroke (Article 1)
   Trauma (Article 2)
   Spine (Article 3)
   Head & neck (Articles 4, 5)
2. *Musculoskeletal emergencies*: More sensitive than X ray or CT for hip fracture detection, infection; otherwise, typically more limited value for acute trauma compared with CT.
   Osteomyelitis (Article 6)
   Hip fracture detection
3. *Liver, gallbladder, bile ducts*: Magnetic resonance cholangiopancreatography; also, penile and scrotal MR imaging less commonly required but can provide more accurate assessment than ultrasound or CT, especially for surgical decisions.
   Hepatobiliary (Article 9)
   Penile / scrotal (Article 7)
4. *Pediatrics and pregnancy*: In these cohorts, where X ray and CT radiation dose should be minimized, MR imaging can provide primary screening.
   Pediatric appendicitis (Article 12)
   Other Gastrointestinal / Genitourinary emergencies (Article 10)
   Obstetrical emergencies (Article 11)
5. *Thoracic emergencies*: Primarily for vascular indications, especially when iodinated CT contrast is contraindicated (eg, history of anaphylaxis); rarely, to rule out pulmonary embolus.
   Aorta evaluation (Article 8)

In conclusion, knowledge of emergency MR imaging indications, pearls, and pitfalls is timely and important, especially in the setting of pregnancy, pediatrics, soft tissue infection, neurologic emergencies, or when iodinated CT contrast is contraindicated. When protocoling, monitoring, or interpreting an emergency MR imaging exam, radiologists should consider the following: (1) What are the critical details from the history and physical exam required to address the clinical question being asked (ie, the "reason for study"); (2) What added value does MR imaging provide, over that of CT, ultrasound, or plain film X rays; and (3) what does the referring provider "need to know," what essential information needs to be included in the report impression, and how will these results change the differential diagnosis, treatment, disposition, or management plan?

Our sincere thanks go to our consulting editors, Drs Suresh K. Mukherji and Lynne S. Steinbach, for inviting us to participate in this *Magnetic Resonance Imaging Clinics of North America* series. We would also like to both acknowledge and thank our authors, the many colleagues, trainees, and friends, who did a phenomenal job in highlighting the essentials of often-nuanced topics. Finally, our heartfelt thanks to our wives, Hyesun Park, MD and Julie M. Goodman, PhD, respectively, for all that they have done to make this work possible.

This issue is dedicated to Bertram Lev (1929–2021).

John Conklin, MD
Director of ED MRI and ED Radiology QA
Massachusetts General Hospital
Harvard Medical School
55 Fruit Street, Boston, MA 02114, USA

Michael H. Lev, MD
Director of Emergency Radiology and
Emergency Neuroradiology
Department of Radiology
Massachusetts General Hospital
Harvard Medical School
55 Fruit Street, Boston, MA 02114, USA

E-mail addresses:
john.conklin@mgh.harvard.edu (J. Conklin)
mlev@partners.org (M.H. Lev)

REFERENCES

1. Röntgen WC. On a new kind of rays. Science 1896; 3(59):227–31.
2. Lauterbur P. Image Formation by Induced Local Interactions: Examples Employing Nuclear Magnetic Resonance. Nature 1973;242(1973):190–1.
3. Wedeen VJ, Meuli RA, Edelman RR, et al. Projective imaging of pulsatile flow with magnetic resonance. Science 1985;230:946–8.

Diffusion MR Imaging of Large Vessel Occlusion Ischemic Stroke for Treatment Selection

Ramon Gilberto González, MD, PhD, FACR

KEYWORDS

• MR imaging • Diffusion • Stroke • Large vessel occlusion • Thrombectomy

KEY POINTS

- Thrombectomy for large vessel occlusions in patients with a major ischemic stroke syndrome has been the most important neurologic therapeutic advance since decades, and making it widely available promises a substantial reduction of major morbidity and death due to stroke.
- Advanced imaging is a key to making this possible in patients treated after 6 hours post-ictus through its ability to estimate the size of the core.
- A higher proportion of favorable outcomes and fewer futile thrombectomies are achieved by using diffusion weighted imaging (DWI) rather than CT perfusion (CTP) because of the higher precision of the former.
- Studies on the dynamics of ischemic core growth indicate that up to half of LVO patients are slow progressors who may be treated up to 24 hours after stroke onset because the ischemic core remains small. These slow progressors may be identified by core measurement by advanced imaging, especially DWI.

HISTORICAL BACKGROUND: FROM TIME IS BRAIN TO PHYSIOLOGIC TIME IS BRAIN

For the treatment of acute ischemic stroke, the goal of thrombectomy is the removal of the thrombus causing a large vessel occlusion (LVO) of the anterior circulation to stop the growth of the ischemic core and maintain it at a size that safeguards a favorable clinical outcome. **Fig. 1** illustrates the basic physiology of acute ischemic stroke of a patient with an occlusion of the M1 segment of the right middle cerebral artery. The irreversibly injured brain (the ischemic core) may be small at first but may grow if the occlusion persists. The rate of growth is highly variable and depends on the strength of the collateral circulation. Some patients have cores that grow rapidly, but many, possibly the majority, have cores that remain small for 24 hours or longer because the collateral circulation is robust.

Previously, a commonly held assumption was that core growth rates in different people were similar and that time was an adequate surrogate for ischemic core size. This assumption is incorrect. Early research on the use of imaging to guide endovascular therapy suggested that visualization of the relevant physiology was a better guide than time.[1,2] More recently, analyses of many prospective thrombectomy trials have confirmed that individual physiology varies widely. The common refrain "time is brain" has evolved to "physiologic time is brain."[3] According to the current American Heart Association Guidelines, the role of imaging is vital, although in patients treated within 6 hours of ictus, only a simple CT scan to exclude hemorrhage is needed. However, in patients beyond 6 hours or with an unknown time of onset, advanced imaging is essential. This is important because most potential patients will be outside the 6-hour threshold.

Division of Neuroradiology, Department of Radiology, Massachusetts General Hospital, 55 Fruit Street, GRB 273A, Boston, MA 02114, USA
E-mail address: RGGONZALEZ@mgh.harvard.edu

Magn Reson Imaging Clin N Am 30 (2022) 363–369
https://doi.org/10.1016/j.mric.2022.04.003
1064-9689/22/Published by Elsevier Inc.

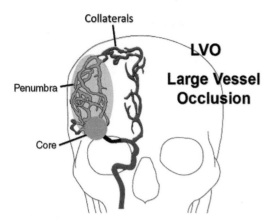

Fig. 1. Basic large vessel occlusion physiology. (*Adapted from* Chapter 2 Figure 2.5 of the book Acute Ischemic Stroke: Imaging and Intervention published by Springer.)

BASELINE CORE VOLUME AND CLINICAL OUTCOMES AFTER THROMBECTOMY

When advanced imaging is used for patient selection, the measurement of the core is essential; direct measurement of the penumbra is not necessary.[4] This was confirmed in the diffusion associated with neurointervention (DAWN) trial, whereby patients were selected if they had a small core and a clinical penumbra, that is, deficits that were unexplained by the core size.[5] This is physiologically reasonable. As shown in **Fig. 1**, the sizes of the core and penumbra are not independent but are linked by the collateral circulation. Thus, in the presence of an LVO, if the core is small, the penumbra is typically large and direct penumbra measurement is unnecessary as first suggested by Copen and colleagues.[4]

There is no single core volume threshold that separates patients with favorable or poor outcomes because of differences in the eloquence of the tissue at risk. For example, a 100 mL infarct in the left middle cerebral artery (MCA) territory may well result in severe paralysis and aphasia with the patient requiring life-long, intensive care. On the other hand, an infarct of 200 mL in the left posterior cerebral artery (PCA) territory may result in visual deficits, but the patient may live fully independently. The relationships between tissue eloquence, infarct size, and outcome were brilliantly illuminated by Boers and colleagues[6] in a meta-analysis of seven prospective thrombectomy trials (**Fig. 2**).

A 3-dimensional plot (see **Fig. 2**) of the probability of a favorable outcome with respect to baseline tissue [National Institutes of Health (NIH) Stroke Scale (NIHSS)] and follow-up infarct volume measured by MR imaging. The blue areas represent the conditions under which the patient has a low probability of a good outcome. Examination of the figure indicates that a patient with a low NIHSS score of 5 could sustain an infarct of 150 mL and still have a favorable outcome after thrombectomy. On the other hand, if the NIHSS is high, greater than 10, reflecting a threatened eloquent cortex, there is a sharp drop from a good to a low probability of favorable outcomes with increasing core size. For example, if someone has an NIHSS of 25, if the follow-up infarct volume is greater than 60 mL, the probability of a favorable outcome is very high. However, the same patient would have a low probability if the follow-up infarct volume is more than 80 mL. These data inform us that the therapeutic window with respect to the final infarct volume is small when the eloquent cortex is involved: a difference between a good and poor outcome may be because of an infarct volume difference of 20 to 30 mL. It is this narrow therapeutic window that requires that we measure the infarct core with high precision and accuracy when eloquence of the threatened brain region is significant.

CORE MEASUREMENT METHOD AND OUTCOMES AFTER THROMBECTOMY

There are four commonly used methods to estimate the size of the ischemic core, two are direct, and the others estimate the core indirectly. The most reliable and accurate method is diffusion MR imaging commonly known as DWI. Severe ischemia produces reduced diffusivity of water in the brain by mechanisms that are not fully understood. Reduced diffusivity is manifest within 30 minutes after the onset of severe ischemia. The other direct method is the identification of an ischemia-induced hypodensity on a non-contrast head computed tomography (CT). Ischemia produces increased local water content and is the physical basis of the hypodensity. However, this process takes hours because the amount of water increase must be greater than 1-2% before it is detectable. This makes non-contrast CT imaging unsuitable in most situations.

The two indirect methods most used to estimate ischemic core volume are CT perfusion and CTA collaterals. CTP is widely used, and it relies on the reduction of the relative cerebral blood volume or blood flow to estimate the core. Participants in nearly all published prospective thrombectomy studies used either CTP or DWI for patient selection. Meta-analysis of these prospective trials provides direct information on the relative efficacy of each method. The results from the Hermes collaboration are shown in **Table 1**.

Eloquence, Final Infarct Volume and 3 Month Outcomes

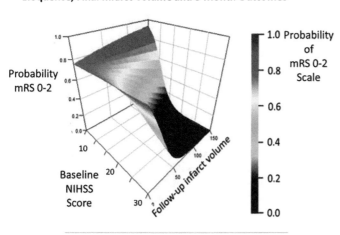

Fig. 2. Probability of a favorable outcome with respect to baseline core volume and baseline eloquence of tissue at risk (NIH Stroke Scale). (*Adapted from* Supplemental Figure 2B of Boers AMM, Jansen IGH, Beenen LFM, et al. Association of follow-up infarct volume with functional outcome in acute ischemic stroke: a pooled analysis of seven randomized trials. J Neurointerv Surg. 2018;10(12):1137-1142.)

The odds ratio for a favorable outcome in patients chosen for thrombectomy using CTP versus DWI was 0.49, meaning that the likelihood of a patient having a good outcome was a factor of 2 better if DWI was used rather than a CTP.[7] This effect was present even though patients selected with DWI, on average, were treated ½ hour later than those selected with CT. These results are best explained by the superior precision of DWI for core measurement: it is more effective in selecting patients more likely to benefit from thrombectomy and excluding those who are not.

Another potential outcome is futile thrombectomy. Futile thrombectomy occurs when the clot is successfully removed, but the patient does poorly. An example would be if the patient died, or from a patient's perspective, if they lived but they were bedridden, incontinent, and completely depend on others thereby being a burden to their family and society. This topic has been specifically examined by a group led by Thomas Meinel and Johannes Kaesmacher.[8] In 2011 patients, they analyzed the occurrence of futile thrombectomy defined as the 90-day modified Rankin Scale

(mRS) score of 4 to 6 despite successful recanalization in patients selected by MR imaging (n = 690) and CT (n = 1321). The results are shown in **Table 2** which clearly shows that CT selection for thrombectomy was associated with an increased risk of futile outcome compared with MR imaging selection. Again, the results are best explained by the superior precision of MR imaging: it more precisely identifies those who are unlikely to benefit from thrombectomy.

ISCHEMIC CORE DYNAMICS AND THROMBECTOMY: IDENTIFYING SLOW PROGRESSORS

Extensive literature to date confirms that baseline ischemic core size has a vital impact on the patient outcome when thrombectomy is considered. A related topic is the growth of the infarct core over time, ischemic core dynamics. This is important because most patients who may potentially benefit from thrombectomy may be situated many hours away from a center that can perform thrombectomy. The critical issue is whether the patient's ischemic core will be suitably small on arrival at a thrombectomy-capable center and such patients are identifiable at the first hospital

Table 1 CTP versus DWI odds ratio of functional independence after thrombectomy		
	OR (95% CI)	P Value
CTP vs DWI	0.49 (0.30–0.72)	.0007
Onset to imaging (per 30 min)	0·89 (0·80–0·99)	·04

This subset analysis involved 778 patients.
Data for table derived from Campbell et al.[7]

Table 2 Imaging modality and probability of futile thrombectomy			
Futile Outcome	MR Imaging	CT	P Value
3-mo mRS 4–6	28.6%	43.8%	<.001
3-mo mRS 5–6	18.6%	30.7%	<.001

Data for table derived from Meinel et al.[8]

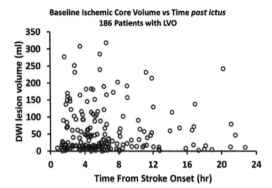

Fig. 3. Admission DWI core infarct volume versus time from stroke onset. Baseline core volumes by DWI in 186 LVO stroke patients. (*Adapted from* Figure 2 of Hakimelahi R, Vachha BA, Copen WA, et al. Time and diffusion lesion size in major anterior circulation ischemic strokes. Stroke; a journal of cerebral circulation. 2014;45(10):2936-2941.)

whereby only CT scanners are available. Let us now consider ischemic core growth.

Ischemic Core at Presentation Does Not Correlate with Time of Onset

Previously, it was assumed that ischemic core growth rates were similar for all patients with an LVO. If true, the prediction is that there is a correlation between the size of the core and the time since occlusion onset. In fact, there is no correlation. This was first shown by Hakimelahi and colleagues[9] from the massachusetts general hospital (MGH) and is illustrated in **Fig. 3**.

In this study, the infarct core was measured using DWI in 186 consecutive patients with an LVO that presented in our ED. Each circle represents a patient. The vertical axis displays the diffusion lesion volume in milliliters. The horizontal axis is the time from stroke onset that extends to 24 hours. There is no correlation between lesion volume and time ($r^2 < 0.0006$ $P > .5$). Assuming linear initial growth, more than half of these patients had cores with an initial growth rate of 4.1 mL per hour or less. The significance of this growth rate is discussed latter.

Slow Progressors and Opportunities for Thrombectomy at 24 Hours

Clearly, the growth of the ischemic core is highly variable and begs the question of how many LVO stroke patients have growth of the core that would permit thrombectomy many hours after presentation. These are the "slow progressors," a term coined by the University of Pittsburgh investigators.[9] We defined slow progressors as those patients that have ischemic cores less than 50 mL 24 hours *post-ictus* (**Fig. 4**). In two investigations, we found that more than half of LVO patients were slow progressors.[10,11]

We performed frequent MR imaging more than 2 days of 38 untreated LVO patients and found logarithmic growth of the ischemic infarct core. In 24 patients with the terminal internal carotid artery or the proximal middle cerebral artery occlusions, we found that an infarct core growth rate (IGR) less than 4.1 mL/h and initial infarct core volumes less than 19.9 mL had accuracies greater than 89% for identifying patients who would still have a core of less than 50 mL 24 hours after stroke onset, a core size that should predict favorable outcomes with thrombectomy even if eloquent tissues were involved. Published initial infarct growth rates from multiple centers[3,9,12–14] indicate that up to half of all LVO stroke patients have an IGR less than 4.1 mL/h. We conclude

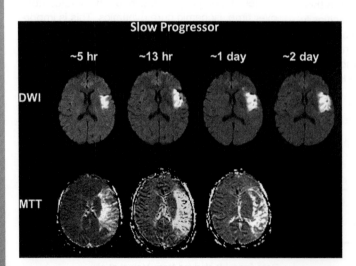

Fig. 4. Example of a slow progressor. The patient was first imaged 5 hours after stroke onset. He had left MCA occlusion. Despite persistence of occlusion and a large mismatch, the core remained under 50 mL for 2 days. MTT, mean transit time. (*Adapted from* Figure 1 of Gonzalez RG, Silva GS, He J, Sadaghiani S, Wu O, Singhal AB. Identifying Severe Stroke Patients Likely to Benefit From Thrombectomy Despite Delays of up to a Day. Sci Rep. 2020;10(1):4008.)

Table 3
Baseline variables to predict ischemic core of less than 50 mL 1 day *post-ictus*

Variables	Criteria	Sensitivity	Specificity	AUC (95% CI)
Infarct growth rate	<4.1 mL/h	89%	100%	0.97 (0.81–1.0)
Initial core volume	<19.9 mL	89%	100%	0.98 (0.82–1.0)
Diff/perf mismatch	<43 mL	44%	92%	0.60 (0.37–0.81)

Receiver operator characteristic (ROC) curves of variables predicting ischemic core volumes less than 50 mL 1 day after stroke onset. Data are from all 25 patients with ICA or M1 LVO identified on CT or MR angiography. AUC, area under curve; ICA, Internal carotid artery.
Adapted from Gonzalez, et al.[11]

that many LVO patients have stroke physiology that is favorable for late intervention, and that imaging biomarkers can accurately identify them at early time points as suitable for transfer for intervention. Baseline variables predictive of an ischemic core of less than 50 mL 1 day post-ictus are shown in **Table 3**.

IDENTIFYING SLOW PROGRESSORS WITHOUT ADVANCED IMAGING

A commonly available method to identify slow progressors would give the benefits of thrombectomy to many more. Slow progressor identification with imaging is possible with advanced imaging such as DWI and CT perfusion, but they are often not readily available. However, CT and CT angiography are widely available. It is possible that the collateral pattern on CTA may be an excellent surrogate marker for identifying slow progressors. The MGH group has previously noted the predictive value of characterizing the collateral pattern on the side of an occlusion.[15–17] Based on this experience, we tested the hypothesis that a pattern of excellent collateral flow could identify slow progressors. We tested this study in the same cohort of patients who underwent multiple MR imaging studies more than 2 days, described above.[18] We defined the excellent collateral flow pattern as an approximately symmetric pattern of the arterial enhancing pattern in both hemispheres. An example is shown in **Fig. 5**. We evaluated 31 patients, and we found that this pattern is highly predictive of a small ischemic core, a core initial growth rate of less than 5 mL/h, and a 24-h core size of less than 50 mL. Symmetric collaterals had a sensitivity of 87% (13 of 15) and a specificity of 94% (15 of 16) for 24-h ischemic core volume less than 50 cm³. We concluded that in patients with LVO, symmetric collateral pattern at CT angiography was common and highly specific for low ischemic core growth rate and small 24-h ischemic core volume as assessed at diffusion-weighted MR imaging. Because CTA is nearly universally available at centers that receive patients with a stroke syndrome, this symmetric collateral pattern identification may ease the timely transfer of patients likely to benefit to thrombectomy-capable centers even if they are located many hours away.

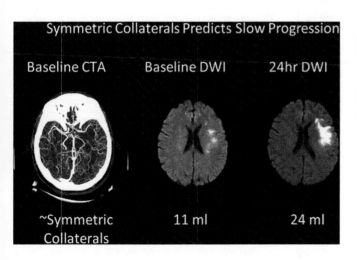

Fig. 5. Slow progressor with symmetric collaterals. The patient was first imaged less than 6 hours after stroke onset. He had left MCA stem occlusion but nearly symmetric collaterals on the left. Despite persistence of the occlusion, the core remained under 25 mL for 24 hours post-ictus (Original Figure).

SUMMARY

Thrombectomy for LVOs in patients with a major ischemic stroke syndrome is the most important neurologic therapeutic advance in decades. Making it widely available promises a substantial reduction of major morbidity and death caused by stroke. Advanced imaging is a key to making this possible in patients treated after 6 hours *post-ictus* through its ability to estimate the size of the core. A higher proportion of favorable outcomes and fewer futile thrombectomies are achieved by using DWI rather than CTP because of the higher precision of the former. Studies on the dynamics of ischemic core growth indicate that up to half of LVO patients are slow progressors who may be treated up to 24 hours after stroke onset because the ischemic core remains small. These slow progressors may be identified by core measurement by advanced imaging, especially DWI. Early evidence suggests that slow progressors may also be identified by a robust collateral pattern on CT angiography.

CLINICS CARE POINTS

- Endovascular thrombectomy has revolutonized the treatment of large vessel occlusion (LVO) ischemic stroke When LVO stroke occurs, time is brain, but each brain has its own time.

- The ischemic core size combined with the eloquence of the tissue at risk is the best predictor of patient outcome after thrombectomy.

- Diffusion MRI is the most sensitive and precise method to measure the core.

- Use of diffusion MRI results in better patient outcomes compared to other imaging methods.

- Slow progressors may be identified with diffuion MRI and they comprise a large number of LVO strokes that may be treated despite long delays.

ACKNOWLEDGMENTS

NIH Grant U01EB025153

REFERENCES

1. Gonzalez RG. Imaging-guided acute ischemic stroke therapy: From "time is brain" to "physiology is brain". AJNR Am J Neuroradiol 2006;27(4): 728–35.
2. Yoo AJ, Chaudhry ZA, Nogueira RG, et al. Infarct volume is a pivotal biomarker after intra-arterial stroke therapy. Stroke 2012;43(5):1323–30.
3. Vagal A, Aviv R, Sucharew H, et al. Collateral clock is more important than time clock for tissue fate. Stroke 2018;49(9):2102–7.
4. Copen WA, Rezai Gharai L, Barak ER, et al. Existence of the diffusion-perfusion mismatch within 24 hours after onset of acute stroke: dependence on proximal arterial occlusion. Radiology 2009;250(3): 878–86.
5. Nogueira RG, Jadhav AP, Haussen DC, et al. Thrombectomy 6 to 24 hours after stroke with a mismatch between deficit and infarct. N Engl J Med 2018; 378(1):11–21.
6. Boers AMM, Jansen IGH, Beenen LFM, et al. Association of follow-up infarct volume with functional outcome in acute ischemic stroke: a pooled analysis of seven randomized trials. J Neurointerv Surg 2018; 10(12):1137–42.
7. Campbell BCV, Majoie C, Albers GW, et al. Penumbral imaging and functional outcome in patients with anterior circulation ischaemic stroke treated with endovascular thrombectomy versus medical therapy: a meta-analysis of individual patient-level data. Lancet Neurol 2019;18(1):46–55.
8. Meinel TR, Kaesmacher J, Mosimann PJ, et al. Association of initial imaging modality and futile recanalization after thrombectomy. Neurology 2020;95(17): e2331–42.
9. Hakimelahi R, Vachha BA, Copen WA, et al. Time and diffusion lesion size in major anterior circulation ischemic strokes. Stroke 2014;45(10):2936–41.
10. Gonzalez RG, Hakimelahi R, Schaefer PW, et al. Stability of large diffusion/perfusion mismatch in anterior circulation strokes for 4 or more hours. BMC Neurol 2010;10:13.
11. Gonzalez RG, Silva GS, He J, et al. Identifying severe stroke patients likely to benefit from thrombectomy despite delays of up to a day. Sci Rep 2020; 10(1):4008.
12. Olivot JM, Sissani L, Meseguer E, et al. Impact of initial diffusion-weighted imaging lesion growth rate on the success of endovascular reperfusion therapy. Stroke 2016;47(9):2305–10.
13. Wheeler HM, Mlynash M, Inoue M, et al. The growth rate of early DWI lesions is highly variable and associated with penumbral salvage and clinical outcomes following endovascular reperfusion. Int J Stroke 2015;10(5):723–9.
14. Desai SM, Rocha M, Jovin TG, et al. High variability in neuronal loss time is brain, requantified. Stroke 2019;50:34–7.
15. Lima FO, Furie KL, Silva GS, et al. The pattern of leptomeningeal collaterals on CT angiography is a

strong predictor of long-term functional outcome in stroke patients with large vessel intracranial occlusion. Stroke 2010;41(10):2316–22.

16. Maas MB, Lev MH, Ay H, et al. Collateral vessels on CT angiography predict outcome in acute ischemic stroke. Stroke 2009;40(9):3001–5.

17. Souza LC, Yoo AJ, Chaudhry ZA, et al. Malignant CTA collateral profile is highly specific for large admission DWI infarct core and poor outcome in acute stroke. AJNR Am J Neuroradiol 2012;33(7): 1331–6.

18. Regenhardt RW, Gonzalez RG, He J, et al. Symmetric CTA Collaterals Identify Patients with Slow-progressing Stroke Likely to Benefit from Late Thrombectomy. Radiology 2022;302:400–7.

MR Imaging for Acute Central Nervous System Pathologies and Presentations in Emergency Department

Damien Galanaud, MD, PhD[a], Rajiv Gupta, MD, PhD[b],*

KEYWORDS

- Emergency department • Brain • Magnetic resonance imaging • Magnetic resonance angiography
- Central nervous system

KEY POINTS

- MR imaging has a role in imaging of acute presentation of many neurologic conditions in emergency department (ED).
- If an MRI is available in an ED, it may be the preferred first-line modality for many central nervous system (CNS) conditions including rapidly progressive headache, acute neurologic deficit, first-time seizure, traumatic brain injury, and CNS infection.
- Since MRI examination takes longer to perfrom than a CT scan, and requires MR safety clearnace, imaging should not delay or hamper emergent treatment.

INTRODUCTION

Although not as commonly used as a computed tomography (CT) scanning, MRI can be extremely useful for the assessment of patients presenting to the emergency department (ED) with neurologic symptoms. MRI can be prescribed either as a first-line examination or as a follow-up examination after a CT scan. In this article, we describe conditions under which an MRI should be ordered and what it can potentially contribute to the diagnostic workup. Most common symptoms that may be assessed using MRI in ED include rapidly progressive headache, acute neurologic deficit, seizure, traumatic brain injury (TBI), and suspected central nervous system (CNS) infection. We consider each of these conditions in the sub-sections that follow.

RAPIDLY PROGRESSIVE HEADACHE

MRI is commonly prescribed in the setting of a rapidly progressive headache to rule out an acute CNS condition, chief among them being cerebral thrombophlebitis. Although MRI is as sensitive as CT angiography for this diagnosis, it does not expose patients to ionizing radiation. In addition, it can detect a wide range of other conditions that are in the differential diagnosis. In the diagnosis of cerebral thrombophlebitis, an MRI scan, however, is more prone to ambiguous results than a CT scan due to anatomic variations and contrast enhancement of the thrombus.

The exact imaging MR protocol used should be adapted to the individual patient and the spectrum of disease conditions that one is interested in exploring. At a minimum, it should include 3D Fluid-attenuated Inversion Recovery (3D-FLAIR), 3D T1-weighted imaging, diffusion weighted imaging (DWI), T2* or susceptibility-weighted imaging (SWI), arterial spin labeling (ASL), and coronal T2 weighted imaging. One should also include an angiography sequence, with or without contrast media injection, to image the venous system. The following subsection describes the multiple

[a] Department of Neuroradiology, Pitié Salpêtrière Hospital, 47 Boulevard de l'hopital, Paris 75013, France;
[b] Department of Radiology, Massachusetts General Hospital, 55 Fruit Street, Boston, MA 02114, USA
* Corresponding author.
E-mail address: rgupta1@mgh.harvard.edu

Magn Reson Imaging Clin N Am 30 (2022) 371–381
https://doi.org/10.1016/j.mric.2022.05.002

Abbreviations	
ED	Emergency Department
CNS	Central Nervous System
MRI	Magnetic Resonance Imaging
CT	Computed Tomography
CTA	CT Angiography
TBI	Traumatic Brain Imaging
DSA	Digital Subtraction Angiography
FLAIR	Fluid Attenuated Inversion Recovery
DTI	Diffusion Tensor Imaging
DWI	Diffusion Weighted Imaging
SWI	Susceptibility Weighted Imaging
ASL	Arterial Spin Labeling
MRA	MR Angiography
ADC	Apparent Diffusion Coifficient
PRES	Posterior Reversible Encephalopathy Syndrome
SAH	Subarachnoid Hemorrhage
RCVS	Reversible Cerebral Vasoconstricton Syndrome
ICH	Intracranial Hemorrhage
AIS	Acute Ischemic Stroke
AVF	Arteriovenous Fistula

conditions that can be diagnosed using an appropriately protocoled MRI scan.

Cerebral Thrombophlebitis

At MR imaging, two elements are present in a cerebral thrombophlebitis:

- The lack of opacification of a venous sinus or cerebral vein on MR angiography;[1]
- A thrombus, whose signal is variable depending on its age. Noticeably, very old thrombi can enhance after contrast media injection. Therefore, a normal-appearing T1 postcontrast MRI does not rule out this diagnosis if specific sequences are not used.[2]

Additionally, secondary signs suggestive of cerebral thrombophlebitis may be present. These include a dilatation of the medullary veins and a venous infarction. The latter condition may include intraparenchymal hemorrhage, areas of restricted diffusion, and of vasogenic edema, as seen in **Fig. 1**.

Aside from cerebral thrombophlebitis, other common causes of rapidly progressive headaches include the following conditions, all of which are diagnosable using an MRI scan.

Posterior Reversible Encephalopathy Syndrome

This syndrome may arise from acute hypertension or may result from complications associated with some treatments such as immunosuppressors (usually at the induction phase) or chemotherapy. Its most characteristic feature is areas of subcortical edema that predominates in the posterior regions. Hence the terminology posterior reversible encephalopathy syndrome (PRES). However, it should be noted that PRES can involve any brain region and is not restricted to the posterior regions.[3,4] Extension to the gray matter including the basal ganglia is also possible although the involvement is usually less extensive. Subtle leptomeningeal enhancement may also be present. Diffusion-weighted imaging should be performed in this setting: although apparent diffusion coefficient (ADC) is increased in most regions, areas of reduced ADC may be present in some patients. These areas are thought to be related to cytotoxic edema, and these patients generally have less favorable prognosis (**Fig. 2**).

Reversible Cerebral Vasoconstriction Syndrome

This syndrome is closely related to PRES. It commonly affects young women and may occur in the postpartum period. It may also be related to drugs (eg, cannabis and cocaine) or vasoactive treatments such as serotonin recapture inhibitors. Typical presenting symptoms include thunderclap headaches, sometimes associated with seizures or stroke. On MRI, reversible cerebral

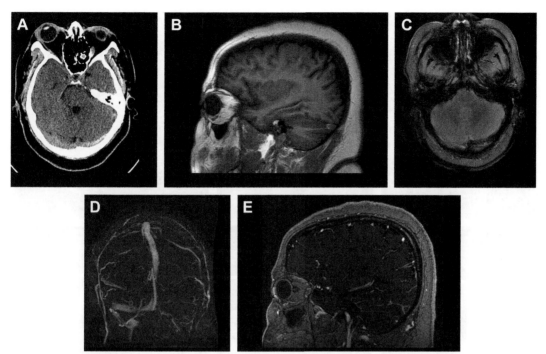

Fig. 1. Progressive headaches in a 34-year-old woman. Nonenhanced CT scan (*A*) MRI with T1-weighted (*B*) T2*-weighted (*C*) sequences and veinous MR angiography with gadolinium injection (*D*, *E*). On the CT scan, there is a spontaneous hyperdensity of the left transverse sinus suggesting a recent thrombosis. This sinus appears in high signal on T1, low signal on SWI and does not fill on the MR angiography confirming the diagnosis of recent thrombosis of the left transverse sinus.

vasoconstriction syndrome (RCVS) is characterized by the presence of multiple short stenosis in mid-sized arteries.[5] Parenchymal involvement is usually minimal and limited to subcortical focal areas of vasogenic edema. In extreme presentations, stroke or intraparenchymal hemorrhage may occur.[6] Hemorrhage in the subarachnoid spaces may also be present. In such presentations, the major difficulty is to rule out an aneurysmal subarachnoid hemorrhage (SAH) as the presenting symptoms are quite similar. On imaging, RCVS may look identical to vasospasm. Therefore, repeated noninvasive vessel imaging or even digitally subtraction arteriography may be required to rule out an aneurysm. Another relatively difficult differential diagnosis is CNS vasculitis. Although the appearance of vessels may be similar in CNS vasculitis and RCVS, in the former condition, the parenchymal signs are much more pronounced and may include large areas of vasogenic edema and intraparenchymal hemorrhage.

Sinusitis

Although a suspicion of sinusitis does not require an MRI in emergency, this condition is frequently discovered in the setting of rapidly progressive headaches. Needless to say, that assessment of

paranasal sinuses should always be performed in this clinical setting irrespective of imaging modality. Sphenoidal sinusitis, in particular, is commonly found during the evaluation of suspected thrombophlebitis. One should also be cognizant of other complications of sinusitis such as periosteal abscess formation and intracranial extension.

Pituitary Necrosis

Pituitary necrosis, although less common than the previous diagnoses, should always be in the search pattern in two specific circumstances: (i) peripartum state and (ii) hypovolemic shock. Sheehan syndrome specifically refers to postpartum pituitary necrosis in the anterior pituitary gland following significant blood loss, hypovolemia, and hypovolemic shock. Necrosis may involve a healthy pituitary or an adenoma. The pituitary or the adenoma appears increased in size, with strong peripheral enhancement. Visual symptoms may occur secondary to compression of the optic chiasm.

Subarachnoid Hemorrhage

MRI is usually not recommended in the diagnostic workup of a patient with a suspicion of SAH, which

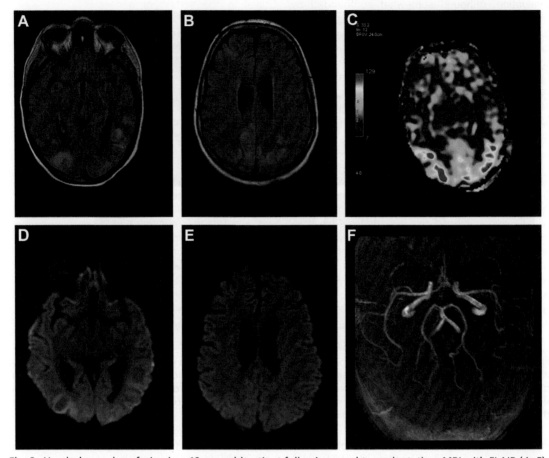

Fig. 2. Headaches and confusion in a 19-year-old patient following renal transplantation. MRI with FLAIR (*A, B*), arterial spin labeling (ASL, *C*), diffusion-weighted (*D, E*) sequences and angiographic MRI of the circle of Willis. (*F*) There are areas of hypersignal in FLAIR, predominating in the posterior, subcortical lesions without increased signal in diffusion suggestive of vasogenic edema. ASL (*F*) shows localized hyperperfusion although the angioMRI of the circle of Willis does not show any sign of vascular occlusion. These MRI findings are highly suggestive of posterior reversible encephalopathy syndrome.

is usually diagnosed using noncontrast CT and CT angiography. If aneurysmal SAH is suspected, CT/CTA may be emergently followed by digital subtraction angiography (DSA) for definitive diagnosis and potential coil embolization. Although the 3DFLAIR sequence is reasonably sensitive for SAH, the diagnostic accuracy of MR angiography of the Circle of Willis to detect intracranial aneurysms is significantly lower than that of CTA and DSA. Nonetheless, MRI does have some niche applications in this setting:

- In a patient presenting to the ED a few days after the acute event, a noncontrast CT may be normal due to the clearance of blood products by the normal flow of the CSF. At MRI, the correct diagnosis can still be made because hyperintensity in the subarachnoid space persists for a longer time.[7]

- Recurring headache in a patient with a history of intracranial aneurysm treated with endovascular coiling may be explored by MRI to assess for coil compaction and recurrence of the aneurysm. MR Angiography may be superior to CT angiography in this setting, as the latter may be significantly degraded by metallic artifacts from the coil mass.
- MRI may be used to detect inflammatory changes in the wall of an intracranial aneurysm.[8] These changes may be responsible for headaches and are considered to be a harbinger of impending aneurysm rupture. A T1-weighted "black blood" sequence with and without contrast is used to assess for enhancement in the wall of the aneurysm. This is particularly useful in patients with multiple aneurysms to determine which one should be treated emergently.

Migraine

Although the diagnosis of migraine is clinical in most cases, MRI can sometimes be used to support it in some atypical cases, especially in patients with aura. Additionally, migraine is a common differential diagnosis in patients explored for a suspicion of acute ischemic stroke (AIS) or thrombophlebitis. The MRI protocol should include 3D-FLAIR, diffusion, MR angiography of the circle of Willis and ASL imaging. The typical imaging pattern observed is normal FLAIR, DWI and angioMRI sequences associated with marked hypo-perfusion of the involved territory on ASL during the aura, followed by hyperperfusion (Fig. 3).[9,10]

ACUTE NEUROLOGIC DEFICIT

MRI is the modality of imaging of choice for patients presenting with acute neurologic deficit at the ER. Its main purpose is to positively diagnose or rule out an AIS. The MR protocol should be fast and simple and includes FLAIR (either axial or 3D), DWI, SWI/T2*, MR angiography of the circle of Willis and most often some kind of perfusion imaging, either dynamic susceptibility contrast or ASL.

Acute Ischemic Stroke

AIS is described in detail in another chapter. An area of reduced ADC in a vascular territory is highly suggestive of this diagnosis (Fig. 4). Further elements to look for are as follows:

- The level of vascular occlusion on the MR angiography and the presence of a thrombus on the SWI/T2* sequence.[11]
- The presence of arteries with hyperintense signal on the FLAIR sequence and veins with the hypointense signal on the SWI/T2* sequence.[12]
- Areas of hyperintense signal in the brain parenchyma on FLAIR, which usually correspond to irreversible ischemia.

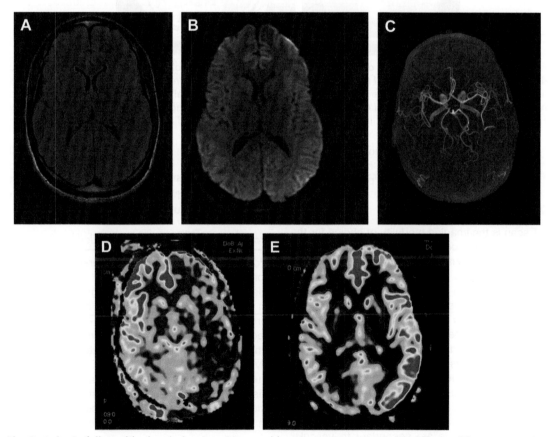

Fig. 3. Aphasia followed by headaches in a 28-year-old patient. MRI in FLAIR (A) diffusion (B) sequences. AngioMRI of the circle of Willis (C). ASL perfusion performed at the acute phase (D) and 12 h later. There is no evidence of acute ischemia in FLAIR and diffusion, and the angioMRI does not show any sign of vessel occlusion. However, there is marked hypoperfusion of the left temporal lobe during the acute event, followed by hyperperfusion on the follow-up examination confirming the diagnosis of migraine (E).

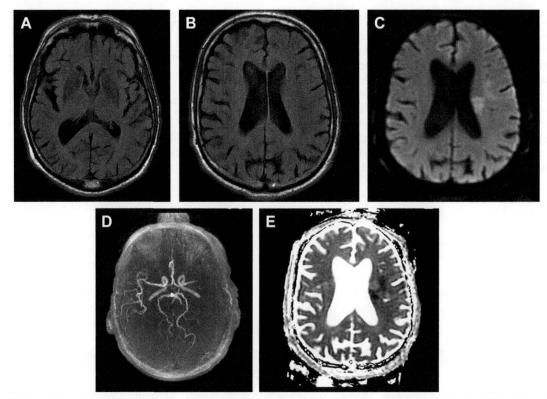

Fig. 4. MRI performed 3 h after the onset of right hemiplegia in an 80-year-old patient. MRI in FLAIR (*A*, *B*) and diffusion (*C*) sequences. AngioMRI of the circle of Willis (*D*). Apparent diffusion coefficient (ADC) map (*E*). There is an occlusion of the distal part of the first segment of the left middle cerebral artery. Diffusion imaging shows a hypersignal of the left centrum semi ovale with a reduced ADC. FLAIR imaging is normal except from some slow flow in the distal branch of the left middle cerebral artery, confirming the diagnosis of acute ischemic stroke.

- Areas of hypoperfusion without changes on diffusion, which usually correspond to salvageable tissue (ischemic penumbra).

Intracerebral Hematoma

CT scan is the imaging modality of choice for the diagnosis of intracerebral hematoma (ICH). However, due to its usual presentation as an acute neurologic deficit, it is a common finding on an MRI performed in search of an AIS. Acute ICH will present as a space-occupying lesion with a variable signal on T1 and a hyperintense signal on FLAIR, hypointense signal on SWI surrounded by a ring of edema after a few hours of evolution. Signal on DWI is usually high, with a falsely reduced ADC due to the hemoglobin-derived products. Small areas of hypointense signal in SWI related to microbleeds and sequela of previous hematomas are also commonly present. Although most ICHs are secondary to vascular risk factors, especially high blood pressure and treatment with anticlotting agents, elements in favor of secondary hematomas must be searched for. Infiltration of the cortex, basal ganglia or

corpus callosum on the FLAIR sequence will strongly suggest the possibility of an underlying brain tumor while the presence of dilated arteries will point toward an arteriovenous malformation or a dural AV fistula as the underlying etiology.

Post-ictal Deficit/Status Epilepticus

Post ictal deficit is a common differential diagnosis for a recurring stroke in a patient with a previous history of AIS. Areas of the high signal of the cortex in the region responsible for the seizure may be present in DWI, which must not be mistaken for a recurring stroke (**Fig. 5**). Arterial blood flow changes are commonly associated, with either hypo- or hyper-perfusion on ASL. Status epilepticus is associated with similar imaging abnormalities; however, the presentation commonly is much more extensive.[13,14] A hyperintense signal in the thalamus may also be present on DWI.

CENTRAL NERVOUS SYSTEM INFECTIONS

Although MRI is usually not indicated in uncomplicated meningitis, it is of major diagnostic and

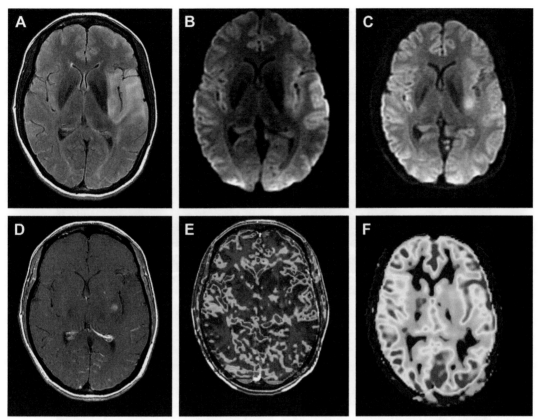

Fig. 5. Generalized seizure in a 45-year-old patient. MRI in FLAIR (*A*) T1 postcontrast injection (*D*). Perfusion imaging using the dynamic susceptibility contrast (relative cerebral blood volume map, *E*) and arterial spin labeling (*F*) sequences. Diffusion imaging performed at admission (*B*) and 24 h later (*C*). There is an infiltration mass of the left temporal lobe and insula, with the presence of a contrast-enhancing nodule, which proved to be an anaplastic glioma. Cortical areas of high signal on diffusion on the initial examination disappear on the follow-up scan, indicating that they were seizure-related, although the hypersignal located in the contrast-enhancing nodule persists, suggesting that it is related to the hypercellularity of this high-grade portion of the tumor.

prognostic value in other less common infectious processes or in complicated cases. As a rule, imaging should never delay the antimicrobial treatment, even if easily and rapidly available. The imaging protocol should include 3D T1 pre- and postcontrast images, 3DFLAIR, diffusion-weighted imaging, and, in some cases, MRA of the circle of Willis.

Bacterial Meningitis

MRI is usually normal in uncomplicated bacterial meningitis. An increased signal of the CSF in the sulci on FLAIR may be observed, which should not be mistaken for a SAH. Leptomeningeal enhancement may also be present (**Fig. 6**). MRI is usually performed in patients with a suspicion of complicated meningitis. The two most common findings are described below.

- *Ventriculitis*: The presence of pus in the ventricles will appear as an increase contrast

enhancement of their walls, associated with a high signal of the CSF on the FLAIR sequence. An area of reduced ADC may also be present. An increase in the size of the ventricles should be assessed as hydrocephalus is an extremely frequent occurrence in this setting.[15]
- *CNS vasculitis* is mostly a complication of pneumococcal meningitis. Multiple areas of ischemic stroke are present, sometimes associated with a "sausage-like" appearance of the major branches of the Circle of Willis.

Brain Abscess

Brain abscesses are rare but require extremely urgent treatment due to their fast growth and evolution toward fistulous egress into the ventricles in a matter of days. MRI scans are quite specific diagnosing this entity and in defining the extent of involvement. Pyogenic abscesses usually appear as cystic lesions with fine, regular walls with low

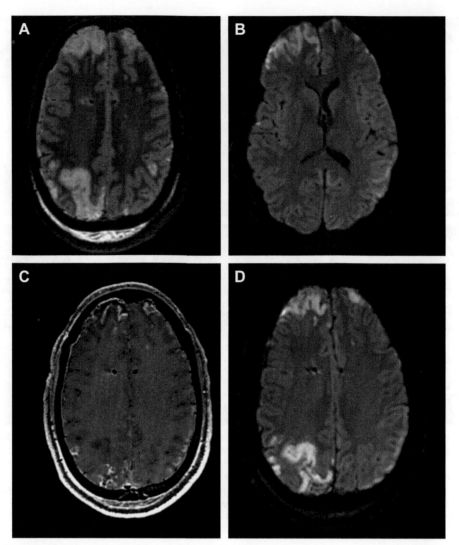

Fig. 6. A 60-year-old patient admitted for confusion followed by coma. *Pneumococcus* meningitis was confirmed on the spinal tap. MRI in FLAIR (*A*) diffusion (*B, D*) T1 postcontrast injection. (*C*) There are areas of cortical and subcortical edema in FLAIR, associated with high signal in diffusion and leptomeningeal enhancement confirming the diagnosis of infectious vasculitis complicating the meningitis.

signal on T2-weighted images, high signal on T1-weighted images, with margins that demonstrate strong enhancement after gadolinium injection. The contents of the cyst usually restrict diffusion leading a high signal on DWI and low signal on ADC images. Amino acids are usually present on MR spectroscopy.[16]

Empyema

Empyema is the presence of pus in the subdural spaces. This diagnosis may be either very easy or very difficult depending on the clinical setting and prior history of the patient.

- *Spontaneous empyema* is usually a complication of dehiscences of the skull base, either at

the level of the frontal sinus or adjacent to the mastoid portion of the temporal bone. The imaging characteristics of a spontaneous empyema are similar to those of a brain abscess: a collection with a high signal on DWI associated with strong enhancement of the adjacent dura.

- *Superinfection of a previous subdural hematoma*, either due to a surgical drainage or an associated fracture of the frontal sinus or mastoid. Diagnosis in this case is extremely difficult as blood products interfere with the signal on DWI rendering this sequence unreliable. In practice, there is no reliable way to differentiate between an infected and a noninfected subdural hematoma with MRI.

Aspergillosis

Aspergillosis is one of the most feared brain infections, with a mortality rate up to 80%. It is most prevalent in immunocompromised patients, especially those undergoing chemotherapy. Its high lethality is due to the angio invasive nature of the fungus and the fragile condition of the subject. Two distinct invasion routes are possible: hematologic or direct spread from the paranasal sinuses. Aspergillosis lesions present as multiple abscesses often located at the cortical and subcortical junction.[17] Intracranial hemorrhage or aneurysms may be present and an MR angiogram of the circle of Willis should be included as part of the MR examination of the patient.

Herpetic Meningoencephalitis

The classical presentation of herpetic encephalitis is the combination of confusion, seizures, and fever. It requires an immediate treatment with acyclovir, and in no case neuro imaging should delay this treatment. The classical pattern of herpetic encephalitis is bilateral but asymmetrical areas of cortical and subcortical swelling, predominating in the frontal and temporal lobes.[18] Areas of contrast enhancement, restricted diffusion, or hemorrhage may be present. The lesions will extend during the first days of follow-up, even if the treatment is successful.

TRAUMATIC BRAIN INJURY

TBI is most commonly evaluated using CT imaging. CT is the first-line examination to rule out intra or extra parenchymal hematomas, skull fractures and for monitoring patients with severe TBI. MRI is typically used to assess the extent of brain damage and evaluate conditions that may be CT occult. However, as discussed below, a few indications of brain MRI in an acute setting of TBI do exist.

Severe Traumatic Brain Injury

MRI is only very rarely performed in the setting of severe TBI. The increased intracranial pressure commonly present in these patients is worsened by the supine position, making this imaging hazardous. However, a very fast examination is doable and may help determine whether the patient may still benefit from decompressive craniotomy (**Fig. 7**). The imaging protocol should include FLAIR, DWI, and SWI sequences. Ischemic or hemorrhagic lesions of the brainstem (especially the mesencephalon and posterior part of the pons), thalami, internal part of the temporal lobes, motor cortices, and language areas will

adversely affect the prognosis and should be carefully assessed.[19]

Minor Trauma

Minor TBI usually does not require MRI. However, a patient with a recent history of TBI may present to the ED with nonspecific and diffuse symptoms compatible with a postconcussion syndrome. MRI may be helpful in this context if it shows areas of cortical and subcortical edema on FLAIR suggesting concussions, or foci of hypointense signal in SWI, usually in the corpus callosum, frontal and temporal lobes related to diffuse axonal injury.

Trauma-Related Skull Base Lesions

Aside from empyema complicating a skull base fracture, other trauma-related injuries may also warrant an emergency MRI. Some of these conditions are described below:

- *Compression of optic nerve* may occur following a fracture of the orbital apex. An MRI may be ordered to assess the extent of the optic nerve damage before a surgical decompression
- *Supra aortic vessels dissection* is a common complication of head trauma, especially in the presence of a skull base fracture. The most common clinical setting is the occurrence of a stroke a few days after a TBI that was not fully investigated with imaging.[20] The imaging protocol should include the standard stroke protocol, with addition of T1-weighted imaging of the cervical region with fat saturation to detect subintimal hematoma in the vessel wall and MRA of the supra-aortic vessels.
- *Dural Sinus Thrombosis* can occur following a fracture going through a venous sinus. Although it is most commonly diagnosed with CT angiography, an MRI may be prescribed to assess a venous infarction. A late complication of dural sinus thrombosis following TBI is the occurrence of an *arteriovenous fistula* (AVF). It should be suspected in a patient presenting to the ER with a pulsatile tinnitus in the weeks and months following a trauma.
- *Cavernous sinus* AVF is another late complication of head trauma. Patient will present at the ER with chemosis and reduced eye motility. MRI will show a dilatation of the ophthalmic vein, and arterial flux in the cavernous sinus.

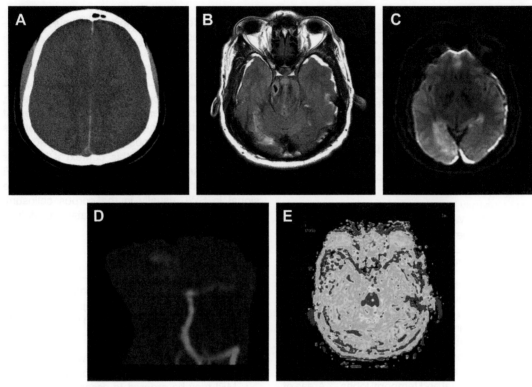

Fig. 7. A 72-year-old patient admitted for agitation and confusion followed by coma. CT scan (*A*), MRI in FLAIR (*B*), diffusion-weighted imaging (*C*) angioMRI of the circle of Willis (*D*). Fractional anisotropy map derived from the diffusion tensor sequence (*E*). A bilateral subdural hematoma induced a left temporal lobe herniation leading to compression and occlusion of the right posterior cerebral artery, leading to an infarction of the right occipital lobe. However, there is no ischemia of the thalami, and the cortico spinal tracks appear preserved in the brainstem, suggesting the absence of irreversible damage of these critical structures. The subdural hematomas were evacuated and the patient made a full recovery, with the exception of a persistent hemianopsia.

SUMMARY

Fast access to MRI is important for the correct assessment of patients presenting to the ED with neurologic symptoms. It is especially critical for acute neurologic deficits, rapidly progressive headache, and suspicion of intracranial infection. It is critical to ensure proper communication between the ER physicians and the radiologist to ensure a timely, appropriately protocoled, and properly focused examination.

- Central Nervous System infections such a bacterial meningitis, brain abscess, empyema, fungal infections, and viral menigoencephalitis require emergent MRI examnination to assess for complications.
- The extent of traumatic brain injury, though most commmonly evaluated using CT/CTA, can be more accurately mapped using MRI.

CLINICS CARE POINTS

- Rapidly progressing headache warrants an appropriately protocolled MRI examination to rule out conditions such as cerebral thrombophlebitis, PRES, RCVS, sinusitis, pituitary necrosis, subarachnoid hemorrhage, and atypical migraines.
- Acute neurological deficit may arise from a number of etiologies that are more sensitively diagnosed by MRI than CT.

DISCLOSURE

RG would like to declare following interests that are not relevant to the current paper: Idorsia, Inc, Consulting/Advising and member of Image Review Committee. "Spectral precision imaging for early diagnosis of colorectal lesions with CT colonography, NIH, 5R01CA212382-05, (PI: Yoshida, Hiroyuki). "Dense array image-compatible EEG for enhanced neonatal care - Administrative Supplement," NIH-National Institutes of Health, 5R01EB024343-04, (PI: Bonmassar, Giorgio). "A Simulation Framework for X-Ray Phase-Contrast

Imaging," (NIH-National Institutes of Health, 1R03EB032038-01, PI: Gupta, Rajiv). Braintale Inc., Scientific Advisory Board. GYS Tech, LLC (now a part of Stryker), Consulting/Advising. Mary Hitchcock Memorial Hospital, Expert testimony. Mosaic Research Management, Consulting/Advising. Siemens Medical Solutions, USA: Speaker honorarium. Samsung: Research Grant. University of Wisconsin: CT Protocols Advisory Board. The Risk Management Foundation of the Harvard Medical Institutions Incorporated (RMF): Legal consulting.

REFERENCES

1. Bonneville F. Imagerie des thromboses veineuses cérébrales. J de Radiologie Diagnostique Interventionnelle 2014;95(12):1130–5.

2. Dormont D, Sag K, Biondi A, et al. Gadolinium-enhanced MR of chronic dural sinus thrombosis. AJNR Am J Neuroradiol 1995;16(6):1347–52.

3. Anderson R-C, Patel V, Sheikh-Bahaei N, et al. Posterior Reversible Encephalopathy Syndrome (PRES): Pathophysiology and Neuro-Imaging. Front Neurol 2020;11:463.

4. Ando Y, Ono Y, Sano A, et al. Posterior Reversible Encephalopathy Syndrome: A Review of the Literature. Intern Med (Tokyo, Japan) 2022;61(2):135–41.

5. Song TJ, Lee KH, Li H, et al. Reversible cerebral vasoconstriction syndrome: a comprehensive systematic review. Eur Rev Med Pharmacol Sci 2021;25(9):3519–29.

6. Pilato F, Distefano M, Calandrelli R. Posterior Reversible Encephalopathy Syndrome and Reversible Cerebral Vasoconstriction Syndrome: Clinical and Radiological Considerations. Front Neurol 2020;11:34.

7. Lummel N, Schoepf V, Burke M, et al. 3D Fluid-Attenuated Inversion Recovery Imaging: Reduced CSF Artifacts and Enhanced Sensitivity and Specificity for Subarachnoid Hemorrhage. AJNR Am J Neuroradiol 2011;32(11):2054–60.

8. Molenberg R, Aalbers MW, Appelman APA, et al. Intracranial aneurysm wall enhancement as an indicator of instability: a systematic review and meta-analysis. Eur J Neurol 2021;28(11):3837–48.

9. Yger M, Villain N, Belkacem S, et al. [Contribution of arterial spin labeling to the diagnosis of sudden and transient neurological deficit]. Rev Neurol (Paris) 2015;171(2):161–5.

10. Law-Ye B, Fargeot G, Leclercq D. Arterial Spin Labeling Hypoperfusion in Migraine Aura. Headache 2017;57(6):935–6.

11. Kang D-W, Jeong H-G, Kim DY, et al. Prediction of Stroke Subtype and Recanalization Using Susceptibility Vessel Sign on Susceptibility-Weighted Magnetic Resonance Imaging. Stroke 2017;48(6):1554–9.

12. Toyoda K, Ida M, Fukuda K. Fluid-attenuated inversion recovery intraarterial signal: an early sign of hyperacute cerebral ischemia. AJNR Am J Neuroradiol 2001;22(6):1021–9.

13. Mendes A, Sampaio L. Brain magnetic resonance in status epilepticus: A focused review. Seizure 2016;38:63–7.

14. Shimogawa T, Morioka T, Sayama T, et al. The initial use of arterial spin labeling perfusion and diffusion-weighted magnetic resonance images in the diagnosis of nonconvulsive partial status epileptics. Epilepsy Res 2017;129:162–73.

15. Hazany S, Go JL, Law M. Magnetic resonance imaging of infectious meningitis and ventriculitis in adults. Top Magn Reson Imaging 2014;23(5):315–25.

16. Grand S, Passaro G, Ziegler A, et al. Necrotic tumor versus brain abscess: importance of amino acids detected at 1H MR spectroscopy–initial results. Radiology 1999;213(3):785–93.

17. Marzolf G, Sabou M, Lannes B, et al. Magnetic Resonance Imaging of Cerebral Aspergillosis: Imaging and Pathological Correlations. PLoS One 2016;11(4):e0152475.

18. Sarton B, Jaquet P, Belkacemi D, et al. Assessment of Magnetic Resonance Imaging Changes and Functional Outcomes Among Adults With Severe Herpes Simplex Encephalitis. JAMA Netw Open 2021;4(7):e2114328.

19. Bigler ED, Abildskov TJ, Goodrich-Hunsaker NJ, et al. Structural Neuroimaging Findings in Mild Traumatic Brain Injury. Sports Med Arthrosc Rev 2016;24(3):e42–52.

20. McFarlane TD, Love J, Hanley S, et al. Increased Risk of Stroke Among Young Adults With Serious Traumatic Brain Injury. J Head Trauma Rehabil 2020;35(3):E310–e319.

Magnetic Resonance Imaging for Spine Emergencies

Jeannette Mathieu, MD[a], Jason F. Talbott, MD, PhD[a,b,*]

KEYWORDS

• MR imaging • Spinal cord • Spinal cord injury • Myelitis • Myelopathy

KEY POINTS

• For traumatic spine emergencies, MR imaging plays a key role in supplementing initial computed tomography in select patients for the evaluation of spinal stability, spinal canal compromise, spinal cord injury, and spinal nerve root injury.
• MR imaging is the initial imaging modality of choice to exclude compressive pathologic condition for nontraumatic spine emergency patients presenting with neurologic deficits.
• In the setting of compressive spinal pathologic condition, the intradural versus extradural location of pathologic condition informs the differential diagnosis.
• Key MR imaging findings, including transverse patterns of spinal cord T2 signal abnormality and enhancement, aid in narrowing the differential diagnosis for emergent noncompressive spinal cord pathologic conditions.

INTRODUCTION

This article is devoted to the MR imaging evaluation of spine emergencies, defined as spinal pathologic conditions that pose an immediate risk of significant morbidity or mortality to the patient if not diagnosed and treated in a timely manner. The spinal cord (SC) is exquisitely sensitive to compression and vascular compromise. Identifying signs of present or impending SC compression and injury is central to the MR imaging search pattern for spine emergencies. In many cases, the cause of imaging findings will be readily apparent, and the focus of spine MR imaging will be to describe and classify the pathologic condition to facilitate appropriate next steps in patient management. To this end, up-to-date evidence-based imaging classification systems will be reviewed. Certain other spine emergencies do not have a clear cause. In these cases, focus shifts to formulating a useful differential diagnosis based on pertinent MR imaging findings and to suggest further evaluations that may yield a definitive diagnosis, such as additional imaging, cerebral spinal fluid (CSF) studies, or biopsy. This article will outline a practical approach to help navigate these various scenarios and highlight key imaging features that can aid in narrowing the differential diagnosis for commonly encountered spine emergencies. We begin with a summary of MR imaging indications and MR imaging protocols tailored for a variety of spinal emergencies. A review of key imaging findings for the most common emergent spine pathologic conditions will follow. Pathologic conditions will be broadly grouped into traumatic and nontraumatic pathologic conditions. For traumatic injuries, an algorithmic diagnostic approach based on the AO Spine injury classification system will be presented. Nontraumatic spinal emergencies will be dichotomized

[a] Department of Radiology and Biomedical Imaging, UCSF and Zuckerberg San Francisco General Hospital, 1001 Potrero Avenue, Room 1X57C, San Francisco, CA 94110, USA; [b] Brain and Spinal Injury Center, Zuckerberg San Francisco General Hospital, 1001 Potrero Ave Rm 101, San Francisco, CA 94110, USA
* Corresponding author. Department of Radiology, Zuckerberg San Francisco General Hospital, 1001 Potrero Avenue, Room 1X57C, San Francisco, CA 94110.
E-mail address: Jason.talbott@ucsf.edu

Magn Reson Imaging Clin N Am 30 (2022) 383–407
https://doi.org/10.1016/j.mric.2022.04.004
1064-9689/22/© 2022 Elsevier Inc. All rights reserved.

into compressive and noncompressive subtypes. The location of external compressive disease with respect to the thecal sac is fundamental to establishing a differential diagnosis for compressive emergencies, whereas specific patterns of SC involvement on MR imaging will guide the discussion of inflammatory and noninflammatory causes of noncompressive myelopathy.

ROLE OF MR IMAGING IN SPINAL EMERGENCIES

MR imaging is the gold standard imaging technique for many spinal emergencies. In the setting of trauma, MR imaging is complementary to initial first-line computed tomography (CT) evaluation for a subset of patients.[1,2] The American College of Radiology (ACR) has published appropriateness criteria with recommendations for MR imaging as "usually appropriate" in patients with confirmed or suspected SC or nerve root injury.[1] Patients with mechanically unstable spine injury for which surgical treatment is planned should also undergo spine MR imaging for characterization of soft tissue injuries, including unstable discoligamentous disruption, that may aid in surgical planning. Obtunded patients with a negative cervical spine

CT and for whom clinical evaluation is not feasible are also recommended for MR imaging by ACR criteria, although this recommendation is more controversial.[3]

In cases of nontraumatic spinal emergency, MR imaging is usually the preferred initial imaging modality due to its excellent soft tissue contrast and ability to reliably identify compressive SC pathologic condition.[4] The ACR has published appropriateness criteria for MR imaging in patients presenting with low back pain and generally limits imaging to those with red flag signs or symptoms including suspected infection, immunosuppression, chronic steroid use, suspicion for cancer, and patients with persistent or progressive symptoms following 6 weeks of conservative therapy.[5] MR imaging is also recommended for any patient with progressive neurologic deficits localized to the SC, conus, or nerve roots/cauda equina.

MR IMAGING PROTOCOL FOR SPINAL EMERGENCIES

The ideal MR imaging protocol for patients with spine emergencies will vary depending on the clinical scenario. Neurologically unstable patients for whom emergent surgical intervention is needed may require an abbreviated examination tailored to address only emergent surgical questions, such as localizing the level of SC compression with a rapid T2-weighted (T2W) sagittal survey of the spine and limited axial imaging at selected levels. Patients with suspected inflammatory, infectious, or neoplastic conditions may need more thorough imaging with inclusion of T1W precontrast and postcontrast sequences. Fat suppression (FS) with T2W and T1W-post contrast sequences is advised whenever spinal pathologic condition may involve extramedullary structures of the spine, such as vertebral bodies, ligaments, or paraspinous tissues. When a purely noncompressive myelopathy is suspected, FS may be unnecessary and only impair signal-to-noise ratio or introduce unwanted artifacts for detailed SC evaluation.[6]

Increasingly, diffusion weighted imaging (DWI) has been incorporated into spine MR imaging protocols and is generally helpful whenever clinical indications would suggest a need for postcontrast imaging. This includes evaluation of the spine for infection and neoplastic pathologic conditions. Just as in the brain, DWI may also be helpful for diagnosing patients with acute SC infarcts. In the setting of traumatic spinal cord injury (SCI), many studies have evaluated diagnostic and neuroprognostic roles of DWI.[7,8] Despite intense investigation, applications for DWI in daily clinical practice for spine trauma remain lacking and future studies are needed to validate utility of DWI beyond standard conventional sequences.[9]

When spinal vascular pathologic condition is suspected, time-resolved MR angiography (MRA) techniques may be useful for characterizing the nature of the vascular malformation and for potentially identifying levels of arterio-venous shunting lesions. Fat-suppressed T1W sequences are particularly useful for diagnosing acute cervical arterial dissections. T2*W and susceptibility weighted imaging techniques can be useful for delineation of gray–white matter contrast and to identify intramedullary SC blood products.[2]

MR imaging for Spine Trauma

A thorough physical examination and comprehensive clinical history remain the gold standard for the initial assessment of patients with acute blunt spine trauma. However, comorbid conditions such as traumatic brain injury, severe pain, obtunded state, and sedative medications among others may interfere with clinical assessment in the acute stage of injury. In selected patients, MR imaging thus plays a crucial role in diagnosing and characterizing the extent of spinal trauma. As a complement to CT, MR imaging is most useful when further imaging characterization for spinal stability and/or neural element compromise is needed. MRA and vessel wall imaging techniques may also be indicated for diagnosing blunt traumatic cerebrovascular injury when CTA findings are equivocal.[10]

A-P-C: a practical approach to MR imaging evaluation for spinal trauma

In this section, we introduce an algorithmic approach to MR imaging interpretation for subaxial spine trauma while highlighting key MR imaging sequences and findings for each of 3 anatomic spine regions. Readers are referred to other excellent reviews for traumatic injuries of the craniocervical junction.[11] As a framework, this algorithmic approach to subaxial spine trauma incorporates nomenclature and concepts from the AOSpine thoracolumbar injury classification[12] and AOSpine subaxial cervical spine injury models[13] (**Box 1**). Although no classification system for spinal injury has gained universal acceptance, the AOSpine classification systems have become increasingly used for their high interrater reliability, relative simplicity, and ease of clinical application. For the assessment of stability, the spinal column is divided into anterior tension band (ATB) and posterior tension band (PTB) with an intervening spinal canal and its contents. Type A injuries primarily include vertebral body compression fractures.

Box 1
AOSpine thoracolumbar and subaxial cervical spine injury morphologic classification[12,13]

Type A: Compression Injuries

- A0: Minor nonstructural fractures (eg, spinous process, transverse process)
- A1: Wedge compression: Single endplate fracture without posterior wall involvement
- A2: Split pincer fracture: vertical fracture in coronal plane through superior and inferior endplates
- A3: Incomplete burst: comminuted fracture of 1 endplate and posterior vertebral wall
- A4: Complete burst: comminuted fracture of both endplates and posterior vertebral wall

Type B: Distraction Injuries

- B1: Trans-osseous posterior tension band (eg, Chance fracture)
- B2: Ligamentous posterior tension band disruption
- B3: Hyperextension anterior tension band disruption

Type C: Translation Injuries

- Combined anterior and posterior tension band disruption with spinal displacement/dislocation

Type F: Facet injuries (subaxial cervical spine)

- F1: Nondisplaced facet fracture
- F2: Facet fracture with potential less than 1 cm in height, less than 40% lateral mass
- F3: Floating lateral mass
- F4: Traumatic perched or jumped facet joints

Modifiers

- M1: Possible/indeterminate posterior capsuloligamentous complex injury
- M2: Critical disc herniation in the presence of facet dislocation (cervical), Bone disease/abnormality (thoracolumbar)
- M3: Bone disease/abnormality (cervical)
- M4: vascular injury/abnormality (cervical)

Type B injuries involve disruption of either the ATB or PTB and are generally considered unstable. Type C injuries are unstable and involve disruption of both ATB and PTB with associated traumatic distraction or translational injuries of the spine.

(A)nterior tension band The ATB is composed of the vertebral bodies and intervertebral discs.

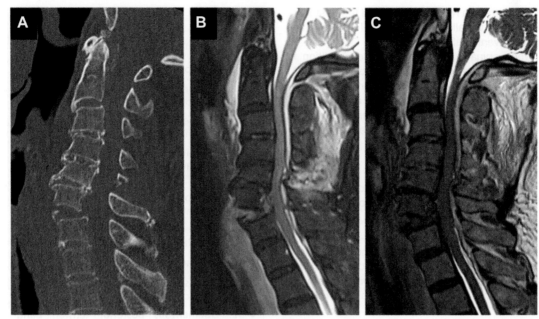

Fig. 1. Hyperextension injury with unstable anterior tension band (ATB) disruption. 85-year-old man presents with left sided weakness after ground level fall and headstrike. Sagittal CT image shows traumatic anterolisthesis at C6-C7 with small anteroinferior avulsion corner fracture of C6 (Arrow in A). Sagittal FS T2W (B) and sagittal T2 SPACE (C) MR images confirm complete disruption of the C6-C7 anterior discoligamentous complex. MRI also reveals long segment severe spinal canal stenosis and cord compression with dorsal epidural hematoma (arrows in C). Focal ligamentum flavum tear at C5-6 is best seen on sagittal T2 SPACE image (arrowhead in C).

Important ligaments stabilizing the ATB also include the anterior and posterior longitudinal ligaments. Traumatic injuries to the ATB are best evaluated with FS T2W sequences, preferably with Dixon or short tau inversion recovery techniques for FS. Prevertebral fluid and hemorrhage are readily identified with FS T2W imaging and absence of prevertebral fluid in the acute stage of injury virtually excludes an unstable ATB injury.[14] When prevertebral fluid is identified, a careful interrogation of anterior ligamentous structures for traumatic disruption is necessary (**Fig. 1**). With hyperextension injuries, there is potential for unstable ATB distraction and resultant disruption of the anterior longitudinal ligament (ALL), PLL, and intervertebral disc (see **Fig. 1**). A partial ATB injury, such as isolated ALL disruption, should be described (**Fig. 2**) but does not qualify as an unstable ATB injury according to AOSpine classification.[12] In addition to ligamentous injuries, MR imaging is also highly sensitive for the detection of ATB vertebral compression fractures, including very mild compression injuries with minimal or no vertebral body height loss, which may be occult on CT (**Fig. 3**). More severe ATB vertebral body injury with hyperflexion injuries, such as flexion teardrop, and burst compression injuries are readily diagnosed with CT. In these cases, MR imaging complements CT in the evaluation of the spinal canal for spinal canal compromise, SCI and for the evaluation of potential concomitant PTB ligamentous injuries (**Fig. 4**).

(P)osterior tension band The PTB similarly includes both osseous and ligamentous components. The posterior elements of each vertebra define the bony contribution while the ligamentum flavum (LF), interspinous ligament, supraspinous ligament, and facet joint capsules constitute the "posterior ligamentous complex" (PLC), the primary soft tissue stabilizers of the PTB. As with the ATB, the initial evaluation of the PTB begins with sagittal FS T2W imaging. Unstable PTB injuries may involve transverse fracture across the bony posterior elements, often as part of a chance type hyperflexion injury, which is readily diagnosed on CT (**Fig. 5**). Alternatively, PTB disruption can involve the soft tissue PLC. MR imaging plays a critical role in diagnosing unstable PLC disruptions. Because the LF is known to be one of the final structures to tear in predictable PLC injury sequence, close attention to LF integrity is key to determining unstable PLC injury[15] (**Fig. 6**). T2 hyperintensity along the LF without clear

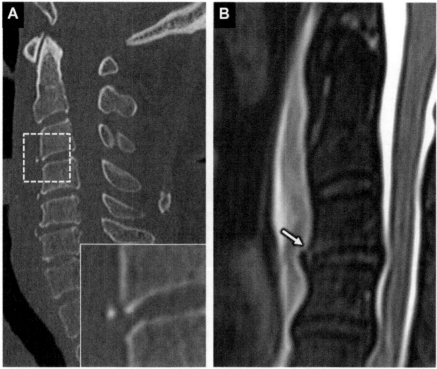

Fig. 2. Hyperextension injury with anterior longitudinal ligament (ALL) disruption. A 70-year-old woman presents with upper extremity paresthesia following low-speed pedestrian vs automobile injury. (*A*) Sagittal CT image of the cervical spine shows a small and minimally displaced anteroinferior avulsion corner fracture at C3 (*dotted square* with zoom in view in the *bottom right inset in A*). (*B*) Sagittal T2 FS MR imaging of the upper cervical spine in the same patient shows prominent prevertebral fluid collection with focal disruption of the ALL (*arrow in B*) with otherwise intact anterior discoligamentous complex.

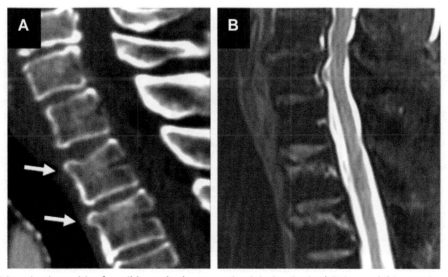

Fig. 3. MR imaging is sensitive for mild vertebral compression injuries. Sagittal CT image (*A*) in a patient who presented with neck pain after a fall reveals mild superior endplate compression fractures at C6 and C7 (*arrows in A*), which are easily seen on sagittal T2W MR imaging (*B*) where linear subchondral marrow edema underlying the superior endplates conspicuously identifies the acute fractures.

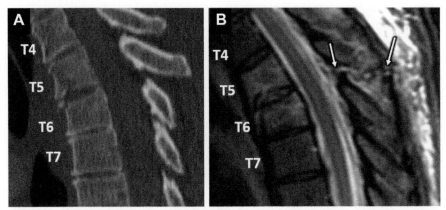

Fig. 4. MR imaging reveals unsuspected ligamentous posterior tension band disruption. Sagittal CT image (A) for a 48-year-old patient suffering a fall reveals mild anterior compression and endplate fractures at T5 and T6 vertebral levels. Sagittal T2W MR image (B) at the same levels reveals complete disruption of the supraspinous ligament, interspinous ligament, and ligamentum flavum at T5-T6 (arrows in B).

disruption of the ligament suggests partial tear or sprain. Definite unstable LF disruption should include unambiguous focal disruption of the ligament with intervening T2 hyperintensity (see **Fig. 6**). High-resolution T2W imaging without FS, such as three-dimensional (3D) T2 SPACE, can be a very useful sequence to complement FS T2W imaging for detailed anatomic delineation of the LF (see **Fig. 6**).

(C)anal and contents MR imaging in spine trauma is arguably of most value for its exquisite evaluation of the spinal canal and its contents, namely the SC and spinal nerve roots. In patients presenting with clinical signs of acute SC or nerve root injury, determination of SC and/or cauda equina compression is the primary focus of the MR imaging examination in preparation for the emergent surgical decompression. The most frequent causes for traumatic spinal canal compromise include herniated disc, bony retropulsion, traumatic spinal malalignment, and extra-arachnoid subdural and epidural space hemorrhages.[3] Preexisting degenerative spondylosis is also a common cause of spinal canal compromise and predisposing risk factor for acute SCI after even mild trauma, particularly common in the elderly population.

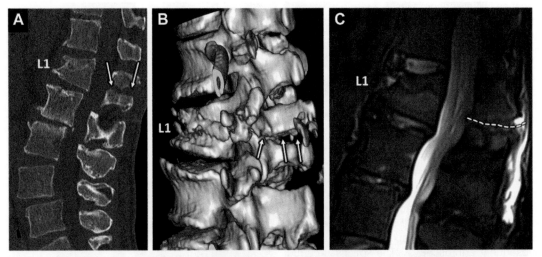

Fig. 5. CT and MRI depictions of Chance fracture. Sagittal CT (A) depicts linear fracture through the spinous process (arrows in A) in a 68-year-old female with seatbelt injury and low back pain. B) 3D reconstruction of the CT images clearly depicts transverse fracture through the entire L1 posterior elements (arrows in B) consistent with an AOSpine type B1 injury. Sagittal T2W MR image in the same patient shows marrow edema and transverse distracted fracture line corresponding to osseous posterior tension band fracture (white dotted line in C).

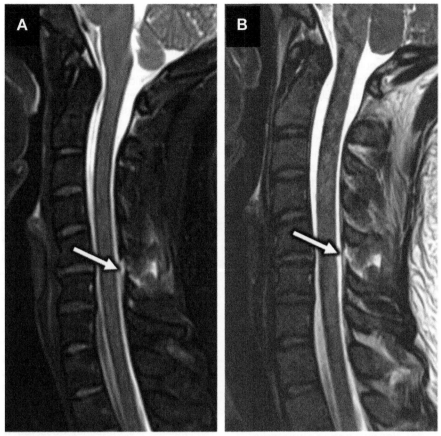

Fig. 6. MR imaging confirms suspected posterior ligamentous complex injury. Sagittal FS T2W (*A*) and T2 SPACE (*B*) MR images obtained for a 33-year-old restrained passenger following motor vehicle collision reveals abnormal edema along the posterior ligamentous complex at C5-C6 (*arrow* in *A, B*).

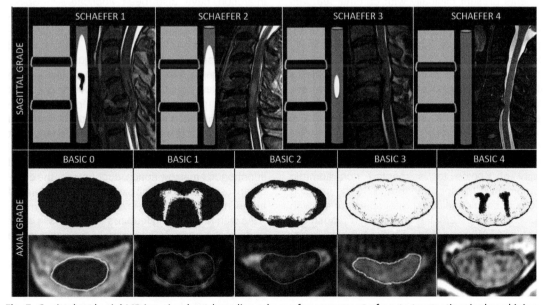

Fig. 7. Sagittal and axial MR imaging-based grading schema for assessment of acute traumatic spinal cord injury.

The most studied and validated MR imaging sequence for SC evaluation is T2W imaging. Axial and sagittal depictions of SC contusion provide complementary information for injury characterization. Schaefer and colleagues first described a sagittal injury classification system based on the relative length of intramedullary T2 hyperintensity and presence or absence of intramedullary blood products[16] (**Fig. 7**). Hemorrhage within contusion injury is defined as circumscribed T2 hypointense foci, often involving central gray matter, related to paramagnetic effects of iron from blood products in the form of deoxyhemoglobin and hemosiderin. Axial-based T2W classification of contusion injury at the epicenter using the BASIC score has also been shown to strongly correlate with initial injury severity and neurologic outcome[17] (see **Fig. 7**). In a large meta-analysis, Fehlings and colleagues concluded that MR evidence of intramedullary hemorrhage was the MR imaging biomarker most strongly associated with injury severity and outcome in acute SCI.[18] In summary, review of axial and sagittal T2W sequences should focus on levels of SC compression, the cranio-caudal and transverse extent of SCI, along with the presence or absence of hemorrhage within the contusion injury.

MR imaging for Nontraumatic Compressive Myelopathy

Compressive myelopathy is a potentially devastating but treatable clinical syndrome of neurologic deficits resulting from SC compression. Patients present clinically with cardinal features of symmetric extremity weakness, urinary retention or incontinence, and a circumferential sensory level, which may assist in spatially localizing the level of compressive pathologic condition.[19] In most patients, the SC terminates at the L1-L2 vertebral level, and lesions compromising the spinal canal below this level may present with a cauda equina syndrome (CES) related to nerve root compression, which includes saddle paresthesia, bowel, bladder, and sexual dysfunction. MR imaging is the initial modality of choice for suspected nontraumatic compressive myelopathy and CES. The imaging protocol should include a total spine survey with inclusion of FS T2, T1 precontrast, T1 postcontrast, and DWI sequences. Dedicated axial imaging may be prescribed based on the sagittal survey or obtained automatically for the entire spine, depending on the institutional workflow. Knowledge of patient's clinical context is of paramount importance for informing the image interpretation. Key risk factors include known malignancy, immunocompromised state, history of intravenous drug use, and use of blood thinning medications. The most common causes of atraumatic compressive myelopathy include extra-arachnoid fluid collections such as epidural abscess and hematoma, degenerative spondylosis, spinal tumors, and spinal webs or adhesions. The MR imaging-based differential diagnosis begins with the determination of the location of offending pathologic condition to either the extramedullary extradural space or extramedullary intradural space (**Box 2**).

Extradural compressive pathologic condition

Spine infection Clinical signs and symptoms of spinal infection are often nonspecific, thus highlighting the critical role for MR imaging in confirming or excluding a suspected diagnosis.[20] Emergent MR imaging is indicated in patients with new or worsening neurologic deficits coupled with clinical suspicion for infection. Notable risk factors include provided clinical history of sepsis, immunosuppression, recent spinal instrumentation such as surgery or percutaneous spinal procedure, and IV drug abuse in patients with back pain and myelopathy. Leukocytosis may be absent. Elevations in erythrocyte sedimentation rate (ESR) and C-Reactive Protein (CRP), while nonspecific, are frequently observed with spinal infection.[21]

Myelopathy from spine infection most frequently relates to mechanical compression of the SC by spinal epidural abscess (SEA) or infectious phlegmon but secondary SC ischemia and vasculitic infarction have also been implicated.[19] Spinal deformity, such as severe kyphosis related to infectious vertebral and discoligamentous destruction, may also contribute to spinal canal compromise and SC or cauda equina compression. Pyogenic spinal infections are most common in the United States, with *Staphylococcus aureus* accounting for 70% of cases.[22] Arterial hematogenous seeding of the spine is the most common route of spinal contamination. The unique vascular supply of the spine, with each segmental spinal artery supplying adjacent vertebral endplates and subchondral marrow space, accounts for the characteristic pattern of discitis osteomyelitis centered at the intervertebral disc level.

As with MR imaging features of abscess in other parts of the body, MR imaging of the spine in the setting of epidural abscess reveals a focal fluid collection in the epidural space with peripheral enhancement and central T2 hyperintensity (**Fig. 8**). DWI may be useful for confirming reduced apparent diffusion coefficient (ADC) measures

Box 2
Common nontraumatic compressive pathologic conditions

Extramedullary and extradural

Spine infection

- Epidural abscess and/or phlegmon
- Bony retropulsion/kyphotic deformity

Neoplasm

- Metastases-most common include breast, prostate, lung, renal-cell carcinoma
- Primary spinal tumors including multiple myeloma and sarcoma

Other

- Degenerative spondylosis/ossification posterior longitudinal ligament
- Acute disc herniation
- Spontaneous epidural hematoma

Extramedullary and intradural

Developmental cystic lesions

- Dermoid
- Epidermoid
- Arachnoid
- Neuroenteric

Primary tumors

- Meningioma
- Schwannoma
- Neurofibroma
- Lipoma

Leptomeningeal Metastases

- Widely metastatic cancer—most common primaries include breast, lung, melanoma, colon, stomach, leukemia, lymphoma
- Aggressive primary CNS tumors—most common tumors include medulloblastoma, glioblastoma, ependymoma, germinoma, pineoblastoma, choroid plexus carcinoma

Other

- Arachnoid web
- Arachnoid cyst

centrally within the epidural collection consistent with purulent contents[23] (see **Fig. 8**). Compressive myelopathy may also result from exuberant epidural phlegmon, without frank abscess. In such cases, solid epidural soft tissue enhancement is present without rim-enhancing fluid collection[21] (**Fig. 9**). SEA is associated with a primary

discitis-osteomyelitis (DOM) in more than 80% of cases.[24] Associated findings of adjacent discitis osteomyelitis thus help confirm the diagnosis. In the absence of imaging findings suggestive of associated DOM, or other primary musculoskeletal spinal infection such as adjacent septic facet arthritis or septic costovertebral arthritis, alternative diagnostic considerations should be also considered because isolated epidural abscess without primary musculoskeletal spinal infection is rare.[25]

Vertebral osteomyelitis with the involvement of multiple nonadjacent vertebral bodies (skip lesions) and relative preservation of the disc space is more characteristic of tuberculous spondylitis.[26] TS is a granulomatous bacterial infection caused by *Mycobacterium tuberculosis* that often presents with a more insidious and chronic clinical presentation compared with pyogenic DOM.[21,25,26] Thoracolumbar spinal involvement is most common, and the natural history of this disease includes vertebral body collapse, kyphotic deformity, and resulting Gibbus deformity with potential cord compression due both to kyphosis and granulation tissue/bony retropulsion into the epidural space. Contiguous paravertebral and epidural phlegmon and abscess may also be seen in the setting of tuberculosis infection with anterior subligamentous extension of infection aiding in distinction from pyogenic DOM[26] (**Fig. 10**). Intramedullary spinal infections are rare and will be considered separately in more detail in the section covering noncompressive myelopathies.

Neoplasm Metastases are the most common symptomatic tumors of the spinal column.[27] Spinal metastases may spread hematogenously into the epidural space but, more commonly, epidural spread is via direct extension of tumor from primary osseous spinal or paraspinous sites. Primary neoplasms arising in the epidural space are exceedingly rare and include angiolipoma, lymphoma, and sarcoma. Multiple myeloma is the most common primary bone malignancy to present with compressive myelopathy.[27]

In the setting of spinal metastatic disease with emergent clinical presentation, MR imaging is indicated for identifying levels of epidural tumor encroachment and spinal canal compromise (**Fig. 11**). Distinguishing acute osteoporotic and malignancy related pathologic vertebral fractures can be difficult. Useful imaging features to favor pathologic fracture include erosive bone destruction with fracture, marrow signal replacement with lower ADC values suggesting cellularity, convex bulging of the posterior vertebral wall into the spinal canal, and associated epidural or

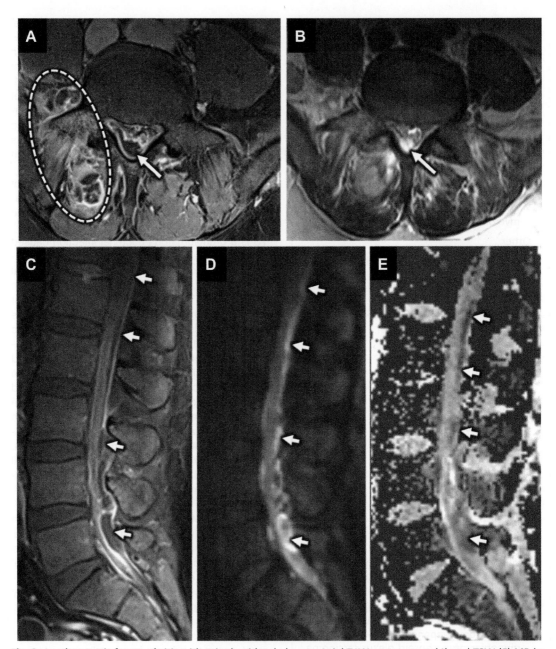

Fig. 8. Lumbar septic facet arthritis with spinal epidural abscess. Axial T1W postcontrast (*A*) and T2W (*B*) MR images from a 54-year-old man with diabetes mellitus type 2 reveals right L5-S1 peri-facet joint soft tissue enhancement and multiloculated abscess (*dotted circle*) consistent with septic facet arthritis. There is associated peripherally enhancing and T2 hyperintense fluid collection in the dorsal epidural space of the lower lumbar spine (*arrow* in *A* and *B*). Sagittal T1W postcontrast MR image shows longitudinal extension of this collection to upper lumbar levels (*arrows* in *C*). Sagittal diffusion weighted (*D*) and apparent diffusion coefficient (*E*) images confirm abnormal reduced diffusion corresponding to the fluid collection consistent with purulent abscess (*arrows* in *D* and *E*).

paraspinal mass (see **Fig. 11**). Assessment for neoplasm-related spinal instability should also be addressed in the diagnostic interpretation of the MR imaging. The spine instability neoplastic score is a simple point-based scoring system that incorporates many MR imaging features of spinal involvement to determine an overall risk of malignancy-related instability.[28] The Bilsky epidural spinal cord compression scale is also a standardized classification system for reporting

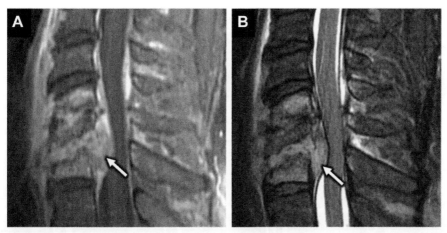

Fig. 9. DOM with epidural phlegmon resulting in spinal canal narrowing and spinal cord compression. Sagittal T1W-post contrast (A) and T2W (B) MR images centered at the midcervical spine show characteristic features of C4-C5 and C5-C6 DOM with prominent, solidly enhancing ventral epidural phlegmon (arrow in A and B).

spinal canal compromise related to spinal metastatic disease.[29] Because medical oncologists, radiation oncologists, and spinal surgeons use these systems to plan patient management, familiarity with and incorporation of these classifications in the MR imaging interpretation for patients with spinal tumors will enhance timely and appropriate care for patients.

Other extradural compressive pathologic conditions In the absence of primary spinal column infection, noninfectious causes for isolated epidural fluid collection should be considered, the most common of which is epidural hematoma (EDH). Nontraumatic EDHs typically result from venous plexus hemorrhage in the setting of

anticoagulation or coagulopathy.[30] Acute hemorrhage in the epidural space characteristically presents as a T1 isointense or hyperintense and T2 hyperintense collection that subtends the dura[30] (Fig. 12). The uplifted dura can be seen as a hypointense membrane containing the hematoma on T2W imaging (see Fig. 12). In the absence of findings suggestive of underlying spinal vascular pathologic condition, such as dilated pial vessel flow voids or enhancing vascular nidus, conventional digital subtraction angiography is likely not necessary for further workup.[31] When there is SC compression and clinical evidence of myelopathy, emergent surgical decompression is indicated.

Cervical spondylotic myelopathy is the most common cause of spinal injury in the United States

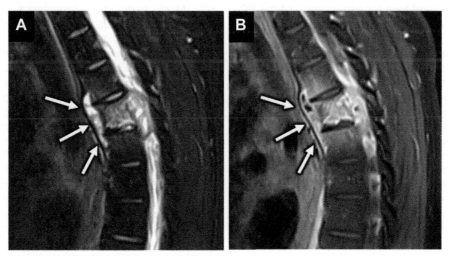

Fig. 10. Tuberculous spondylitis. Sagittal T2W FS (A) and T1W-post contrast MR images from a 31-year-old man with insidious cough, fever, and weight loss reveals abnormal edema and enhancement centered at the T5 spinal level notable for anterior subligamentous phlegmon extension (arrows in A and B) and relative preservation of adjacent intervertebral discs. Subsequent percutaneous biopsy confirmed mycobacterial infection.

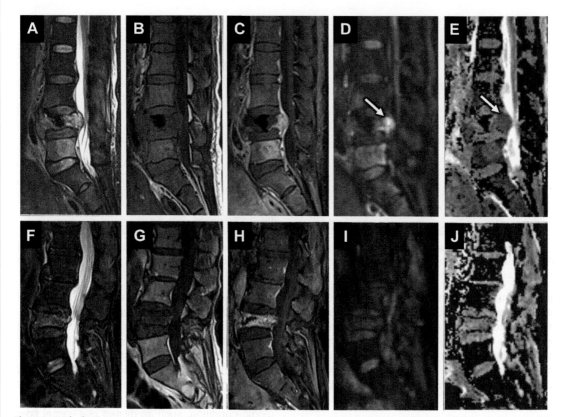

Fig. 11. Pathologic versus osteoporotic compression fractures. Sagittal T2W (*A*), T1W (*B*), T1W-post contrast (*C*), DWI (*D*), and ADC map (*E*) of the lumbar spine from a 59-year-old woman with low back pain and breast cancer show L4 compression deformity with mass-like dorsal bowing of the posterior vertebral wall encroaching on the spinal canal. Mass-like extraosseous enhancement extending from the posterior L4 vertebral body has abnormal reduced diffusion (*arrow* in *D* and *E*) consistent with hypercellular tumor. Similar series of MR images (*F–J*) in a separate 82-year-old osteoporotic woman shows L4 vertebral compression fracture with nonmass-like enhancement, posterior bony retropulsion, and facilitated rather than reduced diffusion within the L4 vertebral body, consistent with osteoporotic fracture.

and is a general term for compression of the SC due to degenerative spinal canal compromise and cord compression.[32] These changes may include not only disc pathologic condition such as herniation and disc osteophyte complex formation but also spondylolisthesis, ossification of the posterior longitudinal ligament or LF, and facet arthropathy are frequently implicated. MR imaging features suggestive of spondylotic myelopathy include variably extensive SC T2 hyperintensity with edema centered in the central gray matter and associated short segment area of pancake-like transverse white matter contrast enhancement centered at the level of maximal cord compression[33] (**Fig. 13**). More acute spondylotic myelopathy may lack associated enhancement.

Intradural Compressive Pathologic Condition

Extramedullary intradural masses arise within the subarachnoid space but are separate from the SC. Most frequently encountered examples include metastatic and primary tumors as well as developmental cystic lesions, such as dermoid, epidermoid, arachnoid, and neurenteric cysts. Metastatic tumors in this location are most frequently the result of leptomeningeal spread in the setting of widely disseminated lung, breast, melanoma, gastrointestinal, or hematologic malignancies, although primary brain neoplasms may also produce intrathecal "drop metastases" to the spine.

The most common extramedullary intradural primary tumors are meningioma, nerve sheath tumor, and lipoma, whereas malignant peripheral nerve sheath tumor, solitary fibrous tumor/hemangiopericytoma, and paragangliomas are additional more rare considerations.[34] Evaluating the MR imaging signal characteristics of extramedullary intradural masses may help narrow the diagnosis. For instance, schwannomas and neurofibromas are more likely than meningiomas to expand and

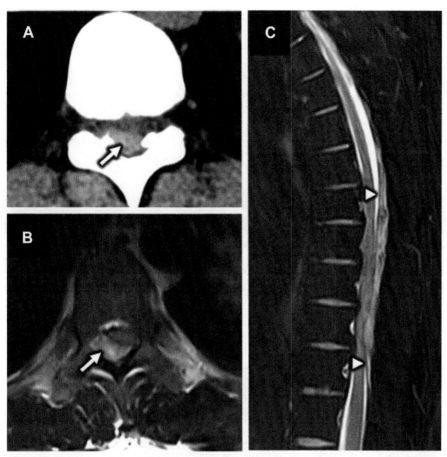

Fig. 12. MR imaging features of spontaneous epidural hematoma. Axial CT (*A*) and T2W MR (*B*) images at the midthoracic level from a 41-year-old man presenting with acute onset loss of sensory and motor function to his bilateral lower extremities immediately following bowel movement reveal intrinsic hyperdense and T2 heterogenous expansion of the right dorsolateral epidural space with resultant severe spinal canal stenosis and spinal cord compression (*arrow* in *A* and *B*). (*C*) Sagittal T2W image from the same patient clearly depicts the dorsal epidural location of this collection with uplifting of the dural membrane (*arrowheads* in *C*). Internal T2 hypointensity within the hematoma corresponds to paramagnetic T2 shortening from blood products.

remodel the neural foramen and may exhibit a characteristic dumbbell morphology with transforaminal extension along the proximal nerve root course.[34] Similar to their intracranial counterparts, meningiomas will demonstrate broad dural attachment and often follow the signal of gray matter on T1W and T2W imaging and enhance avidly and homogeneously (**Fig. 14**). Evidence of tumor mineralization on CT or T2*-weighted MR imaging also favors meningioma.[24]

Spinal arachnoid cysts may be difficult to distinguish from spinal canal webs and SC herniations because all of these lesions tend to displace the SC ventrally. When an arachnoid cyst is suspected, high-resolution 3D T2 or FIESTA imaging sequences of the spine may be useful to resolve thin cyst walls and confirm the diagnosis.[35] The distortion of the SC seen in the setting of arachnoid web or SC herniation tends to be more focal

than that seen with an arachnoid cyst. In the setting of arachnoid webs, there is characteristic focal ventral displacement of the cord with asymmetric posterior cord indentation resembling the profile of the blade of a scalpel (ie, scalpel sign)[36] (**Fig. 15**). This imaging feature is useful in distinguishing from the ventrally tethered SC observed in the setting of cord herniation where the posterior spinal indentation is more symmetric in the craniocaudal axis. With both spinal webs and herniations, there may be an associated intramedullary T2 hyperintensity within the cord and syrinx or presyrinx formation in severe cases.

MR imaging for Noncompressive Spine Emergencies

Noncompressive myelopathy encompasses a vast array of neurologic disorders related to intrinsic SC

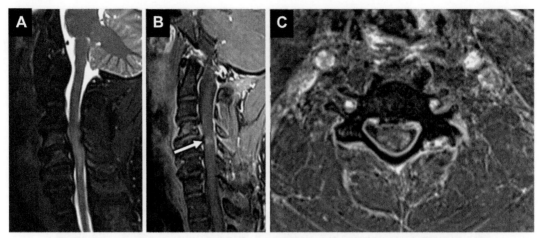

Fig. 13. Spondylotic myelopathy. (A) Sag T2W FS MR image from a 46-year-old man with lower extremity weakness and fall shows severe degenerative spinal canal stenosis at the C4-C5 level with abnormal intramedullary spinal cord T2 hyperintensity centered at this level. Sagittal (B) and axial (C) T1W-post contrast images reveal transverse pattern of "pancake" like enhancement (arrow in B) which primarily involves peripheral white matter columns, consistent with spondylotic myelopathy.

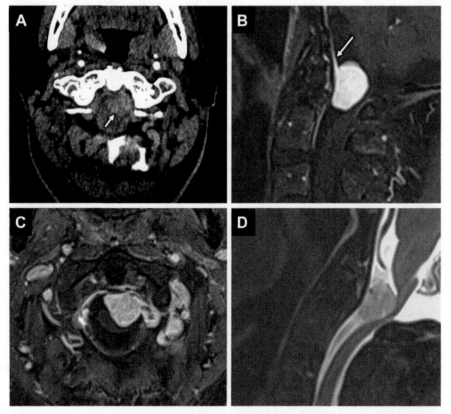

Fig. 14. Intradural compressive meningioma. Axial CT angiogram (A) performed for a 78-year-old man presenting with upper extremity paresthesia and weakness after fall shows subtle enhancing mass within the spinal canal at the C1 level (arrow in A). Sagittal (B) and axial (C) T1W FS-post contrast MR images show an intradural solidly enhancing mass with broad dural attachment and dural tail (arrow in B). Sagittal T2W FS MR image (D) shows severe spinal canal stenosis at C1 with cervicomedullary junction compression.

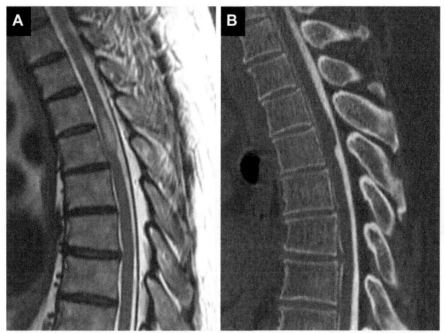

Fig. 15. Arachnoid web with compressive myelopathy. A 54-year-old man presents with severe upper thoracic pain. (*A*) Sagittal T2W MR image centered at the upper thoracic spine reveals concave indentation along the dorsal spinal cord resembling the profile of a surgical scalpel (ie, "scalpel" sign) with intramedullary spinal cord T2 hyperintense edema above the level of spinal cord compression. Subsequent CT-myelogram (*B*) excluded spinal cord herniation and confirmed diagnosis of spinal arachnoid web.

pathologic condition. This includes infectious, inflammatory, and autoimmune diseases, vascular, neoplastic, toxic-metabolic injury, radiation injury, and idiopathic conditions. MR imaging of the spine in these cases is critically important for characterization of the involved areas in both the axial and sagittal dimensions. Distinct patterns of axial SC involvement can help focus a differential diagnosis and include long segment central gray matter/frontal horn predominant, eccentric white matter, dorsal column tractopathy, centromedullary, patchy irregular, and extramedullary distributions[37,38] (**Table 1**). Sagittal SC involvement can be described as either longitudinal extensive, spanning at least 3 sequential vertebral bodies, or short-segment. Although patterns of SC involvement can directly inform the differential diagnosis, it is important to recognize that there is substantial overlap between causes with each of these patterns. In addition to grouping by location and extent, causes of noncompressive myelopathy can also be categorized into inflammatory and noninflammatory causes.[20] In clinical practice, suspicion for an infectious or inflammatory cause may be raised by leukocytosis or elevated serum ESR and CRP levels, elevated WBC, elevated CSF protein, or the presence of immunoglobulins or oligoclonal bands in CSF.[20]

Infectious, parainfectious, and inflammatory myelitis

Primary infections of the SC are fortunately rare, yet critically important due to high associated mortality and morbidity. Causes include viral, bacterial, parasitic, and fungal pathogens.[20] Early recognition and diagnosis are important so immediate antimicrobial therapy can be initiated. Some infections are more common in immune-compromised individuals, and the immune status of the patient should be determined in order to provide the most relevant differential diagnosis. Additional risk factors such as recent travel and IV drug abuse history should be ascertained.

Certain pathogens have characteristic patterns of involvement related to tropism, such as the anterior horn involvement typical of poliovirus, enteroviruses, and West Nile Virus (WNV).[39,40] Acute frontal horn infections can result in the clinical syndrome of acute flaccid myelitis (AFM) characterized by sudden weakness in the extremities and loss of reflexes. Although poliovirus has been largely eradicated, there has been increased recognition of enterovirus A71 and D68 subtypes as the most common causes of modern AFM.[39] Biennial outbreaks of AFM in the Western United States dating back to 2014 have raised awareness of this disease. Most cases involve children with a

Table 1
Transverse patterns of myelopathy on MR imaging

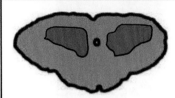

Central gray matter
- Infarct—Anterior spinal artery occlusion
- Infection—Enterovirus 71, Poliovirus, Coxsackie A9 and A23, Coxsackie B, West Nile virus, Japanese Encephalitis virus
- Compressive myelopathy—traumatic or atraumatic

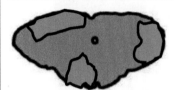

Peripheral white matter predominant
- Demyelinating—multiple sclerosis
- Infection—HIV, HSV, HTLV-1
- Neurodegenerative—ALS
- Neurosarcoidosis

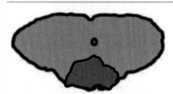

Dorsal column
- Subacute combined degeneration
- Nitrous oxide abuse
- Neurosarcoidosis
- Tertiary neurosyphilis (tabes dorsalis), HIV

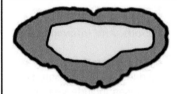

Centromedullary
- Infectious/parainfectious/Acute disseminated encephalomyelitis
- Autoimmune—NMOSD, MOGAD
- Vascular—dural AV fistula
- Radiation
- Idiopathic

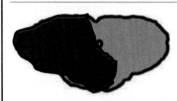

Irregular
- Tumor
- Infection—abscess
- Trauma
- Vascular-cavernous malformation, intramedullary AVM

Abbreviations: AVM, arterovenous malformation; MOGAD, myelin oligodendrocyte glycoprotein antibody disease; NMOSD, neuromyelitis optica spectrum disorders.

median age of 6 years.[41] The associated radiologic pattern of frontal horn-predominant long segment T2 hyperintensity aids in the diagnosis on spine MR imaging for patients presenting clinically with rapid-onset flaccid paralysis of one or more limbs and sensory sparing (**Fig. 16**). Gray matter involvement may be unilateral or bilateral and associated ventral nerve rootlet thickening and hyperenhancement is often observed. WNV-associated

AFM is exceedingly rare but shares many imaging features with enteroviral-related AFM but is more common in adults.[40]

Infectious and postinfectious myelitis presents most often with ellipsoid or patchy long segment centromedullary pattern of SC involvement characteristic of the broad diagnostic category of infectious and noninfectious diseases often grouped under the umbrella term "acute

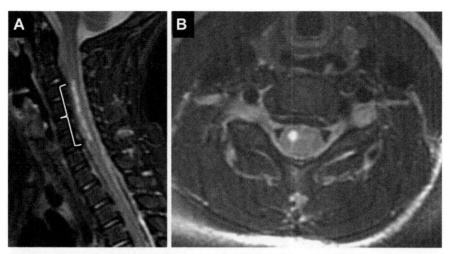

Fig. 16. Enterovirus-related acute flaccid myelitis. A 3-year-old boy with 10-day loss of movement in the right arm in setting of upper respiratory illness. Sagittal (*A*) and axial (*B*) T2W MR images show abnormal T2-hyperintensity spanning multiple cervical vertebral segments centered in the right frontal horn of the spinal cord.

transverse myelitis." Identification of associated nerve root enhancement can be helpful for suggesting an infectious cause in these cases.[37] Patients present clinically with motor, sensory, and autonomic dysfunction. Primary infectious and postinfectious pathologic conditions with this MR imaging pattern include cytomegalovirus (CMV), Epstein-Barr virus (EBV), Lyme disease, hepatitis C, parainfectious transverse myelitis (PITM), and acute disseminated encephalomyelitis. PITM refers to SCI resulting from a postinfectious immune-mediated response.[42] Preceding infections of viral hepatitis, *Mycoplasma pneumoniae*, *Campylobacter jejuni*, CVM, and EBV species among others should trigger consideration of PITM in patients with MR imaging and clinical features of acute transverse myelitis.[42] There are no pathognomonic imaging characteristics that can reliably identify the cause of PITM; therefore, clinical history and laboratory studies are important in confirming a suspected diagnosis.

Noninfectious causes of inflammatory myelitis include autoimmune diseases such as multiple sclerosis (MS), neuromyelitis optica spectrum disorders (NMOSD), and myelin oligodendrocyte glycoprotein antibody disease (MOGAD).[20] Acute treatment of these disorders in the emergent setting is tailored to suppressing the pathologic immune response with steroids, plasmapheresis, and long-acting immunomodulating therapies when necessary. MR imaging in the emergent setting plays a central role in diagnosing these disorders and enabling timely treatment. MS, the most common inflammatory myelitis, is a primary demyelinating disease with white matter predominant involvement. T2-hyperintense MS lesions are

typically short segment, spanning less than 2 vertebral segments, and eccentric. Enhancement is observed in the active stages of inflammatory demyelination. Brain imaging is useful to show associated demyelinating plaques of the brain. NMOSD is an antibody-mediated disease of aggressive spinal demyelination and optic neuritis, which classically presents on MR imaging with long-segment T2 hyperintense spinal edema spanning 3 or more vertebral segments[43] (Fig. 17). Centromedullary T2 hyperintensity of the cord with preferential cervical spine involvement and avid contrast enhancement is typical. Oligoclonal bands are not present in NMO, although immunoglobin G targeting aquaporin-4 is a specific marker for this disease.

MOGAD may present with longitudinally extensive as well as multiple short segment lesions. Central gray-matter T2 hyperintensity on axial imaging has been termed the "H" sign of MOGAD myelitis.[44] Postcontrast enhancement, when present, is usually faint and patchy and may include linear subependymal enhancement paralleling the central canal. There is a predilection for conus involvement with leptomeningeal and cauda equina enhancement.[44]

Other inflammatory causes of myelitis include systemic inflammatory and connective tissue disorders including sarcoidosis, lupus, and Sjögren disease. Theses systemic diseases may present with a transverse myelitis or an irregular pattern of patchy cord involvement. Spinal lesions may enhance in a patchy distribution, "skipping" adjacent portions of the cord and distinguishing these diseases from intramedullary neoplasms, which tend to be continuous and infiltrative. Pial and

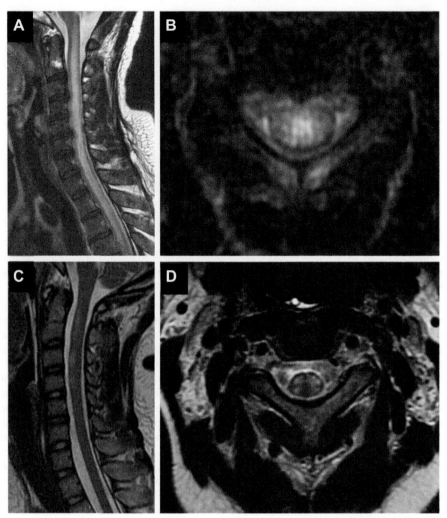

Fig. 17. Neuromyelitis optica spectrum disorder and myelin oligodendrocyte glycoprotein antibody disease-related myelopathies. Sagittal (*A*) and axial (*B*) T2W MR images from a 51-year-old women presenting with acute onset lower extremity weakness and numbness reveals longitudinally extensive centromedullary pattern of spinal cord edema commonly seen with NMO. Sagittal (*C*) and axial (*D*) T2W MR images from a different 15-year-old patient with recurrent hospitalizations for sensory and motor deficits reveals patchy T2 edema in the cervical spine with central gray-matter involvement resembling the letter "H" (*D*).

subpial infiltrative enhancement along the dorsal cord white matter forming a "trident sign" pattern is highly suggestive of neurosarcoidosis[45] (Fig. 18).

Vascular spine emergencies
The most common emergent spine vascular pathologic conditions include acute SC infarct, spinal arteriovenous shunts, and hemorrhagic cavernous malformations.[46] The SC has complex arterial collateralization between a single anterior and paired posterior spinal arteries. Lower thoracic SC infarcts of the anterior spinal artery territory are most common due to the relatively limited

collateralization for the dominant radicular artery of Adamkiewicz territory.[46] Spinal infarcts occur more frequently in women, with an average age of 56 years.[46] Significant risk factors include recent aortic surgery, embolism, vasculitis, dissection, and hypotension. MR imaging may aid in diagnosing acute SC infarct in patients presenting with acute onset weakness, sensory changes, and sphincter dysfunction without antecedent trauma or SC compression. MR imaging signal abnormalities related to acute infarct may be occult for up to 24 hours after symptom onset.[47] Within 2 days, MR imaging usually reveals long segment ventral SC T2 hyperintensity

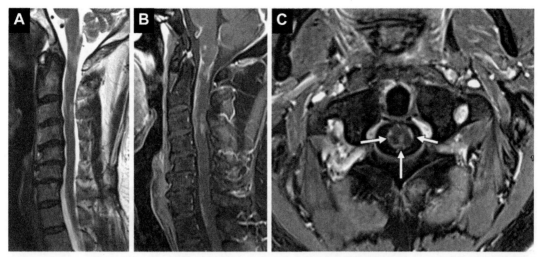

Fig. 18. Spinal neurosarcoidosis. Sagittal T2W (*A*) MR image of the cervical spine from a 51-year-old man with progressive numbness, spasticity, and pain reveals multifocal patchy peripheral spinal cord T2 hyperintensity. Sagittal (*B*) and axial (*C*) T1W-post contrast MR images demonstrate associated "trident" pattern of dorsal pial and infiltrative subpial spinal cord enhancement (*arrows* in *C*), a pattern typical of spinal neurosarcoidosis.

primarily involving the metabolically active frontal horns, termed the "owl's eye" sign of cord infarction[48] (**Fig. 19**). Associated hyperintensity on DWI with reduced ADC values helps confirm the diagnosis of acute SC infarct. Given the shared vascular supply with vertebral bodies, associated vertebral edema at the same level as the cord infarct can help discern from other pathologic conditions that involve the ventral SC[46] (see **Fig. 19**). A less common cause of cord infarction is termed surfer's myelopathy. Underlying pathophysiology is incompletely understood but likely relates to extended cervical hyperextension in novice surfers while paddling their surfboards in the prone position and looking forward, resulting in tension on the SC and surrounding vasculature and avulsion of perforating vessels.[49] Other rare causes include fibrocartilaginous embolism from herniated disc material and decompression sickness.

Among arteriovenous shunting lesions, dural arteriovenous fistulas (dAVFs) are most common, accounting for 60% to 80% of all spinal vascular lesions.[50] The fistulous point most frequently occurs at the dural sleeve within a neural foramen. Spinal dAVFs are more common in middle-aged and older men with insidious clinical symptoms of lower extremity weakness, sensory changes, and sphincter dysfunction. Longstanding venous hypertension from the fistula contributes to perimedullary venous engorgement and congestive venous myelopathy of the SC. On MR imaging, intramedullary SC T2-hyperintense edema with predelection for conus involvement in conjunction with dilated perimedullary vascular flow voids are

characteristic MR imaging features[46] (**Fig. 20**). The cord edema and vascular flow voids may not be located at the same level, and the location of either does not reliably correlate with the location of the fistula. Central cord and cauda equina nerve root enhancement may also be observed. Although conventional digital subtraction angiography of the spine is recommended for diagnostic confirmation and potential treatment, time-resolved MRA may aid in identifying the level of fistulous connection in up to 73% of cases[51] (see **Fig. 20**). Additional more rare spinal arteriovenous shunts include intramedullary glomus arterovenous malformations (AVMs), metameric AVMs, and perimedullary AVMs.

Spinal cord cavernous malformations exhibit many of the same imaging features as seen with cavernous malformations in the brain. T2-hypointense margins with central T1 and T2 heterogenous signal and marked susceptibility artifact within the SC are characteristic MR imaging features. There is no arteriovenous shunt; therefore, MR imaging is superior to spDSA for making the diagnosis. Ventral spinal location is a negative prognostic indicator.[52]

Toxic-Metabolic and Radiation-Related Spine Emergencies

The most common toxic-metabolic cause of emergent myelopathy is Vitamin B12-deficiency, which causes pernicious anemia and subacute combined degeneration. This disease may result from parietal cell autoantibodies, insufficient dietary

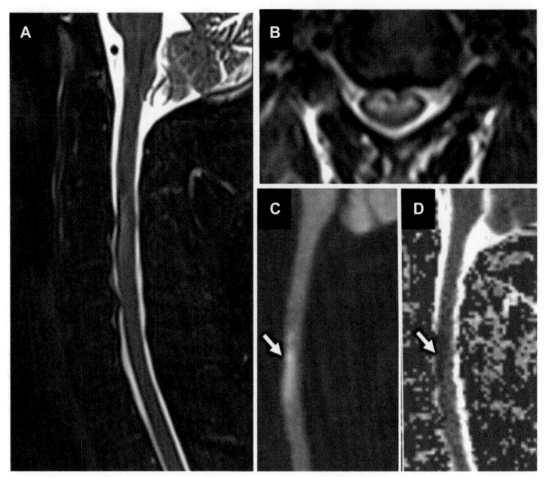

Fig. 19. Acute anterior spinal cord infarct. Sagittal (*A*) and axial (*B*) T2W FS MR images from a 68-year-old man with acute onset upper extremity weakness following aortic aneurysm repair shows ventral frontal-horn predominant T2 hyperintensity. Sagittal DWI (*C*) and ADC map (*D*) from the same examination shows abnormal reduced diffusion (*arrow* in *C* and *D*) corresponding with T2 signal abnormality consistent with acute anterior spinal artery infarct.

intake of Vitamin B12, or intrinsic factor deficiency. Clinical symptoms include spastic paraparesis with distal proprioceptive loss, whereas typical imaging findings include long-segment T2 hyperintensity of the dorsal columns (**Fig. 21**). Associated involvement of the anterolateral columns accounts for the term subacute combined degeneration. Enhancement is unusual. Symptoms and imaging findings may resolve with adequate medical treatment of Vitamin B12 deficiency. Abuse of nitrous oxide, copper deficiency, and zinc toxicity may also cause subacute combined degeneration and thus have identical imaging findings.

Radiation myelopathy can occur either in the immediate aftermath or in a delayed fashion, years after radiation exposure. Radiation myelitis is most often seen after radiation therapy for head and neck cancer and vertebral metastases, usually when patients have received an excess of 4000 rad.[53] Radiation myelopathy may resolve spontaneously or progress insidiously to spinal atrophy and severe disability and death. There is no effective treatment. Early imaging manifestations are nonspecific and include long-segment centromedullary T2 hyperintensity and patchy enhancement.[38] Although SC findings are nonspecific, intrinsic T1 hyperintensity of vertebral bodies corresponding to the radiation field, representing fatty bone marrow replacement, is a useful associated imaging finding to confirm the diagnosis.[54]

Intramedullary spinal cord masses
Intramedullary SC masses and mass-like lesions vary widely in cause and imaging appearance. Patients may present with pain, weakness, and

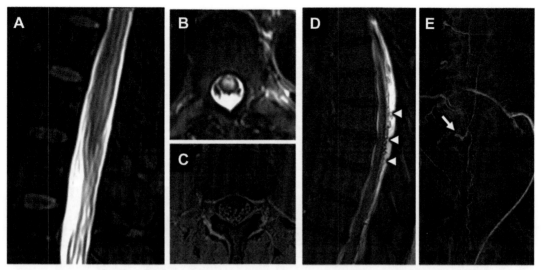

Fig. 20. Spinal dural arteriovenous fistula (sdAVF). Sagittal (*A*) and axial (*B*) T2W MR images from a 52-year-old woman with rapidly progressive bilateral lower extremity weakness and urinary incontinence reveals abnormal centromedullary pattern of T2 hyperintensity in the lower spinal cord and conus. Axial T1W-post contrast image of the cauda equina (*C*) shows abnormal nerve root hyperenhancement. Sagittal T2W image of the thoracic spine (*D*) shows abnormal dilated vascular flow voids along the dorsal surface of the spinal cord (*arrowheads* in *D*). Three-dimensional reconstruction from digital subtraction angiography with selective injection of the right T9 intercostal artery reveals multiple small branches coalescing at a dilated vein within the T10-T11 neuroforamen (*arrow* in *E*) with dilated venous outflow extending cranial and caudal along the dorsum of the spinal cord, consistent with sdAVF.

sensory changes depending on mass location. Causes include primary and metastatic tumors, SC abscess, and cavernous malformations as discussed in the prior section on vascular lesions. Masses should be characterized as circumscribed or infiltrative. The most common primary intramedullary neoplasms include ependymoma, astrocytoma, and hemangioblastoma. Ependymomas are the most common spinal glial tumor in adults and arise from the central canal or from cell rests along the filum terminale.[55] As such, they tend to be centrally located in the SC with symmetric expansion and well-circumscribed margins. Tumor cysts may be seen in up to 22% of ependymomas and adjacent syringohydromyelia is common.[55] Intratumoral hemorrhage can lead to hypointense hemosiderin rim on T2W imaging known as the "cap sign."[55] Avid yet heterogenous tumor enhancement is typical. Astrocytomas are the most common spinal glial tumor in children and are more eccentric, infiltrative, and more likely to involve the entire transverse extent of the cord compared with ependymomas.[55] Hemorrhage is uncommon in astrocytomas. Hemangioblastomas have highly variable MR imaging appearance but often involve multiple vertebral levels with avid enhancement. In large tumors, identification of associated prominent vascular flow voids within the tumor should prompt consideration of spinal hemangioblastoma.[55] Hemorrhage is common and the hemosiderin "cap sign" may also be observed. Multiple spinal hemangioblastomas suggest underlying Von Hippel-Lindau disease.

Intramedullary SC metastases are fortunately rare and clinical history of known widespread malignancy helps favor the diagnosis. On MR imaging, metastases to the SC are expansile with prominent surrounding edema. Following contrast administration, thin linear rim enhancement with more ill-defined enhancement emanating along the superior and inferior margins (rim and flame signs, respectively) have been described as characteristic features.[56]

Intramedullary spinal abscess is rare and may arise from contiguous or hematogenous spread. Congenital dermal sinus tracts may predispose to the development of intramedullary spinal abscesses, particularly in the pediatric population. These lesions have an MR imaging appearance similar to intracranial abscesses, with diffuse or rim enhancement, surrounding edema, and reduced diffusion centrally, although early in the course of the disease the only finding may be ill-defined T2-hyperintensity with or without patchy enhancement.[57] Similar to epidural or intracranial abscesses, the most common causative organisms are *Staphylococcus* and *Streptococcus* species.[37]

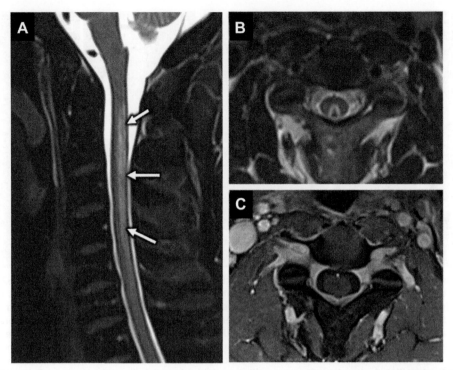

Fig. 21. Dorsal column tractopathy related to Vitamin B12 deficiency. Sagittal (*A*) and axial (*B*) T2W MR images of the cervical spine from a 36-year-old vegetarian woman with low vitamin B12 levels and 1 week history of bilateral hand and lower extremity numbness and gait instability demonstrates longitudinally extensive dorsal column T2 hyperintensity (*arrows* in *A*). Axial postcontrast T1W MR imaging (*C*) shows no associated abnormal enhancement.

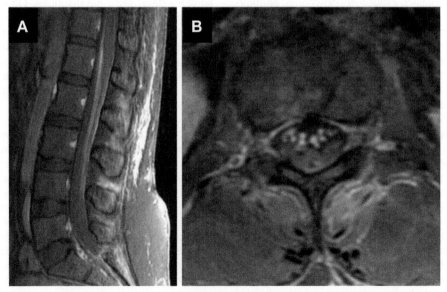

Fig. 22. Guillain Barre syndrome. Sagittal (*A*) and axial (*B*) T1W-post contrast images of the lumbar spine show diffuse thickening and hyperenhancement of the ventral motor nerve rootlets in this 42-year-old woman presenting with 1 month of rapidly progressive ascending weakness following a gastrointestinal illness.

Polyradiculopathies

Guillain Barre syndrome (GBS) is an acute, demyelinating polyneuropathy that is often proceeded by a viral illness, although it may also be associated with vaccine administration and autoimmune disorders. There are several subtypes of GBS, including motor and motor-sensory axonal subtypes and regional GBS (Miller-Fisher variant). The diagnosis is suspected in patients presenting with ascending flaccid paralysis. CSF studies reveal elevated protein without leukocytosis. The diagnosis of GBS may be supported or suggested on MR imaging by smooth enhancement of the cauda equina nerve roots preferentially involving the ventral motor rootlets, although the main purpose of imaging in these patients often serves to exclude other treatable causes of acute paralysis (**Fig. 22**). GBS has recently been reported with COVID-19-related SARS-CoV-2 infection.[58] In a systematic review of 73 patients with GBS associated with COVID-19, neurologic symptoms presented between 2 and 33 days after respiratory symptom onset.[59] Of note, CSF PCR was insensitive and negative for SARS-CoV-2 in all patients tested.

The differential diagnosis for nerve root enhancement is broad and in addition to GBS, includes leptomeningeal carcinomatosis, chronic inflammatory demyelinating polyneuropathy (CIDP), arachnoiditis, sarcoidosis, lymphoma, and infectious radiculitis. Generally, these differential considerations are associated with a nonspecific CSF profile including elevated protein, so clinical presentation and patient history along with imaging findings are usually instrumental in making the final diagnosis. For instance, leptomeningeal carcinomatosis typically occurs in the setting of widespread metastatic disease. CIDP polyneuropathy is a heterogeneous group of demyelinating polyneuropathies that may be antibody mediated or immune cell mediated; regardless of the specific underlying cause and pathophysiology, this syndrome is chronic by definition, with symptoms typically progressing over several months. Arachnoiditis refers to inflammation of the nerves and nerve roots and can be caused by a variety of causes including infection, prior intradural surgical manipulation, and intrathecal drug administration. Patients with neurosarcoidosis causing leptomeningeal inflammation will usually have other stigmata of this disease, even if the neurologic symptoms are the first manifestation. Primary leptomeningeal lymphoma is a rare form of primary CNS lymphoma and a rare cause of leptomeningeal enhancement; the diagnosis is made by identifying malignant lymphocytes on CSF cytology. Finally, AIDS-associated CMV polyradiculopathy and Lyme disease will be associated with specific exposures and/or clinical and laboratory signs of these infections. The radiologist should be prepared to synthesize this clinical data in order to narrow the differential diagnosis.

SUMMARY

MR imaging plays a central role in the timely diagnosis and treatment of spine emergencies. For traumatic emergencies, MR imaging plays a complementary role to CT. Knowledge of the most up-to-date traumatic spine injury classification systems forms a framework for an algorithmic search pattern to best inform treatment decisions. Diagnostic considerations for atraumatic spine emergencies are broad, and MR imaging is the first-line imaging modality for initially determining whether there is compressive pathologic condition. Familiarity with key MR imaging findings along with knowledge of relevant clinical history is necessary for diagnosing both compressive and noncompressive atraumatic spine emergencies.

CLINICS CARE POINTS

- When evaluating for traumatic spinal instability, integrity of the posterior ligamentous complex of the posterior tension band is best evaluated with T2-weighted (T2W) fat-suppressed and high-resolution T2W MR sequences.

- The absence of prevertebral fluid virtually excludes clinically significant traumatic injury to the anterior tension band of the spine.

- The presence of intramedullary spinal cord hemorrhage on MR imaging is the strongest imaging marker of injury severity and neuroprognostication.

- MR imaging is the first-line imaging modality to emergently exclude compressive spinal cord pathologic condition.

DISCLOSURE

The authors have nothing to disclose

REFERENCES

1. Daffner RH, Hackney DB. ACR appropriateness criteria on suspected spine trauma. J Am Coll Radiol 2007;4(11):762–75.

2. Shah LM, Ross JS. Imaging of spine trauma. Neurosurgery 2016;79(5):626–42.

3. Talbott JF, Huie JR, Ferguson AR, et al. MR imaging for assessing injury severity and prognosis in acute traumatic spinal cord injury. Radiol Clin North Am 2019;57(2):319–39.

4. Arce D, Sass P, Abul-Khoudoud H. Recognizing spinal cord emergencies. Am Fam Physician 2001; 64(4):631–8.

5. Expert Panel on Neurological I, Hutchins TA, Peckham M, et al. ACR appropriateness criteria(R) low back pain: 2021 update. J Am Coll Radiol 2021;18(11S):S361–79.

6. Mirowitz SA, Heiken JP, Brown JJ. Evaluation of fat saturation technique for T2-weighted endorectal coil MRI of the prostate. Magn Reson Imaging 1994;12(5):743–7.

7. Lammertse D, Dungan D, Dreisbach J, et al. Neuroimaging in traumatic spinal cord injury: an evidence-based review for clinical practice and research. J Spinal Cord Med 2007;30(3):205–14.

8. Shanmuganathan K, Zhuo J, Chen HH, et al. Diffusion tensor imaging parameter obtained during acute blunt cervical spinal cord injury in predicting long-term outcome. J Neurotrauma 2017;34(21):2964–71.

9. Kurpad S, Martin AR, Tetreault LA, et al. Impact of baseline magnetic resonance imaging on neurologic, functional, and safety outcomes in patients with acute traumatic spinal cord injury. Glob Spine J 2017;7(3 Suppl):151S–74S.

10. Vranic JE, Huynh TJ, Fata P, et al. The ability of magnetic resonance black blood vessel wall imaging to evaluate blunt cerebrovascular injury following acute trauma. J Neuroradiol 2020;47(3):210–5.

11. Riascos R, Bonfante E, Cotes C, et al. Imaging of atlanto-occipital and atlantoaxial traumatic injuries: what the radiologist needs to know. Radiographics 2015;35(7):2121–34.

12. Vaccaro AR, Oner C, Kepler CK, et al. AOSpine thoracolumbar spine injury classification system: fracture description, neurological status, and key modifiers. Spine (Phila Pa 1976) 2013;38(23):2028–37.

13. Vaccaro AR, Koerner JD, Radcliff KE, et al. AOSpine subaxial cervical spine injury classification system. Eur Spine J 2016;25(7):2173–84.

14. Henninger B, Kaser V, Ostermann S, et al. Cervical disc and ligamentous injury in hyperextension trauma: mri and intraoperative correlation. J Neuroimaging 2020;30(1):104–9.

15. Pizones J, Izquierdo E, Sanchez-Mariscal F, et al. Sequential damage assessment of the different components of the posterior ligamentous complex after magnetic resonance imaging interpretation: prospective study 74 traumatic fractures. Spine (Phila Pa 1976) 2012;37(11):E662–7.

16. Schaefer DM, Flanders A, Northrup BE, et al. Magnetic resonance imaging of acute cervical spine trauma. Correlation with severity of neurologic injury. Spine (Phila Pa 1976) 1989;14(10):1090–5.

17. Talbott JF, Whetstone WD, Readdy WJ, et al. The brain and spinal injury center score: a novel, simple, and reproducible method for assessing the severity of acute cervical spinal cord injury with axial T2-weighted MRI findings. J Neurosurg Spine 2015; 23(4):495–504.

18. Fehlings MG, Martin AR, Tetreault LA, et al. A clinical practice guideline for the management of patients with acute spinal cord injury: recommendations on the role of baseline magnetic resonance imaging in clinical decision making and outcome prediction. Glob Spine J 2017;7(3 Suppl):221S–30S.

19. Ropper AE, Ropper AH. Acute spinal cord compression. N Engl J Med 2017;376(14):1358–69.

20. Douglas AG, Xu DJ, Shah MP. Approach to myelopathy and myelitis. Neurol Clin 2022;40(1):133–56.

21. Talbott JF, Shah VN, Uzelac A, et al. Imaging-based approach to extradural infections of the spine. Semin Ultrasound CT MR 2018;39(6):570–86.

22. Hadjipavlou AG, Mader JT, Necessary JT, et al. Hematogenous pyogenic spinal infections and their surgical management. Spine (Phila Pa 1976) 2000; 25(13):1668–79.

23. Dumont RA, Keen NN, Bloomer CW, et al. Clinical utility of diffusion-weighted imaging in spinal infections. Clin Neuroradiol 2018;29(3):515–22.

24. Lavi ES, Pal A, Bleicher D, et al. MR Imaging of the spine: urgent and emergent indications. Semin Ultrasound CT MR 2018;39(6):551–69.

25. Go JL, Rothman S, Prosper A, et al. Spine infections. Neuroimaging Clin N Am 2012;22(4):755–72.

26. Torres C, Zakhari N. Imaging of spine infection. Semin Roentgenol 2017;52(1):17–26.

27. Gibbs WN, Nael K, Doshi AH, et al. Spine Oncology: Imaging and Intervention. Radiol Clin North Am 2019;57(2):377–95.

28. Fisher CG, DiPaola CP, Ryken TC, et al. A novel classification system for spinal instability in neoplastic disease: an evidence-based approach and expert consensus from the Spine oncology study group. Spine (Phila Pa 1976) 2010;35(22): E1221–9.

29. Bilsky MH, Laufer I, Fourney DR, et al. Reliability analysis of the epidural spinal cord compression scale. J Neurosurg Spine 2010;13(3):324–8.

30. Braun P, Kazmi K, Nogues-Melendez P, et al. MRI findings in spinal subdural and epidural hematomas. Eur J Radiol 2007;64(1):119–25.

31. Lonjon MM, Paquis P, Chanalet S, et al. Nontraumatic spinal epidural hematoma: report of four cases and review of the literature. Neurosurgery 1997;41(2):483–6. ; discussion 486-7.

32. Onofrei LV, Henrie AM. Cervical and thoracic spondylotic myelopathies. Semin Neurol 2021;41(3): 239–46.

33. Flanagan EP, Marsh RW, Weinshenker BG. Teaching neuroimages: "pancake-like" gadolinium enhancement suggests compressive myelopathy due to spondylosis. Neurology 2013;80(21):e229.

34. Koeller KK, Shih RY. Intradural extramedullary spinal neoplasms: radiologic-pathologic correlation. Radiographics 2019;39(2):468–90.

35. Li Z, Chen YA, Chow D, et al. Practical applications of CISS MRI in spine imaging. Eur J Radiol Open 2019;6:231–42.

36. Reardon MA, Raghavan P, Carpenter-Bailey K, et al. Dorsal thoracic arachnoid web and the "scalpel sign": a distinct clinical-radiologic entity. AJNR Am J Neuroradiol 2013;34(5):1104–10.

37. Talbott JF, Narvid J, Chazen JL, et al. An imaging-based approach to spinal cord infection. Semin Ultrasound CT MR 2016;37(5):411–30.

38. Lee MJ, Aronberg R, Manganaro MS, et al. Diagnostic approach to intrinsic abnormality of spinal cord signal intensity. Radiographics 2019;39(6):1824–39.

39. Messacar K, Schreiner TL, Maloney JA, et al. A cluster of acute flaccid paralysis and cranial nerve dysfunction temporally associated with an outbreak of enterovirus D68 in children in Colorado, USA. Lancet 2015;385(9978):1662–71.

40. Kraushaar G, Patel R, Stoneham GW. West Nile Virus: a case report with flaccid paralysis and cervical spinal cord: MR imaging findings. AJNR Am J Neuroradiol 2005;26(1):26–9.

41. Ayers T, Lopez A, Lee A, et al. Acute Flaccid Myelitis in the United States: 2015-2017. Pediatrics 2019; 144(5).

42. Beh SC, Greenberg BM, Frohman T, et al. Transverse myelitis. Neurol Clin 2013;31(1):79–138.

43. Wingerchuk DM, Banwell B, Bennett JL, et al. International consensus diagnostic criteria for neuromyelitis optica spectrum disorders. Neurology 2015; 85(2):177–89.

44. Dubey D, Pittock SJ, Krecke KN, et al. Clinical, radiologic, and prognostic features of myelitis associated with myelin oligodendrocyte glycoprotein autoantibody. JAMA Neurol 2019;76(3):301–9.

45. Zalewski NL, Krecke KN, Weinshenker BG, et al. Central canal enhancement and the trident sign in spinal cord sarcoidosis. Neurology 2016;87(7):743–4.

46. McEntire CR, Dowd RS, Orru E, et al. Acute myelopathy: vascular and infectious diseases. Neurol Clin 2021;39(2):489–512.

47. Alblas CL, Bouvy WH, Lycklama ANGJ, et al. Acute spinal-cord ischemia: evolution of MRI findings. J Clin Neurol 2012;8(3):218–23.

48. Weidauer S, Nichtweiss M, Lanfermann H, et al. Spinal cord infarction: MR imaging and clinical features in 16 cases. Neuroradiology 2002;44(10):851–7.

49. Freedman BA, Malone DG, Rasmussen PA, et al. Surfer's myelopathy: a rare form of spinal cord infarction in novice surfers: a systematic review. Neurosurgery 2016;78(5):602–11.

50. Jellema K, Tijssen CC, van Gijn J. Spinal dural arteriovenous fistulas: a congestive myelopathy that initially mimics a peripheral nerve disorder. Brain 2006;129(Pt 12):3150–64.

51. Lee J, Lim YM, Suh DC, et al. Clinical presentation, imaging findings, and prognosis of spinal dural arteriovenous fistula. J Clin Neurosci 2016;26:105–9.

52. Liang JT, Bao YH, Zhang HQ, et al. Management and prognosis of symptomatic patients with intramedullary spinal cord cavernoma: clinical article. J Neurosurg Spine 2011;15(4):447–56.

53. Marcus RB Jr, Million RR. The incidence of myelitis after irradiation of the cervical spinal cord. Int J Radiat Oncol Biol Phys 1990;19(1):3–8.

54. Khan M, Ambady P, Kimbrough D, et al. Radiation-induced myelitis: initial and follow-up MRI and clinical features in patients at a single tertiary care institution during 20 Years. AJNR Am J Neuroradiol 2018;39(8):1576–81.

55. Koeller KK, Rosenblum RS, Morrison AL. Neoplasms of the spinal cord and filum terminale: radiologic-pathologic correlation. Radiographics 2000;20(6): 1721–49.

56. Rykken JB, Diehn FE, Hunt CH, et al. Rim and flame signs: postgadolinium MRI findings specific for non-CNS intramedullary spinal cord metastases. AJNR Am J Neuroradiol 2013;34(4):908–15.

57. Friess HM, Wasenko JJ. MR of staphylococcal myelitis of the cervical spinal cord. AJNR Am J Neuroradiol 1997;18(3):455–8.

58. Moonis G, Filippi CG, Kirsch CFE, et al. The spectrum of neuroimaging findings on CT and MRI in adults with COVID-19. AJR Am J Roentgenol 2021; 217(4):959–74.

59. Abu-Rumeileh S, Abdelhak A, Foschi M, et al. Guillain-Barre syndrome spectrum associated with COVID-19: an up-to-date systematic review of 73 cases. J Neurol 2021;268(4):1133–70.

Magnetic Resonance Imaging of Head and Neck Emergencies, a Symptom-Based Review, Part 1
General Considerations, Vision Loss, and Eye Pain

Paul M. Bunch, MD[a],*, Jeffrey R. Sachs, MD[a], Hillary R. Kelly, MD[b,c,d],
Megan E. Lipford, PhD[a], Thomas G. West, MD[a]

KEYWORDS

• Emergency department • Head and neck • Magnetic resonance imaging • Vision loss • Eye pain

KEY POINTS

- Diagnostic accuracy and timeliness are essential to minimize the risk of morbidity and death among patients with acute head and neck pathologic conditions.
- Although head and neck magnetic resonance (MR) imaging intimidates many, radiologists interpreting emergency studies must be familiar with the relevant anatomy, pathologic conditions, and acute management considerations to meet the needs of their patients and referring physicians.
- Abbreviated or focused MR imaging protocols for emergency department patients are intended to quickly and efficiently address the acute presentation while minimizing image acquisition time and maximizing patient throughput. Essential MR imaging sequences for the evaluation of most head and neck emergencies include small field of view T1, short tau inversion recovery (STIR), and gadolinium-enhanced T1 (with or without fat suppression depending on local preferences), as well as diffusion-weighted and fluid-attenuated inversion recovery (FLAIR) imaging of the brain.

INTRODUCTION

During the past 2 decades, emergency department (ED) magnetic resonance (MR) imaging utilization has considerably increased.[1–4] Access has also expanded with some institutions installing MR imaging systems within EDs to meet critical and time-sensitive patient needs.[5,6] In light of data associating MR imaging use with increased ED length of stay,[7] there have been concerted efforts to develop "abbreviated" or "focused" MR protocols designed to quickly and efficiently answer clinical questions specifically relevant to the ED evaluation while minimizing image acquisition time and maximizing patient throughput. Accurate and timely diagnosis of acute head and neck disease is particularly important because improper or delayed diagnosis places the patient at risk for substantial morbidity and even death.[8,9] Computed tomography (CT) remains the first-line imaging modality for evaluation of most traumatic and infectious head and neck emergencies; however, MR is diagnostically superior in certain

a Department of Radiology, Wake Forest School of Medicine, Medical Center Boulevard, Winston Salem, NC 27157, USA; b Department of Radiology, Massachusetts General Hospital, 55 Fruit Street, Boston, MA 02114, USA; c Department of Radiology, Massachusetts Eye and Ear, 243 Charles Street, Boston, MA 02114, USA; d Harvard Medical School, 25 Shattuck Street, Boston, MA 02115, USA
* Corresponding author.
E-mail address: paul.m.bunch@gmail.com

Magn Reson Imaging Clin N Am 30 (2022) 409–424
https://doi.org/10.1016/j.mric.2022.04.005
1064-9689/22/© 2022 Elsevier Inc. All rights reserved.

scenarios (eg, when intracranial complications are suspected) with the added benefit of no ionizing radiation. As such, ED patients with head and neck pathologic conditions are increasingly being evaluated with MR imaging.

Although head and neck imaging intimidates many, radiologists interpreting ED MR studies should be familiar with the relevant anatomy, pathologic conditions, and acute management considerations to meet the needs of their patients and referring physicians. Acknowledging that a comprehensive discussion of all head and neck pathologic conditions that may be encountered in the ED setting is not possible with a single article, our purpose is to provide an accessible, practical, symptom-based approach to some of the nontraumatic head and neck pathologic conditions most relevant to emergency head and neck MR and with which readers may not already be familiar. We emphasize relevant anatomy, "do not miss" findings, findings affecting clinical management, and clinical and imaging features facilitating differentiation of discussed pathologies

from potential mimics. We also share perspectives on essential sequences to include if considering an "abbreviated" or "focused" protocol (**Table 1**), potential trade-offs and pitfalls, and strategies for obtaining diagnostic information when faced with patient motion and other technical challenges. For more information on emergent clinical presentations (eg, acute neck pain) and associated pathologic conditions (eg, peritonsillar abscess, lymphadenitis, sialoadenitis) for which CT evaluation is most often adequate, we refer the reader to several recent excellent reviews.[10–14]

SAFETY AND TECHNICAL CONSIDERATIONS

Patients undergoing emergency MR imaging must possess a protected airway and be sufficiently medically stable to tolerate the duration of the examination. Many referring physicians consider MR to be "safe" because there is no associated ionizing radiation. However, if patients are not appropriately screened[15] or if proper environmental precautions are not observed,[16–18] patients can be harmed or even fatally injured. As

Table 1
Summary of essential magnetic resonance sequences used to evaluate common indications for emergency head and neck magnetic resonance imaging

Indication	Essential Sequences	Primary Evaluation Purposes
Vision loss	Orbit:	
	• Cor STIR/T2 FS	Optic nerve, orbital fat, fluid collections
	• Cor T1	Orbital fat, extraocular muscles
	• Ax and Cor T1 C+[a]	Abnormal enhancement, blood vessel patency
	Brain:	
	• Ax DWI	Abscess, empyema, ischemia
	• Ax or Cor FLAIR	Demyelinating disease, meningitis, cerebritis
Ear pain	Temporal bone:	
	• Ax T1	Normal fat pads, particularly along the facial nerve and within the deep spaces of the suprahyoid neck
	• Ax SSFP	Internal auditory canal and membranous labyrinth structures
	• Ax and Cor T1 C+[a]	Abnormal enhancement, blood vessel patency
	Brain:	
	• Ax DWI	Abscess, empyema, ischemia
	• Ax or Cor FLAIR	Meningitis, cerebritis
Face pain	Face:	
	• Ax T1	Normal fat pads, particularly along the trigeminal nerve divisions and their branches
	• Ax or Cor STIR/T2 FS	Inflammatory edema, fluid collections
	• Ax and Cor T1 C+[a]	Abnormal enhancement (including loss of normal enhancement as seen in acute invasive fungal sinusitis), blood vessel patency
	Brain:	
	• Ax DWI	Abscess, empyema, ischemia
	• Ax or Cor FLAIR	Meningitis, cerebritis

[a] May be performed with or without fat suppression and as a 2D or 3D acquisition, depending on local preferences. We find 3D postcontrast sequences helpful for evaluating patency of the dural venous sinuses, particularly the cavernous sinuses. DWI, diffusion-weighted imaging; FS, fat-suppressed; SSFP, steady-state free precession.

such, MR safety screening is necessary for all patients and *cannot* be skipped in the emergent setting. Although patient interview by the MR technologist is the quickest and easiest method for completing the MR safety screen, acute illness may prevent some ED patients from participating in this process. To minimize unnecessary delays in the MR safety screening of altered or incapacitated patients, the screening process is best instituted by the referring physician at the time the MR order is placed by either (1) providing the name and contact information for the patient's health-care proxy to the MR technologist or (2) notifying the MR technologist that no health-care proxy is available and that radiographic clearance will be required. By educating ED physicians about the importance of initiating MR safety screening at the time of order entry and by encouraging them to directly connect with MR technologists regarding all altered or otherwise incapacitated patients, radiologists facilitate timely patient care and minimize delay-related frustrations among all stakeholders.

Once the patient has been determined safe for MR imaging, the next task is to acquire images of satisfactory quality to enable accurate and efficient diagnosis. For sequences focusing on a specific region of the head and neck (eg, orbit, temporal bone), a small field of view (eg, 15–20 cm) is often most appropriate. A large matrix (eg, 400 × 400) will yield very high-resolution images in cooperative patients. However, large matrices result in longer acquisition times with increased risk for patient motion, which can in turn necessitate repeat acquisitions. As such, large acquisition matrices may not be feasible in many ED settings. In our experience, a matrix size of 250 × 250 combined with a 15 to 20 cm field of view is often adequate for diagnosis.

The anatomy of the head and neck presents several challenges to MR imaging. Bone–air interfaces create artifacts related to magnetic field inhomogeneity, and swallowing, breathing, and vascular pulsation introduce unavoidable motion artifacts. The susceptibility artifacts caused by bone–air interfaces are of greater magnitude at higher field strengths, with longer echo time, and with gradient echo sequences. Thus, to minimize these artifacts, fast spin echo sequences with minimum echo time should be used.[19] Susceptibility artifacts are also diminished at lower magnetic field strength (eg, 1.5 vs 3.0 T) and with reduced slice thickness.[19] Fat suppression of postcontrast images is helpful to maximize conspicuity of abnormal enhancement. However, failure of fat suppression can obscure or even mimic (**Fig. 1**) pathologic conditions. Spectral fat suppression techniques have a high risk of failure in the head and neck due to susceptibility artifacts at the bone–air interfaces. Although not using fat suppression on gadolinium-enhanced images is one option to avoid associated artifacts potentially obscuring pathologic conditions,[20] the benefits of fat suppression are also lost with this approach. Utilization of Dixon fat suppression[21] is an alternative strategy to reduce fat suppression failure that has recently gained popularity in the head and neck.[22,23] The Dixon sequence generates fat, water, and in-phase and out-of-phase images and can be T1-weighted (**Fig. 2**) or T2-weighted. The water image is fat-suppressed, and the in-phase image can be reviewed if one desires postcontrast images without fat suppression. To similarly minimize failure of fat suppression related to magnetic

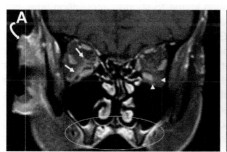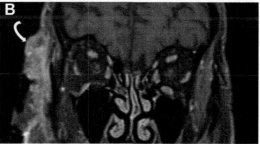

Fig. 1. Failure of spectral fat suppression mimicking a pathologic condition. Coronal gadolinium-enhanced, spectral fat-suppressed (*A*) and Dixon fat-suppressed (*B*), T1-weighted images obtained in an 87-year-old male with a cutaneous squamous cell carcinoma of the right face (*curved arrow, A and B*). The spectral fat-suppressed image (*A*) demonstrates ill-defined apparent T1 hyperintensity in the right orbit (*arrows, A*) that could be easily misinterpreted as enhancement related to right orbital invasion by the adjacent malignancy. However, this finding is not present on the Dixon fat-suppressed image (*B*), consistent with failure of fat suppression at the air–bone interface on the spectral fat-suppressed image (*A*) rather than true orbital invasion. Also note the presence of similar fat-suppression failures in the left orbit (*arrowheads, A*) and associated with the maxillary alveoli (*oval, A*) on the spectral fat-suppressed image (*A*) that are not present on the Dixon fat-suppressed image (*B*).

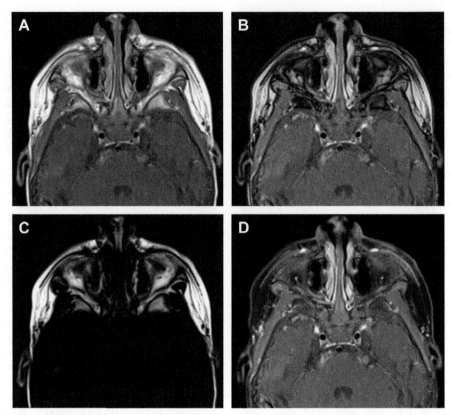

Fig. 2. Dixon method T1-weighted images. Water and fat have different resonance frequencies, which means that, depending on magnetic field strength and echo time, water and fat can be in-phase or out-of-phase. With the Dixon method, in-phase (*A*) and opposed-phase (*B*) images are acquired as part of the same sequence. The in-phase images consist of water + fat signal, and the opposed-phase images consist of water–fat signal. Through subtraction and addition of the acquired in-phase and opposed-phase image sets, respectively, fat only (*C*) images (average of in-phase minus opposed phase) and water only (*D*) images (average of in-phase plus opposed-phase) are generated. The water only image (*D*) represents the fat-suppressed image.

susceptibility artifacts on fluid-sensitive sequences, we favor STIR and T2-weighted Dixon sequences over spectral fat-suppressed T2. Although two-dimensional (2D) and three-dimensional (3D) postcontrast sequences each have value in head and neck imaging, we find 3D postcontrast sequences to be most helpful for evaluating patency of the dural venous sinuses, particularly the cavernous sinuses.

Many patients have difficulty remaining motionless for long periods. In such cases, motion artifacts can be mitigated with faster acquisition. Parallel imaging techniques are widely available as a tool to shorten scan time in head and neck protocols.[24] Although not as widely used, compressed sensing has been shown useful in the clinical setting of head and neck MR imaging to reduce scan time.[25,26] Simultaneous multislice acquisition (also called multiband) is another acceleration technique available on some clinical scanners. This technique is best applied to the diffusion acquisition[27] and requires head coils with a larger number of elements

(ie, at least 20 channels). Finally, there are emerging machine learning applications for "upscaling" a low-resolution image or acquisition to a higher resolution image to shorten acquisition time, improve image quality, or both.[28]

Some patients are unable to hold still for any length of time, in which case fast acquisition will not eliminate motion artifacts. In these cases, a radial acquisition can be used to decrease sensitivity to motion.[29] Vessel pulsation artifacts are also common in head and neck MR imaging. These ghost artifacts occur in the phase-encoding direction, and their spacing is related to the repetition time, number of excitations, and temporal frequency of the motion.[19] By switching the phase-encoding and frequency-encoding directions, the artifact may be moved to avoid overlap with anatomy of greatest interest. Alternatively, spatial presaturation pulses may be used upstream of the imaging volume to saturate the flowing signal.[19] Swallowing artifacts can be mitigated by putting the phase encoding in the anterior–posterior

Table 2
Characteristic features of pathologic conditions presenting with acute vision loss

Pathologic Conditions	Clinical Features	Imaging Features
Optic neuritis	Young adult (aged 20–40 years) females Often in association with multiple sclerosis Most commonly unilateral Pain exacerbated by eye movement	Increased fluid signal within the optic nerve on T2 and STIR sequences Gadolinium enhancement of the involved optic nerve segment
Anterior ischemic optic neuropathy	Nonarteritic: • Far more common • Adults older than 50 years • Typically painless • Idiopathic but most patients have hypertension, diabetes, and other vascular risk factors Arteritic: • Adults older than 70 years • Often painful • Jaw claudication • Proximal myalgias and arthralgias • Fatigue • Elevated erythrocyte sedimentation rate and C-reactive protein	Central bright spot sign observed in both arteritic and nonarteritic anterior ischemic optic neuropathy Absence of central bright spot sign specific for nonarteritic disease
Optic nerve sheath meningioma	Adult (aged 30–40 years) female predilection Painless and progressive More often unilateral Proptosis	Thickening and enhancement of the optic nerve sheath "Tram-track" calcifications
Orbital cellulitis	Most frequently affects children Recent upper respiratory infection Pain, fever, erythema, swelling, proptosis, ophthalmoplegia Leukocytosis	Inflammatory changes of the orbital fat and adjacent structures Coexisting rhinosinusitis Subperiosteal abscess may be present
Idiopathic orbital inflammation	Most frequently affects adults Abrupt onset of pain Proptosis, swelling, erythema Elevated erythrocyte sedimentation rate and C-reactive protein	Unilateral, ill-defined, mass-like tissue with low T2 signal and surrounding fat infiltration Tendon enlargement when extraocular muscles involved (medial rectus most commonly) No orbital fat proliferation
IgG4-related orbital disease	Typically painless Systemic disease, often with multiorgan manifestations Normal serum immunoglobulin G4 (IgG4) levels do not exclude disease, and elevated serum	Bilateral Lacrimal gland and extraocular muscle enlargement (lateral rectus most commonly) Infraorbital nerve enlargement (~30%) No orbital fat proliferation

(continued on next page)

Table 2
(continued)

Pathologic Conditions	Clinical Features	Imaging Features
	IgG4 levels do not confirm it Low threshold to biopsy	
Thyroid eye disease	Occurs in conjunction with autoimmune thyroiditis (Graves, most frequently) Adult females most commonly affected Proptosis, lid retraction, lid lag, periorbital swelling Pain may be present but is not typically the dominant feature	Characteristic pattern of extraocular muscle enlargement (I'M SLO) with sparing of tendinous insertions Orbital fat proliferation Findings typically bilateral but may be asymmetric No lacrimal gland involvement

direction for axial and sagittal images, by using phase oversampling, and with radial sampling.[30,31]

Small anatomy near the neck–chest junction can be difficult to image. The air in the lungs is a source of susceptibility artifacts. Additionally, head–neck coils may not provide sufficient coverage close to the surface of the patient, resulting in lower signal-to-noise. The use of a body coil over the upper torso in addition to a head–neck coil is one mitigation strategy. Alternatively, newer flexible coils can be placed closer to the patient's skin and contoured to fit each patient. These flexible coils have been shown to produce higher signal-to-noise images in this difficult to image region.[32]

VISION LOSS ± EYE PAIN

Acute, nontraumatic vision loss may be caused by ocular, orbital, and intracranial pathologic conditions. Ocular and orbital causes of vision loss are typically unilateral, whereas intracranial causes are typically bilateral with clinical history and physical examination informing further localization. Suspected ocular causes are generally best evaluated by ophthalmologic examination, and intracranial causes are best assessed with brain MR imaging. Causes of acute vision loss for which orbital MR imaging aids diagnosis include optic neuritis, ischemic optic neuropathy, optic nerve sheath meningioma, orbital cellulitis, and orbital inflammatory processes (**Table 2**). Essential orbit MR sequences for this evaluation include the following: (1) coronal STIR or fat-suppressed T2, (2) coronal T1 without fat suppression, and (3) and axial and coronal gadolinium-enhanced T1 (with or without fat suppression, depending on local preferences). Essential brain MR sequences include (1) diffusion-weighted imaging and (2) FLAIR. Ordering providers may request a brain MR for vision loss rather than focused orbital imaging. To increase sensitivity for detecting orbital inflammatory processes in these situations, routine fat-suppression of brain MR T2-weighted images can be helpful.

Optic Neuritis

Optic neuritis refers to inflammation of the optic nerve and typically presents with vision loss and painful eye movement. One in 3 cases of optic neuritis is caused by multiple sclerosis.[33] Alternative causes include other demyelinating diseases (eg, myelin oligodendrocyte glycoprotein [MOG] antibody-associated disease, neuromyelitis optica spectrum disorders [NMOSDs]), autoimmune disorders (eg, sarcoidosis, lupus, Behçet disease, Sjögren syndrome), and infection (eg, Lyme, toxoplasmosis, human immunodeficiency virus [HIV]).[33] On MR imaging, optic neuritis manifests as increased T2 and STIR signal within the involved portions of the optic nerve, most commonly with corresponding gadolinium enhancement (**Fig. 3**).

Among patients with demyelinating disease as the underlying cause of optic neuritis, detailed descriptions of the optic nerve lesion characteristics may help the neurologists diagnose the underlying disease. For example, optic neuritis in multiple sclerosis (**Fig. 4**A) is most commonly unilateral with short segment enhancement.[34] Bilateral optic neuritis with long segment enhancement (**Fig. 4**B) is common in both MOG antibody-associated disease and NMOSDs. However, MOG antibody-associated disease more commonly involves the anterior optic pathways, exhibits perineural enhancement extending into the surrounding orbital fat, and produces tortuous optic nerves secondary to swelling, whereas NMOSDs more commonly involve the posterior optic pathways without optic nerve tortuosity.[34]

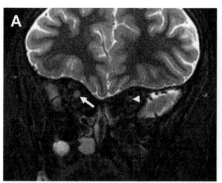
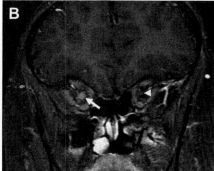

Fig. 3. Optic neuritis. Coronal STIR (*A*) and gadolinium-enhanced, fat-suppressed, T1-weighted (*B*) images obtained in a 9-year-old male with acute onset right vision loss demonstrate abnormal STIR hyperintensity (*arrow, A*) and enhancement (*arrow, B*) of the right optic nerve. The normal left optic nerve (*arrowhead, A and B*) is isointense to the cerebral white matter on the STIR image and does not enhance.

Ischemic Optic Neuropathy

Ischemic optic neuropathy is the most common optic nerve disorder in adults aged 50 years and greater,[35] generally categorized as anterior (involving the optic nerve head) versus posterior (involving the remainder of the optic nerve) and as arteritic (due to giant cell arteritis and often painful) versus nonarteritic (due to other causes and typically painless).[36] Nonarteritic anterior ischemic optic neuropathy (NA-AION) is far more common than arteritic anterior ischemic optic neuropathy (A-AION). The clinical presentation of A-AION most closely overlaps with optic neuritis, and differentiating between these 2 possibilities is a common indication for imaging. A-AION is an ocular emergency requiring prompt work-up for giant cell arteritis and immediate treatment with corticosteroids to prevent further vision loss. The clinical presentation of NA-AION can overlap with compressive optic neuropathy (eg, optic nerve sheath meningioma). Thus, in the setting of suspected NA-AION, imaging may be requested to exclude a compressive mass lesion. The "central bright spot sign" is a recently described imaging finding that is hypothesized to indicate damage to the anterior optic nerve microcirculation (**Fig. 5**). This finding may be useful in differentiating between nonarteritic and arteritic causes of anterior ischemic optic neuropathy to identify patients not requiring emergent corticosteroid therapy.[37] Among a cohort of 15 A-AION patient, 15 NA-AION patients, and 15 healthy subjects, the "central bright spot sign" was observed in all A-AION patients, 7/15 (47%) NA-AION patients, and no healthy controls.[37] Thus, the absence of the "central bright spot sign" suggests that A-AION is very unlikely and that emergent corticosteroids may not be required. Restricted diffusion of the optic nerve can be seen in posterior ischemic optic

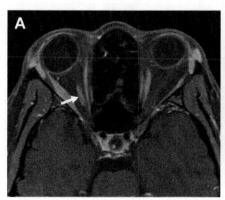
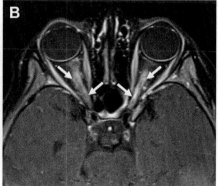

Fig. 4. Optic neuritis. Axial gadolinium-enhanced, fat-suppressed T1-weighted images in 2 different patients with acute optic neuritis. The patient shown in image A is a 30-year-old female with multiple sclerosis and short segment right optic neuritis (*arrow, A*). The patient shown in image B is a 6-year-old male with MOG antibody-associated disease and long segment bilateral optic neuritis (*arrows, B*).

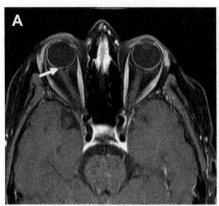
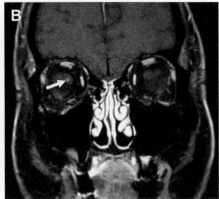

Fig. 5. Central bright spot sign. Axial (*A*) and coronal (*B*) gadolinium-enhanced, fat-suppressed, T1-weighted images obtained in a 67-year-old female with right vision loss attributed to nonarteritic anterior ischemic optic neuropathy demonstrate focal enhancement (*arrow, A* and *B*) of the right optic nerve head—the "central bright spot sign." Among patients with anterior ischemic optic neuropathy, this finding may be seen in both arteritic and nonarteritic disease. However, its absence strongly favors the nonarteritic subtype.

neuropathy; however, the orbits are prone to distortion and artifacts on echo planar diffusion-weighted imaging of the brain, such that caution in attributing significance to apparent optic nerve findings on these images is prudent.

Optic Nerve Sheath Meningioma

Meningiomas of the optic nerve sheath are estimated to account for 1% to 2% of all meningiomas and one-third of all primary optic nerve tumors.[38] Although optic nerve sheath meningiomas most commonly manifest with painless, slowly progressive vision loss, acute presentations have been reported.[39,40] These tumors are benign but they may lead to blindness if untreated. As such, timely diagnosis and appropriate management are necessary to achieve a favorable vision outcome.

On MR imaging, optic nerve sheath meningiomas are most readily identified on gadolinium-enhanced T1-weighted images with fat suppression, where they will exhibit homogeneously enhancing thickening of the optic nerve sheath. In the axial plane, the appearance is described as a "tram-track" configuration and in the coronal plane as a "donut" appearance (**Fig. 6**A, B). In 20% to 50% of cases,[41] calcifications are present and best seen with CT (**Fig. 6**C). Although the characteristic imaging features typically do not warrant biopsy, there are reports of metastatic disease, lymphoma, sarcoid, and idiopathic orbital inflammation (IOI) mimicking the clinical and imaging features of optic nerve sheath meningiomas. However, "tram-track" calcifications would be very unusual with these reported mimics.

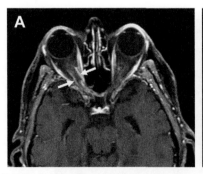
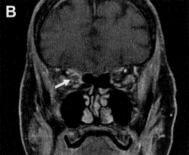
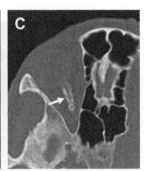

Fig. 6. Optic nerve sheath meningioma. Axial (*A*) and coronal (*B*) gadolinium-enhanced, fat-suppressed, T1-weighted images obtained in a 77-year-old female with progressive right vision loss demonstrate abnormal thickening and enhancement of the right optic nerve sheath compatible with optic nerve sheath meningioma. The nerve sheath thickening and enhancement produce a "tram-track" configuration (*arrows, A*) in the axial image and a "donut" configuration (*arrow, B*) in the coronal image. Axial CT image (*C*) obtained in a 45-year-old female with neurofibromatosis type 2 demonstrates the "tram-track" calcifications (*arrow, C*) present in 20% to 50% of these tumors.

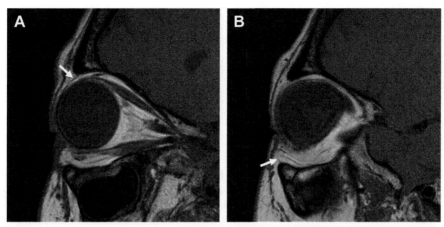

Fig. 7. Orbital septum. Sagittal T1-weighted images demonstrate the superior (*arrow, A*) and inferior (*arrow, B*) attachments of the orbital septum. Periorbital cellulitis involves the tissues anterior to this landmark (ie, "preseptal"), whereas orbital cellulitis involves the posterior structures (ie, "postseptal"). Although visible in these images, the orbital septum is not typically identifiable with routine clinical CT and MR. As such, for practical purposes its location is most often approximated by the orbital rim.

Orbital Cellulitis

Orbital (postseptal) cellulitis refers to a soft tissue infection of the intraorbital structures deep to the orbital septum (**Fig. 7**) and must be differentiated from the more common periorbital (preseptal) cellulitis that is limited to the subcutaneous tissues superficial to the orbital septum. Although uncommon in all age groups, orbital cellulitis most frequently affects children, typically as a complication of acute sinusitis.[42] Both orbital and periorbital cellulitis may present with fever, edema, erythema, and pain; however, vision loss, proptosis, and limited ocular motility are clinical features indicating orbital involvement.[42] Prompt diagnosis, initiation of intravenous antibiotic therapy, and drainage of orbital abscess (if present) are critically important to preserve vision and avoid potentially life-threatening complications, including superior ophthalmic vein (**Fig. 8**) and cavernous sinus thrombosis, meningoencephalitis (see **Fig. 8C**), intracranial abscess, and sepsis.

In most cases, CT is sufficient to differentiate orbital and periorbital cellulitis based on the location of fat stranding and other inflammatory changes (**Fig. 9**). Imaging may also provide valuable information on the underlying cause (eg, acute sinusitis, orbital foreign body, and dental

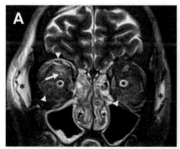
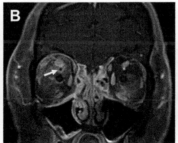
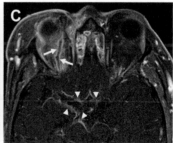

Fig. 8. Superior ophthalmic vein thrombosis in the setting of orbital cellulitis. Coronal STIR image (*A*) obtained in a 60-year-old female with acute sinusitis complicated by right greater than left orbital (postseptal) and periorbital (preseptal) cellulitis demonstrates abnormal fluid signal and fat stranding (*arrowheads, A*) within the right greater than left orbits as well as right greater than left periorbital soft tissue swelling and edema (*asterisks, A*). Also note the abnormally increased signal indicating slow flow versus thrombosis associated with the right superior ophthalmic vein (*arrow, A*) along the inferior aspect of the enlarged right superior rectus muscle. Coronal (*B*) and axial (*C*) gadolinium-enhanced, fat-suppressed, T1-weighted images demonstrate a filling defect consistent with thrombus in the right superior ophthalmic vein (*arrows, B and C*) as well as abnormal enhancement within the right greater than left orbits. The axial postcontrast image also demonstrates abnormal leptomeningeal enhancement (*arrowheads, C*) within the right greater than left basal cisterns consistent with meningitis.

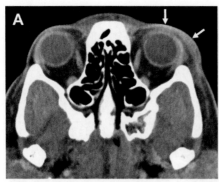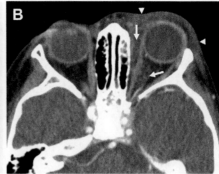

Fig. 9. Periorbital (preseptal) versus orbital (postseptal) cellulitis. Axial contrast-enhanced CT images obtained in 2 different patients demonstrate preseptal soft tissue thickening (*arrows, A*) in a 35-year-old female with left periorbital cellulitis and postseptal fat stranding (*arrows, B*) and left globe proptosis in a 2-year-old male with left orbital cellulitis. Periorbital cellulitis (*arrowheads, B*) is often also present in patients with orbital cellulitis.

disease, all of which the interpreting radiologist should specifically search for in the setting of orbital cellulitis) and the presence or absence of a drainable abscess. However, MR imaging may be useful when CT findings are equivocal or to provide a more sensitive assessment for associated vascular or intracranial complications. Typical MR findings of orbital cellulitis include abnormal fluid signal and stranding within the orbital fat. Extraocular muscle enlargement (ie, myositis) may also be seen. A rim-enhancing fluid collection with central restricted diffusion is consistent with abscess, most commonly subperiosteal as a complication of acute sinusitis (**Fig. 10**). Because wood is an organic material, wooden foreign bodies are particularly high-risk for superimposed infection. Additionally, wooden foreign bodies can be very difficult to identify on CT and MR imaging (**Fig. 11**) unless the radiologist is familiar with their appearance and specifically looks for them.

Inflammatory Diseases of the Orbit

IOI, also known as "orbital pseudotumor," is a non-granulomatous inflammatory process of unknown cause that accounts for 8% to 10% of all orbital masses.[43,44] In adults, the disease is typically unilateral, and pain—often accompanied by impaired ocular motility and/or decreased visual acuity—is a characteristic feature. In children, IOI is uncommon but usually bilateral.[44] IOI may involve any structure within the orbit with recognized anatomic patterns including myositis and dacryoadenitis as well as anterior, apical, and diffuse disease.[44] On MR imaging, IOI most often manifests as ill-defined, mass-like enhancing soft tissue with low T2 signal and surrounding fat infiltration. When the extraocular muscles are affected, fusiform tendon enlargement is expected, and the medial rectus is the most commonly involved muscle (**Fig. 12**). When suspected clinically, a trial of therapeutic corticosteroids is often initiated with subsequent

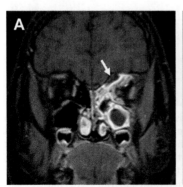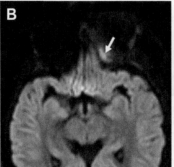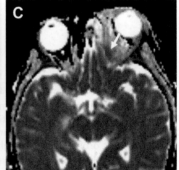

Fig. 10. Subperiosteal orbital abscess. Coronal gadolinium-enhanced, fat-suppressed, T1-weighted image (*A*) obtained in a 7-year-old male with acute sinusitis complicated by left orbital cellulitis demonstrates a rim-enhancing collection (*arrow, A*) along the superomedial aspect of the left orbit. Axial diffusion-weighted image (*B*) and corresponding ADC map (*C*) demonstrate central low diffusivity material associated with the rim-enhancing collection (*arrow, B* and *C*), consistent with abscess.

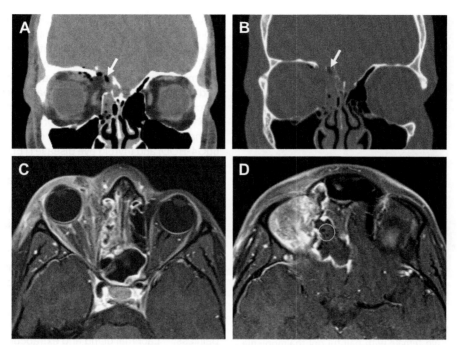

Fig. 11. Undetected wooden foreign body resulting in orbital cellulitis and intracranial abscess. Coronal soft tissue (*A*) and bone (*B*) reconstruction CT images obtained in an 18-year-old male patient who fell out of a tree stand while deer hunting demonstrate multiple right orbital fractures with small volume orbital hemorrhage. On the soft tissue image, all of the orbital and intracranial low attenuation foci could be easily mistaken for post-traumatic gas; however, on the bone window image, one of these foci (*arrow, A* and *B*) exhibits attenuation greater than air but lower than fat. Air-filled interstices in dry wood account for this CT appearance in the acute setting. This wooden foreign body was not identified at the time of CT imaging, and an orbit MR was performed 5 days later when the patient developed vision loss, difficulty with extraocular movements, and chemosis. Axial gadolinium-enhanced, fat-suppressed, T1-weighted images (*C, D*) demonstrate findings of right orbital and peri-orbital cellulitis (*C*) as well as an intracranial abscess surrounding the retained wooden foreign body (*circle, D*). Because of the air-filled interstices, wooden foreign bodies will be hypointense on all MR sequences in the acute setting but will increase in signal over time with the absorption of fluid and blood products. The patient underwent craniotomy for abscess drainage, and the intracranial wooden foreign body was confirmed at surgery.

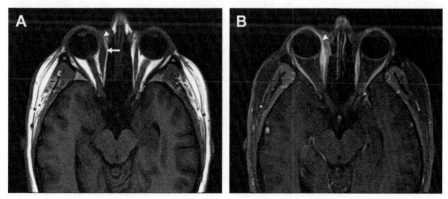

Fig. 12. Idiopathic orbital inflammation. Axial T1-weighted image (*A*) obtained in a 28-year-old female with acute onset right orbital pain and decreased visual acuity demonstrates fusiform enlargement of the right medial rectus muscle with indistinctness of the adjacent fat (*arrow, A*). Axial gadolinium-enhanced, fat-suppressed, T1-weighted image (*B*) demonstrates corresponding hyperenhancement of the affected muscle and fat. Note the involvement of the tendinous insertion (*arrowhead, A* and *B*). Symptoms improved after corticosteroids, and a presumptive diagnosis of idiopathic orbital inflammation was given.

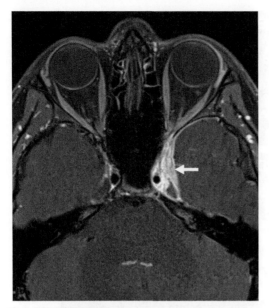

Fig. 13. Tolosa-Hunt syndrome. Axial gadolinium-enhanced, fat-suppressed, T1-weighted image obtained in a 23-year-old female with painful ophthalmoplegia and decreased visual acuity demonstrates abnormal enhancing soft tissue (*arrow*) centered in the left cavernous sinus. Clinical symptoms and imaging findings resolved after corticosteroids, and a presumptive diagnosis of Tolosa-Hunt syndrome was made.

improvement supporting the presumptive diagnosis of IOI. Biopsy is indicated when symptoms persist or if there is evidence of disease progression. Tolosa-Hunt syndrome (**Fig. 13**) is a related condition of idiopathic steroid-responsive cavernous sinus inflammation manifesting as painful ophthalmoplegia with or without vision loss.

The orbit can also be involved by many systemic inflammatory diseases, including autoimmune thyroid disease, IgG4-related disease (IgG4-RD), sarcoidosis, Sjögren syndrome, lupus, and granulomatosis with polyangiitis.[45] Of these, we will further discuss IgG4-related orbital disease (IgG4-ROD) and thyroid eye disease (TED). Recognized as a distinct disease entity in 2003, IgG4-RD is characterized by IgG4-positive plasma cell infiltration and sclerosing inflammation.[46,47] Although IgG4-RD can involve virtually any organ, there is a strong predilection for several head and neck structures, including the orbits and lacrimal glands, the major salivary glands, and the thyroid gland.[47] IgG4-ROD represents a substantial proportion of patients previously diagnosed with IOI because some clinical and imaging features overlap and both are steroid-responsive. However, unlike IOI, IgG4-ROD is typically bilateral and painless.[48] Lacrimal gland and extraocular muscle enlargement are common IgG4-ROD findings with the lateral recti most often involved and with sparing of the tendinous insertions. Infraorbital nerve enlargement (**Fig. 14**) is reported in approximately 30% of IgG4-ROD cases and can be a clue to diagnosis[48]; however, a low threshold to biopsy accessible sites is recommended, particularly because malignancy (eg, lymphoma, metastasis) is often a differential consideration. Importantly, normal serum IgG4 levels do *not* exclude this

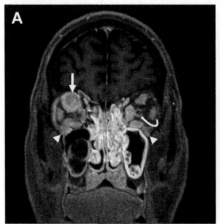

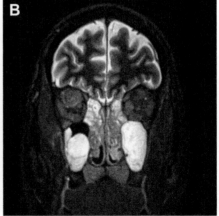

Fig. 14. IgG4-related orbital disease. Coronal gadolinium-enhanced, fat-suppressed, T1-weighted image (*A*) obtained in a 62-year-old male with biopsy-proven IgG4-related disease demonstrates enlargement of the right greater than left extraocular muscles with most severe involvement of the right superior muscle complex (*straight arrow, A*). The right greater than left infraorbital nerves are enlarged and abnormally enhancing (*arrowheads, A*), and there is abnormal enhancement of the left optic nerve sheath (*curved arrow, A*) suggesting perineuritis. Note the hypointensity of the abnormally enlarged extraocular muscles and infraorbital nerves on the coronal STIR image (*B*), consistent with the fibrosing nature of this disease. There is also evidence of paranasal sinus and nasal cavity inflammation, a common finding in IgG4-related disease.

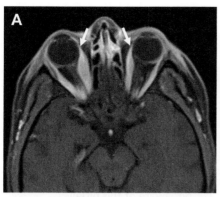 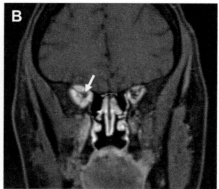

Fig. 15. Optic nerve crowding in thyroid eye disease. Axial gadolinium-enhanced, fat-suppressed, T1-weighted image (A) obtained in a 46-year-old female with history of Graves disease presenting to the emergency department with right vision loss demonstrates enlargement of the right greater than left extraocular muscles. The medial recti are affected more than the lateral recti, and the tendinous insertions (arrows, A) are relatively spared. The coronal gadolinium-enhanced, fat-suppressed, T1-weighted image (B) demonstrates marked crowding of the right optic nerve (arrow, B) at the orbital apex, likely accounting for vision loss.

disease, and elevated serum IgG4 levels do *not* confirm it.

TED is caused by orbital and periorbital inflammation in association with autoimmune thyroiditis, most commonly Graves disease.[45] The disease most often affects adult females and is rare in children. Proptosis, lid retraction, and periorbital

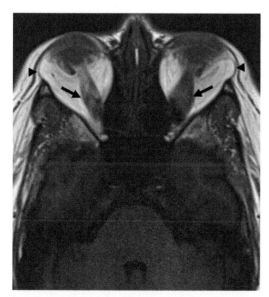

Fig. 16. Orbital fat proliferation in thyroid eye disease. Axial T1-weighted image obtained in a 51-year-old female with Graves disease demonstrates enlargement of the left greater than right inferior rectus muscles (arrows) as well as abundant orbital fat contributing to proptosis and resulting in subconjunctival fat prolapse (arrowheads). Orbital fat proliferation may be the sole manifestation of thyroid eye disease in some patients.

swelling are the most common presenting symptoms. Pain may or may not be present. Crowding of the optic nerve at the orbital apex by the enlarged extraocular muscles may produce vision loss (**Fig. 15**). As such, the imaging assessment of TED should always include the presence or absence of orbital apex crowding. In addition to extraocular muscle enlargement, TED also produces increased orbital fat (**Fig. 16**), which is not seen with IOI or IgG4-ROD. The pattern of extraocular involvement is also useful for distinguishing among these inflammatory diseases of the orbit. Although the medial rectus is most commonly affected in IOI and the lateral rectus in IgG4-ROD, the pattern of involvement (decreasing order of frequency) in TED is captured by the mnemonic "I'M SLO"— inferior rectus, medial rectus, superior rectus, lateral rectus, and oblique muscles. Unlike IgG4-ROD, there is no lacrimal gland involvement, and, unlike IOI, findings are typically bilateral. Increased T2 signal within the involved extraocular muscles is expected in the acute phase.

CLINICS CARE POINTS

Head and neck emergency magnetic resonance (MR) imaging: pearls

- MR safety screening is necessary for <u>all</u> patients, even in the emergent setting. For altered or otherwise incapacitated patients who are unable to complete the MR safety questionnaire, unnecessary delays are minimized if the referring physician at the time of order entry provides the name and contact information for the patient's health-care proxy to the MR technologist or notifies the MR technologist that radiographic clearance will be required because no health-care proxy is available.

- If patient motion is a problem, a radial acquisition may yield diagnostic images.
- Flexible coils placed close to the skin and contoured to fit each patient can improve signal-to-noise at the neck–chest junction, a technically challenging area to image.
- Although 2D and 3D postcontrast sequences each have value in head and neck imaging, we find 3D postcontrast sequences to be most helpful for evaluating patency of the dural venous sinuses, particularly the cavernous sinuses.
- Optic neuritis in multiple sclerosis is most commonly unilateral with short segment enhancement as opposed to myelin oligodendrocyte glycoprotein antibody-associated disease and neuromyelitis optica spectrum disorders where bilateral involvement with long segment enhancement is common.
- Nonarteritic anterior ischemic optic neuropathy is far more common and typically painless. Arteritic anterior ischemic optic neuropathy (A-AION) is often painful.
- If a patient is being worked up for possible A-AION, absence of the "central bright spot sign" suggests that A-AION is very unlikely and that emergent corticosteroids may not be required.
- Relation to the orbital septum differentiates periorbital (preseptal) and orbital (postseptal) cellulitis. Because the orbital septum is not typically identifiable with routine imaging, its location is most often approximated by the orbital rim.
- Lacrimal gland and infraorbital nerve enlargement can be a clue to the diagnosis of IgG4-related orbital disease.
- Among diseases causing extraocular muscle enlargement, only thyroid eye disease produces orbital fat proliferation.

Head and neck emergency MR imaging: pitfalls

- Although a very large image matrix (eg, 400 × 400) will yield exquisite images in ideal conditions (eg, cooperative outpatient, anesthesia case), very large acquisition matrices may not be feasible in many emergency department settings with acutely ill patients because of the associated longer acquisition times with increased risk for patient motion, potentially requiring repeat acquisitions.

- Spectral fat suppression techniques have a high risk of failure in the head and neck due to susceptibility artifacts at bone–air interfaces, and these failures of fat suppression can obscure or mimic pathologic condition. We use Dixon fat suppression to reduce the risk of fat suppression failure.
- Exercise caution in attributing significance to apparent optic nerve findings on echo planar diffusion-weighted imaging of the brain. The orbits are prone to distortion and artifacts on these images, which can be mistaken for a pathologic conditions if the radiologist is not aware of this pitfall.
- Because wood is an organic material, failing to identify a wooden foreign body places the patient at particularly high risk for superimposed infection. Air-filled interstices in dry wood account for its difficult to detect imaging appearance—hypoattenuating on computed tomography (ie, greater than air but less than fat) and hypointense on all MR sequences.
- When considering the diagnosis of IgG4-related disease, the radiologist should not be influenced by serum IgG4 levels because normal serum IgG4 levels do *not* exclude the diagnosis, and elevated serum IgG4 levels do *not* confirm it.

DISCLOSURE

J.R. Sachs is a paid consultant for GE Healthcare, not related to the subject material presented here. H.R. Kelly has served as a Principal Investigator with clinical trial funding provided to her institution by Bayer AG (no personal compensation or salary support). All other authors have nothing to disclose.

REFERENCES

1. Rankey D, Leach JL, Leach SD. Emergency MRI utilization trends at a tertiary care academic medical center: baseline data. Acad Radiol 2008;15(4):438–43.
2. Korley FK, Pham JC, Kirsch TD. Use of advanced radiology during visits to US emergency departments for injury-related conditions, 1998-2007. JAMA 2010;304(13):1465–71.
3. Ahn S, Kim WY, Lim KS, et al. Advanced radiology utilization in a tertiary care emergency department from 2001 to 2010. PLoS One 2014;9(11):e112650.
4. Levin DC, Rao VM, Parker L, et al. Continued growth in emergency department imaging is bucking the overall trends. J Am Coll Radiol JACR 2014;11(11):1044–7.

5. Redd V, Levin S, Toerper M, et al. Effects of fully accessible magnetic resonance imaging in the emergency department. Acad Emerg Med 2015; 22(6):741–9.

6. Buller M, Karis JP. Introduction of a Dedicated Emergency Department MR Imaging Scanner at the Barrow Neurological Institute. AJNR Am J Neuroradiol 2017;38(8):1480–5.

7. Kocher KE, Meurer WJ, Desmond JS, et al. Effect of testing and treatment on emergency department length of stay using a national database. Acad Emerg Med 2012;19(5):525–34.

8. Cramer JD, Purkey MR, Smith SS, et al. The impact of delayed surgical drainage of deep neck abscesses in adult and pediatric populations. Laryngoscope 2016;126(8):1753–60.

9. Fernandez IJ, Crocetta FM, Demattè M, et al. Acute invasive fungal rhinosinusitis in immunocompromised patients: role of an early diagnosis. Otolaryngol Head Neck Surg 2018;159(2):386–93.

10. Kamalian S, Avery L, Lev MH, et al. Nontraumatic head and neck emergencies. Radiographics 2019; 39(6):1808–23.

11. Cunqueiro A, Gomes WA, Lee P, et al. CT of the neck: image analysis and reporting in the emergency setting. Radiographics 2019;39(6):1760–81.

12. Loureiro RM, Naves EA, Zanello RF, et al. Dental emergencies: a practical guide. Radiographics 2019;39(6):1782–95.

13. Vaughn J. Emergency imaging of the nontraumatic pediatric head and neck. Semin Ultrasound CT MR 2019;40(2):147–56.

14. Brucker JL, Gentry LR. Imaging of head and neck emergencies. Radiol Clin North Am 2015;53(1): 215–52.

15. Klucznik RP, Carrier DA, Pyka R, et al. Placement of a ferromagnetic intracerebral aneurysm clip in a magnetic field with a fatal outcome. Radiology 1993;187(3):855–6.

16. Chaljub G, Kramer LA, Johnson RF, et al. Projectile cylinder accidents resulting from the presence of ferromagnetic nitrous oxide or oxygen tanks in the MR suite. AJR Am J Roentgenol 2001;177(1):27–30.

17. Landrigan C. Preventable deaths and injuries during magnetic resonance imaging. N Engl J Med 2001; 345(13):1000–1.

18. Beitia AO, Meyers SP, Kanal E, et al. Spontaneous discharge of a firearm in an MR imaging environment. AJR Am J Roentgenol 2002;178(5):1092–4.

19. Stadler A, Schima W, Ba-Ssalamah A, et al. Artifacts in body MR imaging: their appearance and how to eliminate them. Eur Radiol 2007;17(5):1242–55.

20. Curtin HD. Detection of perineural spread: fat suppression versus no fat suppression. AJNR Am J Neuroradiol 2004;25(1):1–3.

21. Dixon WT. Simple proton spectroscopic imaging. Radiology 1984;153(1):189–94.

22. Barger AV, DeLone DR, Bernstein MA, et al. Fat signal suppression in head and neck imaging using fast spin-echo-IDEAL technique. AJNR Am J Neuroradiol 2006;27(6):1292–4.

23. Gaddikeri S, Mossa-Basha M, Andre JB, et al. Optimal Fat Suppression in Head and Neck MRI: Comparison of Multipoint Dixon with 2 Different Fat-Suppression Techniques, Spectral Presaturation and Inversion Recovery, and STIR. AJNR Am J Neuroradiol 2018;39(2):362–8.

24. Fruehwald-Pallamar J, Szomolanyi P, Fakhrai N, et al. Parallel imaging of the cervical spine at 3T: optimized trade-off between speed and image quality. AJNR Am J Neuroradiol 2012;33(10): 1867–74.

25. Sartoretti E, Sartoretti T, Binkert C, et al. Reduction of procedure times in routine clinical practice with Compressed SENSE magnetic resonance imaging technique. PLoS One 2019;14(4):e0214887.

26. Ikeda H, Ohno Y, Murayama K, et al. Compressed sensing and parallel imaging accelerated T2 FSE sequence for head and neck MR imaging: comparison of its utility in routine clinical practice. Eur J Radiol 2021;135:109501.

27. Hoch MJ, Bruno M, Pacione D, et al. Simultaneous Multislice for Accelerating Diffusion MRI in Clinical Neuroradiology Protocols. AJNR Am J Neuroradiol 2021;42(8):1437–43.

28. Montalt-Tordera J, Muthurangu V, Hauptmann A, et al. Machine learning in Magnetic Resonance Imaging: Image reconstruction. Phys Med 2021;83:79–87.

29. Schäffter T, Rasche V, Carlsen IC. Motion compensated projection reconstruction. Magn Reson Med 1999;41(5):954–63.

30. Block KT, Chandarana H, Milla S, et al. Towards routine clinical use of radial stack-of-stars 3D gradient-echo sequences for reducing motion sensitivity. J Korean Soc Magn Reson Med 2014;18(2):87.

31. Wu X, Raz E, Block TK, et al. Contrast-enhanced radial 3D fat-suppressed T1-weighted gradient-recalled echo sequence versus conventional fat-suppressed contrast-enhanced T1-weighted studies of the head and neck. AJR Am J Roentgenol 2014;203(4):883–9.

32. Sneag DB, Queler S. Technological advancements in magnetic resonance neurography. Curr Neurol Neurosci Rep 2019;19(10):75.

33. Braithwaite T, Subramanian A, Petzold A, et al. Trends in optic neuritis incidence and prevalence in the UK and Association with systemic and neurologic disease. JAMA Neurol 2020;77(12):1514–23.

34. Server Alonso A, Sakinis T, Pfeiffer HCV, et al. Understanding pediatric neuroimmune disorder conflicts: a neuroradiologic approach in the molecular era. Radiographics 2020;40(5):1395–411.

35. Rucker JC, Biousse V, Newman NJ. Ischemic optic neuropathies. Curr Opin Neurol 2004;17(1):27–35.

36. Hayreh SS. Ischemic optic neuropathy. Prog Retin Eye Res 2009;28(1):34–62.

37. Remond P, Attyé A, Lecler A, et al. The central bright spot sign: a potential new MR imaging sign for the early diagnosis of anterior ischemic optic neuropathy due to giant cell arteritis. AJNR Am J Neuroradiol 2017;38(7): 1411–5. https://doi.org/10.3174/ajnr.A5205.

38. Miller NR. New concepts in the diagnosis and management of optic nerve sheath meningioma. J Neuroophthalmol 2006;26(3):200–8.

39. Alroughani R, Behbehani R. Optic nerve sheath meningioma masquerading as optic neuritis. Case Rep Neurol Med 2016;2016:5419432.

40. Holan C, Homer NA, Epstein A, et al. Atypical acute presentation of an optic nerve sheath meningioma. Am J Ophthalmol Case Rep 2020;20:100951.

41. Tailor TD, Gupta D, Dalley RW, et al. Orbital neoplasms in adults: clinical, radiologic, and pathologic review. Radiographics 2013;33(6):1739–58.

42. Tsirouki T, Dastiridou AI, Ibánez Flores N, et al. Orbital cellulitis. Surv Ophthalmol 2018;63(4):534–53.

43. Nguyen VD, Singh AK, Altmeyer WB, et al. Demystifying orbital emergencies: a pictorial review. Radiographics 2017;37(3):947–62.

44. Yeşiltaş YS, Gündüz AK. Idiopathic Orbital Inflammation: Review of Literature and New Advances. Middle East Afr J Ophthalmol 2018;25(2):71–80.

45. Kahana A. Orbital inflammatory disorders: new knowledge, future challenges. Curr Opin Ophthalmol 2021;32(3):255–61.

46. Kamisawa T, Funata N, Hayashi Y, et al. A new clinicopathological entity of IgG4-related autoimmune disease. J Gastroenterol 2003;38(10):982–4.

47. Wallace ZS, Naden RP, Chari S, et al. The 2019 American College of Rheumatology/European League Against Rheumatism Classification Criteria for IgG4-Related Disease. Arthritis Rheumatol 2020;72(1):7–19.

48. Tiegs-Heiden CA, Eckel LJ, Hunt CH, et al. Immunoglobulin G4-related disease of the orbit: imaging features in 27 patients. AJNR Am J Neuroradiol 2014;35(7):1393–7.

Magnetic Resonance Imaging of Head and Neck Emergencies, a Symptom-Based Review, Part 2
Ear Pain, Face Pain, and Fever

Paul M. Bunch, MD[a],*, Jeffrey R. Sachs, MD[a], Hillary R. Kelly, MD[b,c,d], Megan E. Lipford, PhD[a], Thomas G. West, MD[a]

KEYWORDS

- Emergency department • Head and neck • Magnetic resonance imaging • Ear pain • Face pain

KEY POINTS

- Diagnostic accuracy and timeliness are essential to minimize the risk of morbidity and death among patients with acute head and neck pathologic conditions.
- Although head and neck magnetic resonance (MR) imaging intimidates many, radiologists interpreting emergency studies must be familiar with the relevant anatomy, pathologic conditions, and acute management considerations to meet the needs of their patients and referring physicians.
- Abbreviated or focused MR imaging protocols for emergency department patients are intended to quickly and efficiently address the acute presentation while minimizing image acquisition time and maximizing patient throughput. Essential MR imaging sequences for the evaluation of most head and neck emergencies include small field of view T1, short tau inversion recovery (STIR), and gadolinium-enhanced T1 (with or without fat suppression depending on local preferences) as well as diffusion-weighted and fluid-attenuated inversion recovery (FLAIR) imaging of the brain.

EAR PAIN ± FEVER

Local causes of acute, nontraumatic ear pain include acute mastoiditis, necrotizing otitis externa, cholesteatoma, and herpes zoster oticus (Ramsay Hunt syndrome) (**Table 1**). Essential temporal bone magnetic resonance (MR) sequences for this evaluation include (1) axial T1 without fat suppression, (2) axial high-resolution steady-state free precession (eg, fast imaging employing steadstate acquisition [FIESTA], constructive interference in steady state (CISS)), and (3) axial and coronal gadolinium-enhanced T1 (with or without fat suppression, depending on local preferences).

Essential brain MR sequences include (1) diffusion-weighted imaging and (2) FLAIR. Although beyond the scope of this article, there are also myriad causes of referred otalgia with which radiologists should be familiar[1] and for which neck computed tomography (CT) is often performed.

Acute Mastoiditis

Acute mastoiditis is a clinical diagnosis, typically manifesting with otalgia, fever, posterior auricular swelling, erythema, and mastoid tenderness. A bulging tympanic membrane is commonly seen

[a] Department of Radiology, Wake Forest School of Medicine, Medical Center Boulevard, Winston Salem, NC 27157, USA; [b] Department of Radiology, Massachusetts General Hospital, 55 Fruit Street, Boston, MA 02114, USA; [c] Department of Radiology, Massachusetts Eye and Ear, 243 Charles Street, Boston, MA 02114, USA; [d] Harvard Medical School, 25 Shattuck Street, Boston, MA 02115, USA
* Corresponding author.
E-mail address: paul.m.bunch@gmail.com

Magn Reson Imaging Clin N Am 30 (2022) 425–439
https://doi.org/10.1016/j.mric.2022.04.006
1064-9689/22/© 2022 Elsevier Inc. All rights reserved.

Table 1
Characteristic features of pathologic conditions presenting with ear pain

Pathologic Conditions	Clinical Features	Imaging Features
Acute mastoiditis	Most frequently affects children as a complication of acute otitis media Fever, posterior auricular swelling, erythema, mastoid tenderness Bulging tympanic membrane	Opacified mastoid air cells sensitive but not specific Loss of normal mastoid septa (coalescence) on CT Inflammatory changes of soft tissues overlying mastoid Complications include epidural or subperiosteal abscess, subdural empyema, dural sinus thrombosis, labyrinthitis, meningitis, brain abscess
Necrotizing otitis externa	Elderly diabetic or otherwise immunocompromised patients Severe pain disproportionate to physical examination findings Fever and leukocytosis often absent	External auditory canal thickening and adjacent fat stranding Skull base soft tissue and osseous involvement common, sometimes mimicking nasopharyngeal malignancy
Cholesteatoma	Chronic otitis media and Eustachian tube dysfunction White mass behind the tympanic membrane Conductive hearing loss, ear drainage	Rounded soft tissue Osseous erosion Restricted diffusion No enhancement
Herpes zoster oticus (Ramsay Hunt syndrome)	Older adults (aged older than 50 years), commonly immunocompromised Characteristic erythematous papular and vesicular rash involving the ear and external auditory canal Facial paralysis, vertigo, altered hearing and taste, lacrimation	Abnormal ipsilateral facial nerve enhancement, often involving the internal auditory canal and typically not masslike Membranous labyrinth enhancement may also be seen Asymmetric enhancement of the ipsilateral ear and external auditory canal

on otoscopy. In most cases, imaging is not required. However, imaging is indicated when there is suspicion for coalescent mastoiditis, intracranial complications, or underlying chronic pathologic conditions such as cholesteatoma. Acute mastoiditis, which is relatively uncommon, should not be confused with incidental mastoid opacification, which is estimated to be present on 10% of MR examinations.[2] Importantly, a recent meta-analysis found that among 9 studies reporting clinical outcomes of patients with incidental mastoid opacification, *none* reliably reported any clinical cases of mastoiditis.[2] As such, it is most appropriate for radiologists to suspect acute mastoiditis (1) when the referring physicians are concerned for acute mastoiditis based on clinical symptoms and (2) when there is imaging evidence of mastoiditis complications (eg, epidural or subperiosteal abscess, adjacent dural sinus thrombosis, meningitis, cerebritis, parenchymal abscess, labyrinthitis,

Bezold abscess, or petrous apicitis[3]), even in the absence of clinical concern (**Fig. 1**). Inflammatory changes in the subcutaneous tissues overlying the mastoid are also a helpful clue. It is certainly worthwhile for radiologists to specifically look for evidence of coalescence or other mastoiditis complications when faced with incidental middle ear and mastoid opacification on imaging. However, in their absence, we suggest merely describing the presence of "opacification" and not ascribing clinical significance with terms such as "mastoiditis" and "otomastoiditis."

Necrotizing Otitis Externa

Necrotizing otitis externa, also referred to as malignant otitis externa, is an invasive infection of the external auditory canal occurring primarily in elderly diabetic or otherwise immunocompromised patients. *Pseudomonas aeruginosa* is the most common causative organism. Severe ear

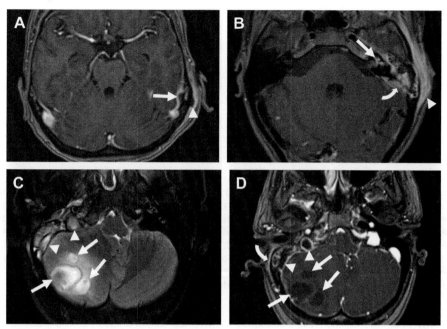

Fig. 1. Complications of acute mastoiditis. Selected MR images (*A, B, C, D*) from 3 different patients with acute mastoiditis. Axial gadolinium-enhanced, T1-weighted image (*A*) obtained in a 41-year-old female with acute left mastoiditis demonstrates small epidural (*arrow, A*) and subperiosteal (*arrowhead, A*) abscesses adjacent to the left mastoid temporal bone. Notice the soft tissue swelling and enhancement surrounding the subperiosteal abscess. Axial gadolinium-enhanced, fat-suppressed, T1-weighted image (*B*) obtained in a 19-year-old female with acute left mastoiditis demonstrates abnormal enhancement of the left cochlea (straight *arrow, B*) and vestibule, consistent with acute labyrinthitis. There is also abnormal enhancement of the left internal auditory canal, of the dura along the left posterior petrous ridge (curved *arrow, B*), and of the soft tissues overlying the infected left mastoid air cells (*arrowhead, B*). Axial fat-suppressed, T2-weighted (*C*) and gadolinium-enhanced, T1-weighted (*D*) images obtained in a 35-year-old female with acute right mastoiditis demonstrate thrombosis of the right sigmoid sinus (*arrowheads, C and D*) and multiple right cerebellar abscesses (straight *arrows, C and D*) with surrounding edema and associated mass effect producing midline shift and partial effacement of the fourth ventricle. Finally, note the soft tissue thickening and enhancement (curved *arrow, D*) overlying the infected right mastoid air cells.

pain disproportionate to the clinical examination is typical, and purulent ear discharge may also be present. Notably, fever and leukocytosis are often absent.[4] Prompt initiation of intravenous antibiotics is required to minimize the risk of skull base osteomyelitis, a life-threatening complication of necrotizing otitis externa. The infection is believed to gain access to the deep spaces of the neck via the vertically oriented fissures of Santorini located within the cartilaginous portion of the external auditory canal. Cranial nerve palsies represent clinical evidence of extension beyond the external auditory canal to involve the skull base, and vascular complications (eg, arterial or venous thrombosis) may also occur.

The initial imaging study is most commonly CT, which will show thickening of the external auditory canal and inflammatory fat stranding. To identify early signs of osteomyelitis, the radiologist should scrutinize the bone for erosive changes, which are often subtle, paying particular attention to the osseous external auditory canal, mastoid tip, temporomandibular joint, petrous apex, jugular foramen, and clivus.[5] MR imaging is superior for depicting soft tissue extent and marrow involvement, and the unenhanced T1-weighted images without fat suppression are particularly useful for these purposes (**Fig. 2**). MR imaging is also more sensitive than CT for detecting intracranial complications. When there is extension of disease to involve the skull base, asymmetric soft tissue fullness of the ipsilateral nasopharynx is common and may mimic nasopharyngeal carcinoma (**Fig. 3**). In this setting, a normal mucosal examination by a consulting otolaryngologist would strongly favor necrotizing otitis externa with skull base involvement over nasopharyngeal carcinoma; however, tissue sampling is typically warranted for definitive

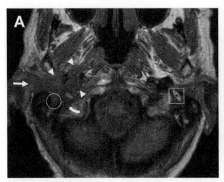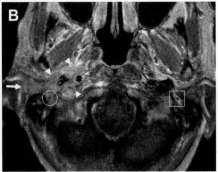

Fig. 2. Necrotizing otitis externa. Axial T1-weighted (*A*) and gadolinium-enhanced, T1-weighted (*B*) images obtained in a 79-year-old male with poorly controlled diabetes demonstrate abnormal soft tissue thickening (straight *arrow*, *A*) and enhancement (*arrow*, *B*) of the right external auditory canal. The soft tissue abnormality extends medially to involve the right prestyloid and poststyloid parapharyngeal spaces (*arrowheads*, *A* and *B*) as well as the right stylomastoid foramen (*circles*, *A* and *B*). The normal left stylomastoid foramen is marked with a square for comparison. When postcontrast fat suppression is not applied, the extent of soft tissue involvement is more easily appreciated on the unenhanced T1-weighted image, and the right occipital bone involvement (*curved arrow*, *A*) consistent with osteomyelitis is only detectable on the unenhanced image.

determination and to isolate the causative pathogen.

Cholesteatoma

A cholesteatoma is a keratin-filled cystic mass lined by stratified squamous epithelium that can be conceptualized most simply as skin in the wrong place. Although congenital cholesteatomas rarely occur, the vast majority (98%) of cholesteatomas are acquired, typically resulting from Eustachian tube dysfunction and chronic otitis media.

The hallmark of cholesteatoma is osseous erosion, which accounts for many of the associated symptoms (eg, conductive hearing loss from ossicular erosion) and complications (eg, cephalocele from tegmen erosion). Presenting features of cholesteatoma vary. The diagnosis is most commonly made by otoscopy when a white mass is seen behind the tympanic membrane. Common clinical symptoms are conductive hearing loss, drainage from the ear, and ear pain. However, some patients are entirely asymptomatic, in which case CT or MR imaging

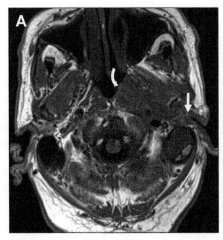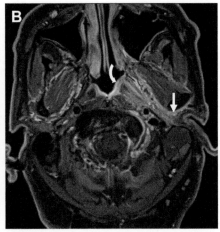

Fig. 3. Necrotizing otitis externa and skull base infection mimicking nasopharyngeal carcinoma. Axial T1-weighted (*A*) and gadolinium-enhanced, fat-suppressed, T1-weighted (*B*) images obtained in a 71-year-old immunocompromised male with left ear pain demonstrate soft tissue thickening and enhancement extending from the left external auditory canal (*straight arrow*, *A* and *B*) to the left nasopharynx with associated masslike left nasopharyngeal soft tissue asymmetry (*curved arrow*, *A* and *B*). Although nasopharyngeal carcinoma can have a similar appearance and biopsy is often warranted for diagnostic certainty, the mucosal examination was normal, and the findings resolved after antibiotic therapy.

may first identify the cholesteatoma as an incidental finding. Cholesteatoma is treated with complete surgical removal and will recur if any squamous epithelium is left behind during or introduced at surgery.

Temporal bone CT is useful to delineate extent of disease as well as to assess for complications (eg, lateral canal fistula) and surgical pitfalls (eg, dehiscent facial nerve canal, cephalocele). On MR imaging, cholesteatomas restrict diffusion (**Fig. 4**). As such, diffusion-weighted imaging is highly sensitive and specific for both initial diagnosis and detecting recurrence. Although not typically performed in the ED setting, coronal nonecho planar and coronal multishot (readout segmented) echo planar acquisitions diminish artifacts at the air–bone interface compared with a standard echo planar axial diffusion-weighted acquisition with the coronal nonecho planar technique outperforming the coronal multishot echo planar technique in 2 comparative studies.[6,7] Unlike granulation tissue, cholesteatoma *does not enhance* on gadolinium-enhanced T1-weighted images (see **Fig. 4**).

Herpes Zoster Oticus (Ramsay Hunt Syndrome)

Herpes zoster oticus, also known as Ramsay Hunt syndrome, results from reactivation of the varicella zoster virus in the facial nerve geniculate ganglion. The risk increases with age and with immune suppression. The classic clinical triad is ear pain, facial nerve palsy, and vesicles involving the auricle and external auditory canal.[8] Vertigo and ipsilateral hearing loss, taste alterations, and lacrimation may also occur.[8] On MR imaging, abnormal enhancement of the cranial nerve VII and VIII complex within the internal auditory canal should raise suspicion, and enhancement of the membranous labyrinth may also be seen (**Fig. 5**). Importantly, these imaging findings may precede the vesicular rash.[9] Abnormal labyrinthine enhancement may also be seen with acute labyrinthitis and with labyrinthine schwannoma; however, ear pain and vesicular rash would not be expected with these pathologic conditions. Finally, MR imaging may be performed for some patients with facial paralysis and a suspected clinical diagnosis of Bell palsy. Although abnormal (eg, involving the labyrinthine segment) or asymmetric enhancement of the ipsilateral facial nerve can be seen in the clinical setting of Bell palsy, we caution against confidently attributing these imaging findings to Bell palsy until the clinical symptoms have resolved and encourage careful assessment of the parotid gland for possible underlying mass. If the facial weakness persists or worsens, repeat imaging is indicated because

perineural tumor spread from an occult malignancy is a differential consideration.

FACE PAIN ± FEVER

Causes of acute, nontraumatic face pain relevant to emergency MR imaging include bacterial sinusitis, invasive fungal sinusitis, and petrous apicitis (**Table 2**). Essential face MR sequences for this evaluation include (1) axial T1 without fat suppression, (2) axial or coronal STIR or fat-suppressed T2, and (3) axial and coronal gadolinium-enhanced T1 (with or without fat suppression, depending on local preferences). Essential brain MR sequences include (1) diffusion-weighted imaging and (2) FLAIR.

Acute Bacterial Sinusitis

Acute (<4 weeks duration) bacterial sinusitis is diagnosed clinically, typically from fever, pain, and purulent nasal discharge following a viral upper respiratory infection. The presence of air-fluid levels on imaging can raise suspicion but is not diagnostic. The primary role of imaging in acute sinusitis is to assess for complications resulting from spread of infection beyond the paranasal sinuses. Intracranial complications of bacterial sinusitis include epidural abscess, subdural empyema, venous thrombosis, and meningoencephalitis (**Fig. 6**). Frontal sinusitis (**Fig. 7**) and sphenoid sinusitis warrant particular scrutiny for intracranial complications, given anatomic proximity. Although patients with suspected complicated sinusitis are more commonly imaged with CT, we suggest a low threshold for MR imaging to maximize sensitivity for detection, particularly in patients with suspected acute frontal or sphenoid sinusitis. An additional complication unique to frontal sinusitis is extracranial extension of infection with formation of a subperiosteal abscess (**Fig. 8**), the so-called Pott puffy tumor. Orbital complications include subperiosteal abscess, orbital cellulitis, and superior ophthalmic vein thrombosis, which have been previously discussed in Part 1.

Odontogenic infection is an important cause of sinusitis that may not be readily apparent on clinical examination. Patients with odontogenic sinusitis will experience recurrent sinus infections until the diseased tooth is addressed. As such, radiologists add value in the imaging of patients with acute sinusitis by specifically assessing the maxillary teeth with special attention to the roots for possible periapical infection. Periapical enhancement on MR imaging (**Fig. 9**) corresponds to periapical lucency on CT. When ipsilateral to sinus disease, these findings raise suspicion for odontogenic sinusitis and warrant dental consultation.

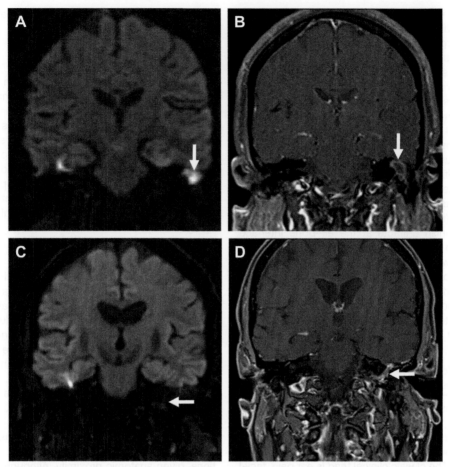

Fig. 4. Cholesteatoma. Coronal diffusion-weighted (*A*) and gadolinium-enhanced, fat-suppressed, T1-weighted (*B*) images obtained in a 50-year-old female with left ear pain, otorrhea, and hearing loss demonstrate a low diffusivity (*arrow, A*), nonenhancing (*arrow, B*), rounded lesion within the left mastoid air cells consistent with cholesteatoma. In contrast, avidly enhancing soft tissue (*arrow, D*) without low diffusivity (*arrow, C*) is most consistent with granulation tissue.

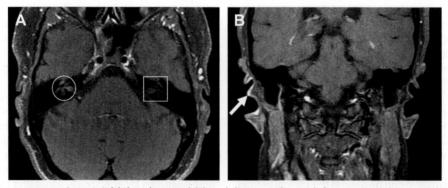

Fig. 5. Herpes zoster oticus. Axial (*A*) and coronal (*B*) gadolinium-enhanced, fat-suppressed, T1-weighted images obtained in a 54-year-old female with vertigo, ear pain, and right facial paralysis demonstrate abnormal enhancement of the right cranial nerve VII/VIII complex within the right internal auditory canal and of the right membranous labyrinth (*circle, A*). The normal left internal auditory canal, membranous labyrinth, and facial nerve tympanic segment are marked with a square for comparison. There is also asymmetric enhancement of the right facial nerve tympanic segment (*circle, A*) and of the skin of the right ear (*arrow, B*). Right ear vesicles were noted on physical examination, consistent with herpes zoster oticus (Ramsay Hunt syndrome).

Table 2
Characteristic features of pathologic conditions presenting with acute face pain

Pathologic Conditions	Clinical Features	Imaging Features
Acute bacterial sinusitis	Recent viral upper respiratory infection Nasal congestion, obstruction, purulent discharge Fever, headache	Air-fluid levels sensitive but not specific Low diffusivity luminal material Orbital and intracranial complications Periapical lucency (CT) or enhancement (MR) suggest dental infection as underlying cause
Acute invasive fungal sinusitis	Immune compromised Neutropenic fever	Loss of normal mucosal enhancement Infiltration of fat and involvement of structures surrounding the paranasal sinuses Bone destruction
Acute petrous apicitis	Recent or active middle ear infection Diplopia secondary to abducens palsy	Opacified petrous apex air cells sensitive but not specific Loss of normal septa (coalescence) on CT Loss of normal marrow signal on T1 with associated petrous apex enhancement Complications include epidural abscess, subdural empyema, dural sinus thrombosis, internal carotid artery vasospasm and arteritis, meningitis, brain abscess

Abbreviations: MR, magnetic resonance; CT, computed tomography.

Acute Invasive Fungal Sinusitis

Acute invasive fungal sinusitis is a life-threatening, angioinvasive infection affecting immunocompromised patients. Patients typically present acutely with facial pain and swelling, fever, and nasal congestion.[10] Ophthalmoplegia, proptosis, and decreased vision are also commonly present and represent clinical evidence of extension beyond the paranasal sinuses and nasal cavities.[10] Primary risk factors are neutropenia and dysfunctional neutrophils, and the most common predisposing conditions are hematologic malignancies, chemotherapy, organ transplantation, and uncontrolled diabetes mellitus.[11] Although the disease is relatively rare, mortality is approximately 50% and even higher among patients with intracranial involvement and those who do not undergo surgery as a component of their therapy.[10] Rapid and accurate diagnosis is necessary to facilitate prompt surgical debridement, which maximizes chances for survival.

Loss of normal mucosal enhancement (eg, "black turbinate sign") within the paranasal sinuses and nasal cavities (**Fig. 10**) on MR imaging has been described as a specific imaging sign of acute invasive fungal sinusitis.[12] However, in many practice settings pursuing MR imaging of patients with suspected acute invasive fungal sinusitis risks unnecessarily delaying definitive pathologic diagnosis and surgical intervention, which may contribute to a poor patient outcome. In most situations, CT imaging is both sensitive and specific with a 7-variable model (**Table 3**) based on the presence or absence of (1) bone dehiscence, (2) septal ulceration, and (3) soft tissue infiltration at 5 specific sites outside of the paranasal sinus achieving high sensitivity, specificity, positive predictive value, and negative predictive value.[11] Importantly, the paranasal sinus findings (eg, mucosal thickening, fluid) may be minimal in these immunocompromised patients, and any inflammatory changes in the soft tissues surrounding the paranasal sinuses must be viewed with high suspicion and warrant prompt otolaryngology surgical consultation for further evaluation (**Fig. 11**).

There has been recent interest in transcutaneous retrobulbar injection of amphotericin B as an alternative to orbital exenteration for patients

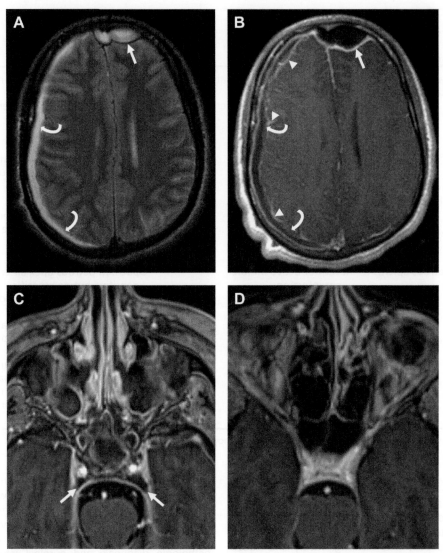

Fig. 6. Intracranial complications of acute sinusitis. Selected MR images (*A, B, C*) from 2 different patients with complicated acute sinusitis. Axial fat-suppressed, T2-weighted (*A*) and gadolinium-enhanced, T1-weighted (*B*) images obtained in a 17-year-old male demonstrate an epidural abscess (*straight arrows, A and B*) overlying the left frontal lobe, a subdural empyema (*curved arrows, A and B*) overlying the right cerebral convexity, and abnormal leptomeningeal enhancement (*arrowheads, B*) consistent with meningitis. The relationship of the epidural abscess to the T2 hypointense dura is best appreciated on the axial T2-weighted image. Axial gadolinium-enhanced, T1-weighted image (*C*) obtained in a 53-year-old female demonstrates thrombosis of the bilateral cavernous sinuses (*arrows, C*). The normal contrast-enhanced appearance of the cavernous sinuses in a different patient (*D*) is shown for comparison.

with orbital involvement by acute invasive fungal sinusitis.[13–15] Further study is needed; however, there may be a role for MR imaging in this setting to determine whether the orbital contents (eg, extraocular muscles) enhance normally and remain viable (**Fig. 12**) versus no longer enhance and are likely not salvageable with retrobulbar amphotericin B injection.

Acute Petrous Apicitis

Up to 35% of patients have pneumatization of the petrous apex.[16] Although this anatomic variant is most often of no clinical relevance, infections from the adjacent middle ear and mastoid air cells rarely (estimated fewer than 1 in 50,000 patients with otitis media[17]) spread to involve the petrous

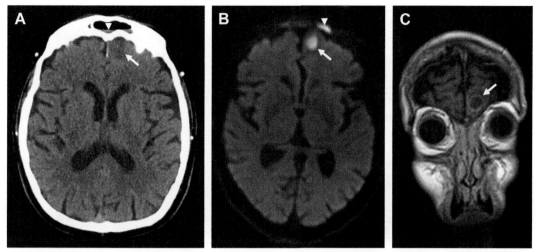

Fig. 7. Undetected left frontal lobe abscess as a complication of acute left frontal sinusitis. Axial noncontrast head CT (*A*) obtained in a 70-year-old male with headache demonstrates a small amount of fluid in the left frontal sinus (*arrowhead, A*) and abnormal hypoattenuation in the subjacent left frontal lobe (*arrow, A*). The left frontal sinus fluid was identified and reported, but the brain parenchymal abnormality was overlooked. Axial diffusion-weighted image (*B*) and coronal gadolinium-enhanced, T1-weighted image (*C*) from brain MR performed 3 days later for altered mental status demonstrate a left frontal lobe abscess (*arrow, B* and *C*) and low diffusivity material consistent with pus in the left frontal sinus (*arrowhead, B*).

apex air cells. Complications of suppurative infection within the petrous apex air cells (petrous apicitis) overlap with the complications of acute mastoiditis, including coalescence of air cells, osseous erosion (**Fig. 13**), and intracranial spread of infection with the risk of vascular thrombosis. Some clinical manifestations of acute petrous apicitis also overlap with acute mastoiditis, including fever and ear pain. However, because of the

petrous apex's proximity to Meckel's cave (cranial nerve V) and Dorello's canal (cranial nerve VI), patients with acute petrous apicitis commonly also experience severe face pain and diplopia.

As with the mastoid air cells, mere opacification of petrous apex air cells does not equate to petrous apicitis. However, in the clinical setting of face pain, abducens palsy, and otitis media (Gradenigo triad), a high index of suspicion for

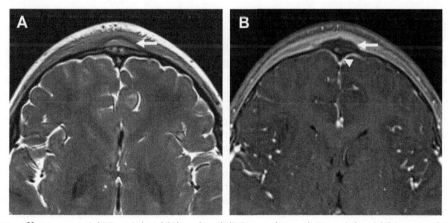

Fig. 8. Pott puffy tumor. Axial T2-weighted (*A*) and gadolinium-enhanced, T1-weighted (*B*) images obtained in a 7-year-old male with acute frontal sinusitis demonstrate a T2 hypointense, rim-enhancing subperiosteal abscess (*arrow, A* and *B*; Pott puffy tumor) with surrounding cellulitis. There is also a filling defect (*arrowhead, B*) within the anterior aspect of the superior sagittal sinus consistent with thrombophlebitis. Similar to the elevated dura shown in Figure 6A, the elevated periosteum can be seen as a hypointense line on the T2-weighted image (*arrow, A*).

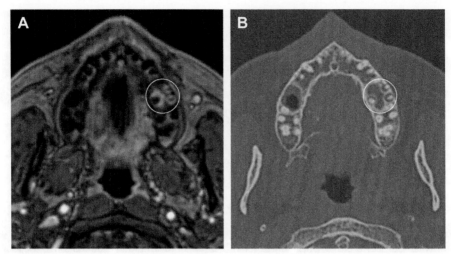

Fig. 9. Odontogenic sinusitis. Axial gadolinium-enhanced, T1-weighted image (*A*) obtained in a 56-year-old male with odontogenic left maxillary sinusitis demonstrates abnormal enhancement associated with the roots of the left first maxillary molar (*circle, A*). Axial CT image (*B*) obtained in the same patient shows the enhancement to correspond to periapical lucency (*circle, B*) consistent with odontogenic infection.

petrous apicitis is appropriate, and a careful search for imaging evidence of complications (eg, osseous erosion, dural thickening and enhancement, intracranial abscess, adjacent dural venous sinus thrombosis) is warranted. The non-pneumatized petrous apex may also be second-arily involved by infection (**Fig. 14**)—either acute mastoiditis or necrotizing otitis externa—in which

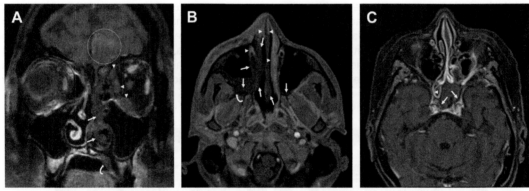

Fig. 10. Absent mucosal enhancement in invasive fungal sinusitis. Selected MR images (*A, B, C*) from 3 different patients with invasive fungal sinusitis. Coronal gadolinium-enhanced, fat-suppressed, T1-weighted image (*A*) obtained in a 36-year-old male with history of acute myeloid leukemia complicated by graft-versus-host disease requiring chronic immunosuppression demonstrates absent left nasal cavity mucosal enhancement (*straight arrows A*). Note the normal enhancement of the right middle and inferior turbinates. Additionally, there is absent enhancement of multiple left extraocular muscles (*arrowheads, A*), the left palate (*curved arrow, A*), and evidence of intracranial extension (*circle, A*). Axial gadolinium-enhanced, T1-weighted image (*B*) obtained in a 26-year-old male with poorly controlled diabetes demonstrates absent mucosal enhancement (*straight arrows, B*) of the right inferior turbinate, the nasal septum, and the right greater than left maxillary sinuses. Additionally, there is abnormal hypoenhancement of the right retroantral fat and adjacent right temporalis muscle (*curved arrow, B*) as well as right periorbital cellulitis. The arrowheads indicate the normal expected mucosal enhancement of the nasal and paranasal sinus mucosa. Axial gadolinium-enhanced, fat-suppressed, T1-weighted image (*C*) obtained in an 87-year-old female with multiple myeloma demonstrates absent enhancement of the left sphenoid sinus mucosa (*arrows, C*). Note the normal mucosal enhancement of the right sphenoid sinus (*arrowheads, C*) and nasal cavity. In a case like this, the otolaryngologist's nasal cavity examination will often be normal, and the radiologist adds value by directing the surgeon to the specific site(s) of nonenhancing mucosa for tissue diagnosis.

Table 3
Acute invasive fungal rhinosinusitis 7-variable computed tomography-based predictive model

Variable	Model Performance Among Immunocompromised Patients
Periantral fat	0 abnormalities present:
Pterygopalatine fossa	• 95% negative predictive value
Nasolacrimal duct	1 abnormality present:
Lacrimal sac	• 95% sensitivity
Orbit	• 86% specificity
Septal ulceration	• 87% positive predictive value
Bone dehiscence	2+ abnormalities present:
	• 88% sensitivity
	• 100% specificity
	• 100% positive predictive value

Data from Middlebrooks EH, Frost CJ, De Jesus RO, Massini TC, Schmalfuss IM, Mancuso AA. Acute Invasive Fungal Rhinosinusitis: A Comprehensive Update of CT Findings and Design of an Effective Diagnostic Imaging Model. *AJNR Am J Neuroradiol.* 2015;36 (8):1529 -1535. doi:10.3174/ajnr.A4298.

case the term "petrous apex osteomyelitis" is preferred.[18] Finally, the most common primary lesion of the petrous apex is cholesterol granuloma,[19] which should not be mistaken for acute petrous apex infection. These gradually enlarging cystic lesions are typically asymptomatic until they reach sufficient size to produce clinical manifestations related to mass effect. An expansile, T1 and T2 hyperintense lesion with rim-enhancement or no enhancement is characteristic (**Fig. 15**).

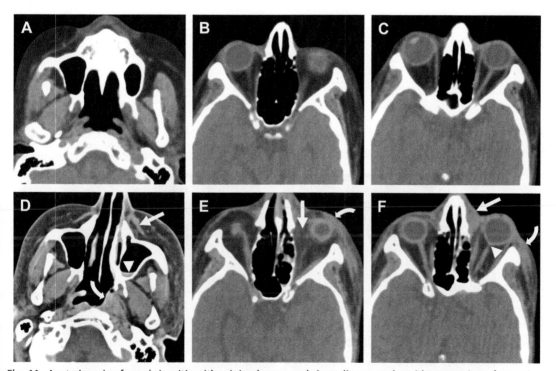

Fig. 11. Acute invasive fungal sinusitis with minimal paranasal sinus disease and rapid progression of extrasinus soft tissue findings. Initial axial noncontrast CT images (*A, B, C*) obtained in the same 36-year-old immunocompromised male patient shown in Figure 10A demonstrate no sinus disease or evidence of extrasinus inflammation. Subsequent axial noncontrast CT images (*D, E, F*) acquired 3 days later demonstrate interval development of a small amount of left maxillary sinus fluid (*arrowhead, D*) as well as interval development of pronounced extrasinus soft tissue abnormalities, including masslike left nasopharyngeal soft tissue (*curved arrow, D*), thickening of the left lip levator muscle (*straight arrow, D*) with subjacent fat stranding, left periorbital (*curved arrow, E, F*) and left orbital (*straight arrow, E*) cellulitis, masslike soft tissue in the left lacrimal sac (*straight arrow, F*), and left globe proptosis with tenting of the posterior globe (*arrowhead, F*).

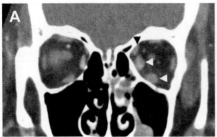
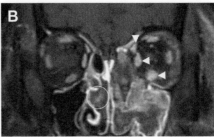

Fig. 12. Orbital involvement by acute invasive fungal sinusitis. Coronal contrast-enhanced CT image (*A*) obtained in a 29-year-old female with neutropenic fever in the setting of acute lymphocytic leukemia demonstrates partial opacification of the left nasal cavity, left ethmoid air cells, and left maxillary sinus with left orbital fat stranding and abnormal enlargement of multiple left extraocular muscles (*arrowheads, A*). Physical examination demonstrated necrotic nasal cavity mucosa consistent with acute invasive fungal sinusitis, and the patient underwent debridement of the left nasal cavity and left paranasal sinuses. Three days later, the patient developed acute onset vision loss. Although the initial CT demonstrated clear evidence of left orbital involvement, an orbit MR was requested to assess the viability of the orbital contents, which would inform decision-making regarding treatment with retrobulbar injection of amphotericin B versus orbital exenteration. Coronal gadolinium-enhanced, fat-suppressed, T1-weighted image (*B*) demonstrates enhancement of the abnormally enlarged extraocular muscles (*arrowheads, B*), suggesting viability. Note the absent mucosal enhancement of the right middle turbinate (*circle, B*) indicating involvement by invasive fungus as well as the interval operative changes related to left nasal cavity and left paranasal sinus debridement. The patient's vision loss resolved following retrobulbar injection of amphotericin B, and orbital exenteration was not required. Unfortunately, the patient died 3 weeks later from multiorgan failure in the setting of bacterial sepsis.

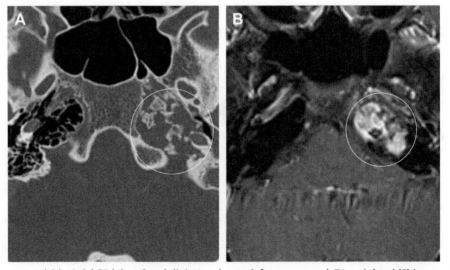

Fig. 13. Petrous apicitis. Axial CT (*A*) and gadolinium-enhanced, fat-suppressed, T1-weighted (*B*) images obtained in a 43-year-old female with left petrous apicitis. The CT image (*A*) demonstrates bilateral petrous apex pneumatization with opacification and coalescence of the left petrous apex air cells (*circle, A*). The MR image (*B*) demonstrates corresponding enhancement (*circle, B*).

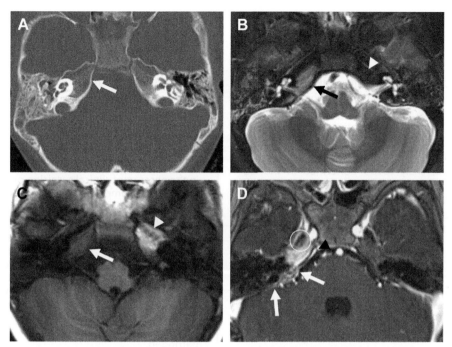

Fig. 14. Petrous apex osteomyelitis. Axial CT (*A*) and MR (*B, C, D*) images obtained in a 6-year-old female with acute right otitis media complicated by right petrous apex osteomyelitis. The CT image (*A*) demonstrates opacification of the right middle ear and right mastoid air cells without petrous apex air cells and without appreciable erosion or sclerosis of the right petrous apex (*arrow, A*). The fat-suppressed, T2-weighted image (*B*) and the T1-weighted image (*C*) demonstrate abnormal marrow T2 hyperintensity and T1 hypointensity, respectively, within the right petrous apex (*arrow, B* and *C*). The normal left petrous apex (*arrowhead, B* and *C*) is marked for comparison. The fat-suppressed, gadolinium-enhanced, T1-weighted image (*D*) demonstrates avid enhancement of the right petrous apex and thickening of the dura along the right posterior petrous ridge consistent with pachymeningitis. Note the close proximity of the right petrous apex infection to the right Meckel's cave (*circle, D*) and the right abducens nerve (*arrowhead, D*) traversing the basilar sinus, which explains the clinical symptoms of face pain and abducens palsy among patients with acute petrous apex infection.

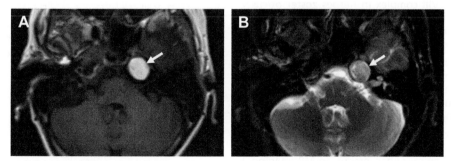

Fig. 15. Cholesterol granuloma. Axial T1-weighted (*A*) and fat-suppressed, T2-weighted (*B*) images obtained in a 59-year-old female undergoing brain MR for breast cancer staging demonstrate an expansile, T1-hyperintense, T2-hyperintense lesion (*arrow, A* and *B*) within the left petrous apex consistent with an incidentally detected cholesterol granuloma.

SUMMARY

Because MR imaging is increasingly used to evaluate emergency department (ED) patients with suspected acute head and neck disease, it is important for radiologists interpreting ED imaging to be familiar with the anatomy, pathologic conditions, and management considerations relevant to common MR imaging indications, such as acute vision loss, ear pain, and face pain, for which MR imaging offers distinct advantages over CT and is, therefore, likely to be performed in the ED setting. By ensuring inclusion of essential MR sequences most relevant to the clinical question, using appropriate strategies for quickly and efficiently obtaining diagnostic information when faced with patient motion and other technical challenges, recognizing and highlighting imaging findings affecting clinical management, and aiding the ED physician in engaging appropriate consult services for further patient evaluation and treatment, the radiologist is well-positioned to meet the emergent needs of ED patients and referring physicians.

CLINICS CARE POINTS

Head and neck emergency magnetic resonance (MR) imaging: pearls

- Severe ear pain disproportionate to the clinical examination in an elderly diabetic or otherwise immunocompromised patient should raise suspicion for necrotizing otitis externa. Notably, fever and leukocytosis are often absent.

- Unlike granulation tissue, cholesteatoma does not enhance.

- Abnormal enhancement of the cranial nerve VII and VIII complex in herpes zoster oticus may precede the vesicular rash. As such, absence of the characteristic rash does not exclude this diagnostic possibility.

- Frontal and sphenoid sinusitis warrant particular scrutiny on computed tomography (CT) for intracranial complications, given anatomic proximity. A low threshold for MR imaging is appropriate.

- Radiologists add value by inspecting the maxillary teeth in patients with acute sinusitis. Periapical enhancement on MR imaging corresponds to periapical lucency on CT. When ipsilateral to sinus disease, these findings raise suspicion for odontogenic sinusitis and warrant dental consultation.

- In the clinical setting of face pain, abducens palsy, and otitis media (Gradenigo triad), a high index of suspicion for petrous apicitis is appropriate.

Head and neck emergency MR imaging: pitfalls

- Acute mastoiditis is a clinical diagnosis, typically manifesting with otalgia, fever, posterior auricular swelling, erythema, and mastoid tenderness. Using terms such as "mastoiditis" and "otomastoiditis" to describe incidental mastoid opacification (ie, in the absence of clinical suspicion or imaging evidence of complications) may lead to unnecessary additional workup and inappropriate antibiotic therapy.

- Nasopharyngeal soft tissue fullness caused by necrotizing otitis externa extending to involve the skull base and deep neck spaces can mimic nasopharyngeal carcinoma. A normal mucosal examination strongly favors necrotizing otitis externa; however, tissue sampling is typically warranted for definitive determination and to isolate the causative pathogen.

- Attributing abnormal or asymmetric facial nerve enhancement to "Bell palsy" can be falsely reassuring. Until the clinical symptoms have resolved, perineural tumor spread from an occult malignancy is a "do not miss" differential consideration.

- Because CT is both sensitive and specific for the diagnosis of acute invasive fungal sinusitis among immunocompromised patients, routinely also performing MR imaging risks delaying definitive pathologic diagnosis and surgical intervention, which may contribute to a poor patient outcome.

DISCLOSURE

J. R. Sachs is a paid consultant for GE Healthcare and is not related to the subject material presented here. H. R. Kelly has served as a Principal Investigator with clinical trial funding provided to her institution by Bayer AG (no personal compensation or salary support). All other authors have nothing to disclose.

REFERENCES

1. Norris CD, Koontz NA. Secondary otalgia: referred pain pathways and pathologies. AJNR Am J Neuroradiol 2020;41(12):2188–98.
2. Mughal Z, Charlton AR, Clark M. The prevalence of incidental mastoid opacification and the need for

intervention: a meta-analysis. Laryngoscope 2021. https://doi.org/10.1002/lary.29581.

3. Sachs JR, Lack CM. Acute otomastoiditis and its complications. Neurographics 2016;6(5):317–27.

4. Mahdyoun P, Pulcini C, Gahide I, et al. Necrotizing otitis externa: a systematic review. Otol Neurotol 2013;34(4):620–9.

5. Chapman PR, Choudhary G, Singhal A. Skull base osteomyelitis: a comprehensive imaging review. AJNR Am J Neuroradiol 2021;42(3):404–13.

6. Dudau C, Draper A, Gkagkanasiou M, et al. Cholesteatoma: multishot echo-planar vs non echo-planar diffusion-weighted MRI for the prediction of middle ear and mastoid cholesteatoma. BJR Open 2019; 1(1):20180015.

7. Benson JC, Carlson ML, Lane JI. Non-EPI versus Multishot EPI DWI in cholesteatoma detection: correlation with operative findings. AJNR Am J Neuroradiol 2021;42(3):573–7.

8. Adour KK. Otological complications of herpes zoster. Ann Neurol 1994;35(Suppl):S62–4.

9. Labin E, Tore H, Alkuwaiti M, et al. Teaching neuroimages: classic ramsay hunt syndrome and associated MRI findings. Neurology 2017;89(7):e79–80.

10. Turner JH, Soudry E, Nayak JV, et al. Survival outcomes in acute invasive fungal sinusitis: a systematic review and quantitative synthesis of published evidence. Laryngoscope 2013;123(5):1112–8.

11. Middlebrooks EH, Frost CJ, De Jesus RO, et al. Acute Invasive fungal rhinosinusitis: a comprehensive update of CT findings and design of an effective

diagnostic imaging model. AJNR Am J Neuroradiol 2015;36(8):1529–35.

12. Safder S, Carpenter JS, Roberts TD, et al. The "Black Turbinate" sign: an early MR imaging finding of nasal mucormycosis. AJNR Am J Neuroradiol 2010;31(4):771–4.

13. Kalin-Hajdu E, Hirabayashi KE, Vagefi MR, et al. Invasive fungal sinusitis: treatment of the orbit. Curr Opin Ophthalmol 2017;28(5):522–33.

14. Ashraf DC, Idowu OO, Hirabayashi KE, et al. Outcomes of a modified treatment ladder algorithm using retrobulbar amphotericin B for invasive fungal rhino-Orbital sinusitis. Am J Ophthalmol 2021. https://doi.org/10.1016/j.ajo.2021.05.025.

15. Arreenich P, Saonanon P, Aeumjaturapat S, et al. Efficacy and safety of retrobulbar amphotericin B injection in invasive fungal rhinosinusitis with orbital invasion patients. Rhinology 2021;59(4):387–92.

16. Virapongse C, Sarwar M, Bhimani S, et al. Computed tomography of temporal bone pneumatization: 1. Normal pattern and morphology. AJR Am J Roentgenol 1985;145(3):473–81.

17. Gadre AK, Chole RA. The changing face of petrous apicitis-a 40-year experience. Laryngoscope 2018; 128(1):195–201.

18. Jackler RK, Parker DA. Radiographic differential diagnosis of petrous apex lesions. Am J Otol 1992; 13(6):561–74.

19. Chapman PR, Shah R, Curé JK, et al. Petrous apex lesions: pictorial review. AJR Am J Roentgenol 2011; 196(3 Suppl):WS26–37. Quiz S40-43.

Musculoskeletal Trauma and Infection

Jacob C. Mandell, MD[a],*, Bharti Khurana, MD[b]

KEYWORDS

- Hip fracture • Pelvic fracture • Trauma • Musculoskeletal infection • Septic arthritis • Osteomyelitis
- Pyomyositis

KEY POINTS

- MR Imaging is the most sensitive imaging modality to assess for occult hip and pelvic fracture because radiographs may be falsely negative in a substantial minority of radiographs performed for trauma. However, computed tomography (CT) is a reasonable alternative modality if magnetic resonance (MR) is not readily available or if there are contraindications.
- An abbreviated MR protocol is equivalent in sensitivity to a complete MR protocol to assess for hip/ pelvic trauma.
- MR is the optimal imaging modality to evaluate for musculoskeletal infection, including septic arthritis, osteomyelitis, and soft tissue infection.
- For MR evaluation of osteomyelitis, if the fluid-sensitive sequences are normal then osteomyelitis is very unlikely. If the T1-weighted images are abnormal, osteomyelitis *may* be present, depending on the pattern of T1 signal change. The confluent intramedullary pattern is most strongly associated with osteomyelitis.
- To differentiate between Charcot arthropathy and diabetic pedal osteomyelitis, the two most helpful imaging features are the *distribution* of signal abnormality, and presence of a *sinus tract*. Charcot tends to involve the midfoot, whereas osteomyelitis involves weight-bearing bones and the ends of bones. A sinus tract leading to abnormal bone is seen exclusively in osteomyelitis.

INTRODUCTION

MR is often the most definitive imaging for assessment of musculoskeletal trauma and infection. Although it is not possible to address all the intricacies of these complex topics in a single article, this review will attempt to provide a useful toolbox of skills by discussing several common clinical scenarios faced by emergency radiologists in interpretation of adult trauma and infection. These scenarios include MR assessment of hip and pelvic fracture, traumatic soft tissue injuries, septic arthritis, soft tissue infection, and osteomyelitis.

Hip fractures, often defined as fractures of the proximal femur, impose a large financial burden on the global health-care system and can substantially decrease healthy life-years,[1] with the overall mortality rate ranging from 14% to 36%.[2] Most hip fractures are treated surgically. Although most nonfemoral pelvic and sacral fractures are treated conservatively, these fractures do contribute to morbidity with potentially prolonged recovery and are thus important to identify. Hip and pelvic fractures are predominantly a disease of the elderly with concomitant osteoporosis, which is an independent risk factor for increased mortality and failure of surgical fixation.[3]

The evaluation of acute musculoskeletal infection in the emergent setting can be a vexing clinical challenge and often requires synthesis of the imaging findings as well as a comprehensive clinical and laboratory evaluation. MR plays a key role in

[a] Musculoskeletal Imaging and Intervention, Division of Musculoskeletal Radiology, Harvard Medical School, Brigham and Women's Hospital, 75 Francis Street, Boston, MA 02115, USA; [b] Division of Emergency Radiology, Brigham and Women's Hospital, Trauma Imaging Research and Innovation Center, Harvard Medical School, 75 Francis Street, Boston, MA 02115, USA
* Corresponding author.
E-mail address: jmandell@bwh.harvard.edu

Magn Reson Imaging Clin N Am 30 (2022) 441–454
https://doi.org/10.1016/j.mric.2022.04.007
1064-9689/22/© 2022 Elsevier Inc. All rights reserved.

mri.theclinics.com

guiding clinical management of suspected musculoskeletal processes, with this article focusing on septic arthritis, soft tissue infection, and osteomyelitis.

Traumatic Injuries

Hip fractures

Anatomy of the hip The hip is a highly stable articulation, with greater than 80% of the femoral head cartilage articulating with the acetabulum.[4] Several strong ligaments coalesce into a fibrous capsule to provide additional support and increase the passive stability of the hip. Fractures of the hip and/or acetabulum tend to occur with a bimodal age distribution; younger patients with traumatic injuries and older patients with fragility fractures. In general, due to the extensive osseoligamentous supporting structures, hip dislocations occur primarily in high-velocity trauma.[5] In contrast, the elderly population is more susceptible to femoral neck fractures.[6] Fractures of the intracapsular proximal femur are at increased risk of avascular necrosis due to either disruption of the arterial vascular supply or increased venous pressures.[7] The medial femoral circumflex artery provides the sole clinically significant blood supply to the subchondral bone of the femoral head,[8] and therefore, if this critical vessel is kinked, thrombosed, or transected, then the risk of subsequently developing avascular necrosis is increased.

Imaging of hip fracture: radiography, CT, or MR imaging? Although the focus of this article is on MR imaging, it is important to understand the imaging workup of suspected hip fracture including appropriate use of radiography and CT, as well as the optimal and appropriate use of MR imaging in the emergent setting. Imaging of hip fracture should begin with conventional radiography, including an anterior-posterior (AP) view of the pelvis and frontal and lateral radiograph of the affected hip.[9] Most hip fractures can be detected and classified on conventional radiography, and advanced imaging is not typically needed if the fracture is clearly seen on radiography. Despite optimal radiographic technique, however, up to 1'0% of hip fractures are not evident on radiography[10–12]; these fractures are called *occult* fractures. In patients with negative radiographs and persistent clinical concern for hip fracture, the incidence of occult proximal femoral fracture has been reported to be as high as 40%.[10,12–15] Importantly, the frequency of occult fracture is higher in elderly patients (80 years or older) or in those with an equivocal (rather than negative) radiographic report.[16] There are several reasons why a fracture may not be able to be seen on radiography,

including overlying soft tissue, nondisplacement, or osseous demineralization. Additionally, the clinical examination and inability to bear weight cannot reliably distinguish patients with hip fracture from those without.[17] Therefore, if there is persistent clinical concern for fracture despite negative radiographs, further imaging evaluation is warranted because prompt treatment of even nondisplaced fractures has been shown to decrease long-term morbidity and mortality.[18] Cross sectional with MR or CT plays a key role in the evaluation of these radiographically occult hip fractures.

In the clinical setting of a suspected occult fracture, either MR or CT are reasonable imaging modalities as the next step in evaluation. Several studies have compared the sensitivity and specificity of CT, using either MR or clinical follow-up as the standard of reference. A meta-analysis comprising 1,248 patients using either clinical follow-up or MR as the standard of reference demonstrated an overall sensitivity of CT of 94% for detecting occult proximal femoral fractures.[19] An additional meta-analysis of 2,992 patients using MR as the standard of reference (including many patients who not have CT) showed a high frequency of occult hip fractures seen on MR, with a total incidence of 39% of occult hip fracture, and a sensitivity of CT of 79%.[16] Both surgical and nonsurgical cases may be missed by CT.[20] In summary, either CT or MR are reasonable imaging modalities to detect nondisplaced hip fracture but if MR is available expeditiously and there are no contraindications, then MR does provide demonstrably higher sensitivity and is generally considered the gold standard.[14,21–23] One may rightfully ask, "why not perform MR imaging in all patients with suspected occult hip fracture?" The answer to that is highly dependent on regional practice patterns, costs, and MR availability; however, recent literature suggests that there may be a cost savings with initial imaging performed by CT, to be followed by MR if CT is negative.[24]

MR imaging protocol for hip/pelvic trauma Several studies have evaluated the feasibility of abbreviated or focused MR imaging for the assessment of radiographically occult hip fractures, which have uniformly demonstrated reduced scanning time (generally <10 minutes), with high diagnostic accuracy.[23,25–28] A recent meta analysis demonstrated that an abbreviated protocol consisting solely of coronal T1-weighted and short-tau inversion recovery (STIR) images was 100% sensitive to detect occult hip fracture.[28] The authors initiated an abbreviated protocol at our institution in 2012, which also includes axial

T2-weighted images with fat suppression in addition to the coronal T1-weighted and STIR sequences described in the literature; we thought that the additional axial sequence allows better characterization of myotendinous injury.

MR imaging of hip fracture Due to typical imaging workup of radiographs followed by MR if negative, the vast majority of fractures seen on MR will be nondisplaced. A fracture will be evident as an irregularly-shaped, "lightning bolt" or linear signal abnormality that may either be low signal intensity (if there is trabecular impaction) or high signal intensity (if there is a fracture gap) on fluid sensitive sequences, and low in signal intensity on T1-weighted images. Surrounding "edema" is manifest on MR as high signal intensity on fluid-sensitive sequences, although the term "edema" should be used with some degree of caution because it likely encompasses a range of osseous injuries including hemorrhage, microinfarction, and microtrabecular impaction in addition to edema.[29]

Femoral head fractures and hip dislocations Due to the strong osseoligamentous supports, femoral head fractures are typically seen in the setting of hip dislocation.[5,30] Usually these types of injuries are evident on radiography or CT but occasionally MR imaging can be used as a problem-solving tool. The joint should be symmetrically reduced, and a careful search should be performed to evaluate for intra-articular bodies or chondral fragments, as well as displaced labral tears. Intra-articular bodies are highly prevalent, seen in up to 89% of patients who had a hip dislocation and subsequent arthroscopy.[31] The soft tissue structures around the hip should be evaluated, with particular attention paid to the sciatic nerve, which can be at risk of injury in the setting of posterior dislocation.

Femoral head fractures should be described relative to the fovea, which is the indentation where the ligamentum teres attaches to the femoral head. Fractures above the fovea are typically treated surgically, whereas fractures located inferior to the fovea have a better prognosis and can be treated conservatively. An often-overlooked injury is an osteochondral impaction injury of the anterior femoral head seen in posterior hip dislocation, which is conceptually similar to a reverse Hill-Sachs lesion.[32]

In addition to acute traumatic injuries, avascular necrosis and subchondral insufficiency fracture may also involve the femoral head and be evident on MR imaging. Morphologically, osteonecrosis is said to have a smooth, low-signal intensity band that is concave (mirror image) to the articular surface, whereas a subchondral insufficiency fracture is irregular, discontinuous, and parallels the curve of the articular surface.[33] Despite these features described in the literature, these entities can have overlapping clinical and imaging features but a subchondral insufficiency fracture should be the primary consideration in an elderly woman without history of alcohol abuse or corticosteroid administration.[34]

Occult femoral neck fractures The specific location within the intracapsular femoral neck does not have any impact on prognosis or surgical management,[35] so terms such as "subcapital" or "transcervical" are generally superfluous. Fractures are evident as linear/irregular low signal on T1-weighted images with surrounding edema (**Fig. 1**). Basicervical fractures, however, are a

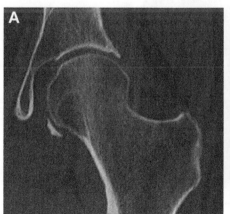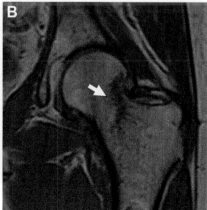

Fig. 1. Nondisplaced occult femoral neck fracture. (*A*) Coronal noncontrast CT of the left hip does not identify a fracture. (*B*) Coronal T1-weighted images demonstrate the low-signal intensity irregular morphology trabecular fracture line through the femoral neck (*arrow*). This patient was treated with surgical fixation.

special type of femoral neck fractures that are extracapsular in location (located just proximal to the intertrochanteric crest). Basicervical fractures deserve special mention in the radiology report because these fractures are treated differently and generally have a favorable outcome with operative management.[36]

Greater and lesser trochanteric fractures In elderly individuals, greater trochanteric fractures are usually due to direct impaction due to fall.[37] Although fractures isolated to the greater trochanter are often treated conservatively,[38] greater trochanter fractures frequently extend into the intertrochanteric region, where they may be treated surgically similar to a nondisplaced intertrochanteric fracture. MR plays an important role in distinguishing isolated greater trochanteric fractures from fractures with trochanteric extension. In fact, up to 90% of greater trochanteric fractures identified on radiography have intertrochanteric extension evident on MR[39] (**Fig. 2**). If linear edema originating from the greater trochanter extends beyond 50% to the medial femoral cortex, then the fracture may be treated surgically as an intertrochanteric fracture.[40]

In adults, isolated fracture or avulsion of the lesser trochanter should be consider a pathologic fracture.[41,42] Although it can be difficult to distinguish traumatic from pathologic fractures on radiography, on MR a pathologic lesion should generally be apparent, and MR imaging can be a helpful problem-solving tool in this circumstance.

Intertrochanteric and subtrochanteric fractures Intertrochanteric fractures can be stable or unstable. A stable fracture is typically a 2-part fracture (although the lesser trochanter can be avulsed), whereas an unstable fracture is more highly comminuted or involves the lateral cortex. Most intertrochanteric fractures detected on MR will be nondisplaced/noncomminuted and therefore stable. The subtrochanteric region extends from the lesser trochanter to 5 cm more distally. There is generally no need to classify subtrochanteric fractures because they are virtually all treated with an intramedullary nail. From an MR imaging perspective, it is important to recognize edema of the lateral femoral cortex, which may signify the presence of an atypical femoral fracture. An atypical femoral fracture is due to osteoclast inhibition due to either systemic factors or long-term bisphosphonate use. These types of fractures may occur with minimal trauma[43] and are important to recognize in order to optimize patient treatment, such as involving the endocrine service and imaging the contralateral hip.

Nonfemoral pelvic/sacral fractures Nonfemoral pelvic/sacral fractures are most commonly treated

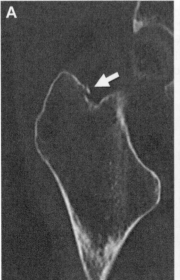 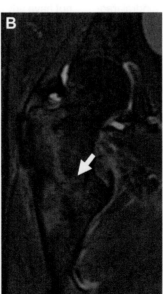 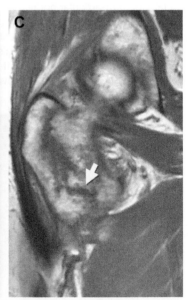

Fig. 2. Greater trochanteric fracture with intertrochanteric extension. (*A*) Coronal CT demonstrates an apparently tiny fracture of the greater trochanter evident as a focus of cortical disruption (*arrow*). (*B*) Coronal STIR image demonstrates edema extending greater than 50% through the intertrochanteric region (*arrow*), and coronal T1 image (*C*) demonstrates that the trabecular fracture line nearly reaches to the lesser trochanter (*arrow*). This patient was treated with surgical fixation.

conservatively but are still important to recognize to optimize patient care. In a study of 263 consecutive patients receiving focused hip MR at our institution,[44] 112 nonfemoral pelvic/sacral fractures were identified, all of which were treated conservatively. In fact, fractures of the pelvis and sacrum were twice as common as proximal femoral fractures in this study: of the 27% patients with occult fractures, one-third were fractures of the proximal femur and two-thirds were pelvic or sacral fractures. In a smaller study of 77 patients receiving CT after negative pelvic or hip radiographs, 40 fractures were present in 25 patients. Of these, pelvic or sacral fractures were far more common than proximal femur fractures, representing 32/40 fractures; all of which were treated conservatively[45] (**Fig. 3**). The most common type of pelvic/sacral fracture is lateral compression,[46] which results on a side-compressive force on the pelvis. Of most relevance to MR imaging, lateral compression 1 fractures include fractures of the inferior and superior pubic rami, with fracture to the ipsilateral sacrum. These sacral fractures are usually not evident on radiography,[46] so MR plays a key role in identifying this pattern of injury.

Soft tissue traumatic injuries about the hip There is a broad range of acute traumatic soft tissue injuries about the hip, including tendon tears, muscle contusion or strain, and Morel-Lavallée lesions. Both gluteus minimus and medius tendons insert onto the greater trochanter of the proximal femur, with gluteus minimus located more anteriorly. Similar to rotator cuff tears, gluteus minimus and medius tendon tearing may be partial or full-thickness.[47] Injury to the hamstring muscle complex is common in athletes, typically occurring at the myotendinous junction in the thigh.[48] The hamstrings originate from the ischial tuberosity, with the semimembranosus arising anteriorly/laterally, and the conjoint semitendinosus and biceps femoris arising posteriorly/medially. Myotendinous junction injuries tend to be treated conservatively, whereas avulsion from the ischial tuberosity may be treated surgically. A Morel-Lavallée lesion is a closed degloving injury caused by disruption of capillaries resulting in a collection containing lymph and necrotic fat. Potential complications include secondary infection or skin necrosis.[47] In contrast to atraumatic greater trochanteric bursitis, Morel-Lavallée lesions are located superficial to the tensor fascia lata. A hallmark-imaging feature of a Morel-Lavallée (although not always present) is globules of fat within the lesion[49] (**Fig. 4**).

Infection

Septic arthritis

Overview of septic arthritis Septic arthritis is bacterial infection of a joint. In the clinical setting of an acute monoarticular arthritis (a single acutely painful joint), septic arthritis should be the primary diagnostic consideration; however, it is often difficult to differentiate acute septic arthritis from a multitude of noninfectious mimics even with MR imaging.[50] Septic arthritis may be present even in the absence of fever, elevated white count, or other system signs of infection. Septic arthritis is a medical emergency, as timely diagnosis and treatment is necessary to prevent cartilage damage and progression of infection. The purulent infection can cause cartilage destruction in as few as 3 days,[51] with rapid joint destruction predominantly mediated by host inflammatory response and synovial ischemia.[52] *Staphylococcus aureus* is the most common causative organism.[52] In patients presenting to the emergency room with an acute monoarticular arthritis, septic arthritis has been reported to be the cause in between 8% and 27% of patients.[53] The differential diagnosis of monoarticular arthritis

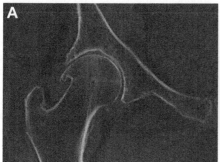
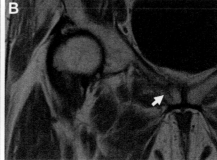

Fig. 3. Occult parasymphyseal fracture. (*A*) Coronal noncontrast CT of the hip does not identify a fracture. (*B*) Coronal T1-weighted images demonstrate the low-signal intensity trabecular fracture line through the right pubic tubercle (*arrow*). This patient was treated conservatively.

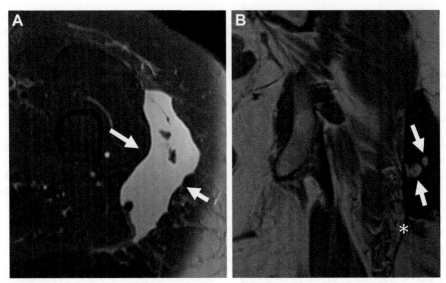

Fig. 4. Morel-Lavallée lesion. (*A*) Axial STIR image demonstrates a large fluid collection of deep subcutaneous tissues of the left proximal thigh (*arrows*). (*B*) Coronal T1-weighted MR shows globules of intralesional fat (*arrows*), which is the hallmark-imaging feature of a Morel-Lavallée degloving lesion. Note that the collection is located superficial to tensor fascia lata (*asterisk*).

includes inflammatory and neoplastic causes, including pigmented villonodular synovitis, avascular necrosis, neuropathic arthropathy, and crystalline arthropathy, among others.[54]

Septic arthritis usually presents with the involvement of a single joint, with risk factors including any structural joint abnormality, intravenous drug abuse, advanced age, diabetes, rheumatoid arthritis, skin infection, prior surgery, and arthroplasty.[55] Hematogenous spread of septic arthritis is approximately twice as common as direct inoculation (such as from prior surgery or penetrating injury).[56] Throughout the body, the knee is by far the most common site (accounting for 48% of infections in one study), followed by the hip (24%), ankle (12%), and elbow (9%).[56] Of note, in patients with a history of intravenous drug abuse, the most commonly involved joints are reported to be the sacroiliac and sternoclavicular joints in a single small study.[57]

MR of septic arthritis Imaging evaluation of suspected septic arthritis should start with radiographs, which can detect soft tissue swelling, joint effusion, or any potentially confounding or alternative diagnoses such as fracture, arthritis, or calcific tendinopathy. Because the radiographic findings of septic arthritis are not reliable, MR plays a key role in suspected septic arthritis, especially for joints where effusion may not be evident clinically, such as the hip, shoulder, sacroiliac joints, and acromioclavicular joints. Additionally, even if radiographs are positive for osteomyelitis,

MR is often performed to evaluate the extent. There is no single optimal MR protocol or commonly performed abbreviated protocol but a combination of fluid-sensitive and T1-weighted sequences should be performed, with ideally at least 2 planes of each. Proton-density sequences are less useful for the evaluation of suspected infection because both fat and fluid can be similar high signal intensity. An optimal selection of imaging planes and sequences should be performed, especially for small joints and the feet when the alignment can vary from patient to patient, and the exact site of involvement may not be known.

For the assessment of suspected septic arthritis and other soft tissue infections, the administration of intravenous Gadolinium-based contrast can be very helpful, especially for the assessment of synovial enhancement, evaluation of peripherally enhancing abscesses, and differentiation of bland subcutaneous edema from enhancing cellulitis. At our institution, postcontrast images are performed in 2 phases to provide a simple type of enhancement kinetics. In the absence of indwelling metallic hardware, postcontrast images should be obtained with fat suppression in at least 2 planes, and a precontrast fat-saturated sequence should also be routinely obtained in the same imaging plane as the postcontrast sequences, using the same tissue weightings so pre-and-post contrast imaging can be directly compared.

The imaging hallmark of septic arthritis is the presence of an effusion; however, effusions are not always present, especially in smaller joints.[58]

In a normal joint, the synovium is barely evident; however, with septic arthritis the synovium may be thickened and enhancing[58] (**Fig. 5**). A *lamellated* appearance of the synovium with whorls of thickened synovium is thought to be highly specific for septic arthritis[58] (**Fig. 7**). If the synovium is not thickened, then the enhancement kinetics of the synovium can be evaluated. Eventually even normal synovium and joint fluid will enhance, but the rate of enhancement is more rapid if the synovium is inflamed.[59]

Definitive diagnosis of suspected septic arthritis is arthrocentesis, which may be performed at the bedside or with imaging guidance, depending on the joint involved and specific skillset of the referring providers. As emphasized previously, septic arthritis may be present even in the absence of an effusion, so aspiration should not be deferred even if no effusion is present (although in the personal experience of the authors, the ability to obtain joint fluid is substantially less if there is no effusion evident on MR).

Periprosthetic joint infection The diagnosis of periprosthetic joint infection is a complex topic often requiring a collaborative approach between the orthopedic surgeon and the radiology team, as well as comprehensive interpretation of multiple imaging modalities including radiography, nuclear medicine, and MR in conjunction with laboratory analysis. However, there are several key features seen on MR imaging that can predict the presence of periprosthetic infection. Specifically, periosteal

edema (sensitivity of 78% and specificity of 90%), capsular edema (sensitivity and specificity of 83% and 95%) and intramuscular edema (sensitivity and specificity of 95% and 86%) are all helpful imaging features to evaluate periprosthetic infection.[57]

Soft tissue infection Soft tissue infection includes cellulitis, infectious tenosynovitis, pyomyositis, septic bursitis, and necrotizing fasciitis.[60] Cellulitis is infection of the subcutaneous tissues and superficial fascia without muscular involvement. MR demonstrates T2-hyperintense thickening and reticulation of the subcutaneous tissues. In contrast to bland edema, cellulitis enhances after administration of contrast.[60] Infectious tenosynovitis is bacterial infection of the synovial membrane surrounding a tendon, with the hand and wrist the most commonly involved sites. Infectious tenosynovitis of the hand and wrist is an emergency because infection can rapidly spread to different compartments, and an urgent surgery may be warranted.[61] MR typically demonstrates a fluid-distended tendon sheath with internal complexity and enhancement.

Pyomyositis is bacterial infection of a muscle, with 3 discrete phases classically described.[62] In the initial phase, MR imaging shows edema of the muscle without discrete fluid collection. The imaging features of this phase are nonspecific and include inflammatory myositis, viral myositis, rhabdomyolysis, contusion, strain, or delayed onset muscle soreness.[63] The second phase is

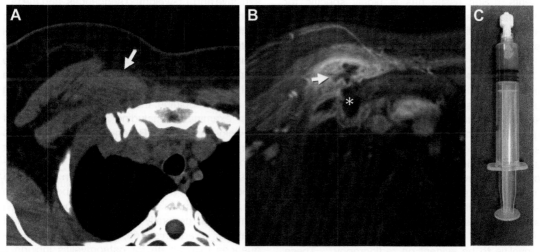

Fig. 5. Costosternal septic arthritis and adjacent abscess. (*A*) Axial noncontrast CT demonstrates extensive soft tissue swelling with apparent expansion of the superior fibers of pectoralis major (*arrow*). (*B*) Axial T1-weighted post-contrast MR with fat suppression demonstrates a large nonenhancing joint effusion (*asterisk*) with adjacent enhancing synovitis. There is a peripherally nonenhancing collection deep to pectoralis major (*arrow*) with thickened surrounding enhancement. Aspiration revealed this collection to be contiguous with the joint and a several cc's of purulent fluid were aspirated (*C*).

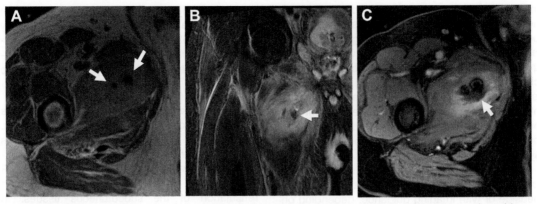

Fig. 6. Pyomyositis. (*A*) Axial T1-weighted MR demonstrates a complex appearing collection in the adductor compartment. There are rounded foci of susceptibility (*arrows*) in the center of the collection corresponding to gas. (*B*) Coronal STIR shows extensive edema and expansion of the adductors with complex fluid signal centrally (*arrow*). (*C*) Axial T1-weighted postcontrast image with fat suppression redemonstrates the susceptibility artifact and confirms the presence of a collection with central nonenhancement (*arrow*). Approximately 10 mL of purulent fluid was aspirated.

characterized by suppuration, and MR imaging may show an intramuscular abscess (**Fig. 6**). The signal characteristics of the abscess may be variable, although the key imaging finding is central nonenhancement.[60] If gas is present, this will be evident on MR as foci of susceptibility artifact. The third stage of myositis is characterized by sepsis and multiorgan failure.

Necrotizing fasciitis is an infection of the deep soft tissues that can have a rapidly progressive course. The key MR imaging finding of necrotizing fasciitis is edema-like signal along the deep intermuscular fascia, fascial thickening of 3 mm or more, and involvement of 3 or more compartments.[60] Soft tissue gas is highly specific for necrotizing fasciitis, although this is a rare finding, and nonvisualization of soft-tissue gas does not exclude necrotizing fasciitis.[64]

Osteomyelitis

Imaging of osteomyelitis Similar to the evaluation of suspected septic arthritis, imaging evaluation of suspected osteomyelitis should begin with radiographs.[65,66] These are often negative but may offer an alternative diagnosis, provide insights as to the status of prior surgeries, and can visualize changes of advanced osteomyelitis. Early imaging findings of osteomyelitis are evident as soft tissue swelling, which may be seen with 2 to 3 days of symptoms onset[67,68]; however, it generally takes up to 10 to 12 days for the bony changes of osteomyelitis to be evident on radiography.[67] These bony changes are first evident as focal osteopenia and periosteal mineralization. After 2 to 3 weeks, cortical erosions may be evident,[69] and frank bony destruction can be seen in advanced disease.

MR of osteomyelitis Although it is important to maintain a systematic approach and keen eye when assessing radiographs in suspected osteomyelitis, MR remains the most definitive imaging modality, with a sensitivity of 90% and specificity of 79%.[70] In distinction to the imaging evaluation of suspected septic arthritis, the role of intravenous Gadolinium-based contrast for the evaluation of osteomyelitis remains controversial. Contrast can aid in differentiating necrotic from viable bone,[71] and can increase confidence in diagnosing soft tissue abscesses. However, the disadvantage of administering contrast include less available scanner time to obtain multiple fluid sensitive and T1-weighted sequences, and the potential risk for causing harm by administering contrast. Especially in patients with reduced estimated glomerular filtration rate (eGFR), intravenous Gadolinium-based contrast must be administered with caution. For MR imaging of the foot, many experts feel that contrast is helpful. In the authors' opinion, the advantages of a noncontrast examination including additional planes of T1-weighted and STIR sequences outweigh the marginal benefit of contrast for the assessment of pedal osteomyelitis, although this is a controversial topic. For other body parts in suspected infection, especially where there may be a concern for septic arthritis or soft tissue abscess, then contrast is generally preferred. Regardless if contrast is administered, the primary MR sequences to evaluate for osteomyelitis include a fluid-sensitive sequence (either STIR or T2-weighted with fat suppression) and T1-weighted nonfat suppressed sequences. These should be obtained in as many planes as feasible (generally, at least 2 planes, and optimally 3 planes) to allow best assessment of curved, small, or irregular structures. Additional sequences such as diffusion may be helpful,[72,73] although these are not performed routinely at the authors' institution.

Interpretation of the MR imaging of osteomyelitis generally starts with the fluid-sensitive sequences. If these are normal, osteomyelitis is very unlikely. If these show bone marrow edema in the area of clinical concern, then osteomyelitis *may* be present, and the T1-weighted images are used to improve specificity. If the T1-weighted images remain normal (even in the presence of edema evident on the fluid-sensitive sequences), then osteomyelitis is probably not present, although there are rare reports of biopsy-proven osteomyelitis with normal T1-weighted images,[74,75] possibly due to marrow necrosis. However, as a general rule, if T1-weighted images are negative, then osteomyelitis is unlikely. Despite this, it is important to keep in mind that in the setting of normal T1-weighted images, if an ulcer is present immediately subjacent to the region of edema, 61% of patients eventually develop osteomyelitis,[76] so it is the authors' practice in this scenario to recommend continued clinical follow-up with reimaging if the patient does not improve with conservative management.

If the T1-weighted images show decreased signal intensity to correspond with the high signal on fluid-sensitive sequences, then the morphology of the T1 signal changes should be carefully described because not all signal changes correspond to osteomyelitis. Three distinct patterns of signal change on T1-weighted images are *confluent intramedullary*, *subcortical*, and *hazy reticular*.[77] Of these 3 patterns, only the confluent intramedullary pattern is highly associated with osteomyelitis, with a reported sensitivity and specificity of 95% and 91%, respectively[74] (**Figs. 7** and **8**). This confluent intramedullary pattern shows a geographic contiguous region of decreased signal intensity on T1-weighted images progressing from the end of the bone. The subcortical pattern shows decreased signal intensity on T1-weighted images isolated to the subcortical region, and the hazy reticular pattern demonstrates interspersed preserved marrow fat. Diffusion-weighted imaging may also be helpful in differentiating osteomyelitis from Charcot arthropathy.[73]

Diabetic pedal osteomyelitis The incidence of diabetic foot complications continues to increase with potential for amputation, sepsis, and even mortality.[78] Foot ulcers are seen in up 5.8% of patients with diabetes and greatly contribute to the US health-care burden.[79] Of those patients with ulcers, osteomyelitis has been reported in up to 15%.[79] Ulcers tend to develop over weight-bearing regions, including the fifth metatarsal, first metatarsal, calcaneus, and great toe distal phalanx as the 4 most common sites.[80]

Imaging of diabetic pedal osteomyelitis and differentiation from neuropathic arthropathy Distinguishing between osteomyelitis and neuropathic arthropathy (synonymous with Charcot arthropathy when involving the foot) can strike fear into the hearts of many radiologists, possibly exacerbated by the sometimes conflicting and often overlapping imaging findings described in the literature.[81–83] Additionally, the imaging hallmarks of osteomyelitis including bone marrow edema and abnormal signal intensity on T1-weighted images are seen in both neuropathic arthropathy and osteomyelitis. However, despite

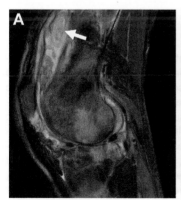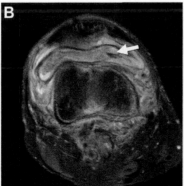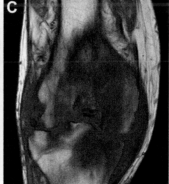

Fig. 7. Septic arthritis and osteomyelitis. (*A*) Sagittal and axial (*B*) T2-weighted MR with fat suppression demonstrates a large effusion with a complex, lamellated appearance (*arrows*). There is extensive bone marrow edema about the knee. (*C*) Coronal T1-weighted MR with fat suppression demonstrates multifocal confluent intramedullary signal change of the distal femur and proximal tibia with cystic change and erosion, in keeping with osteomyelitis.

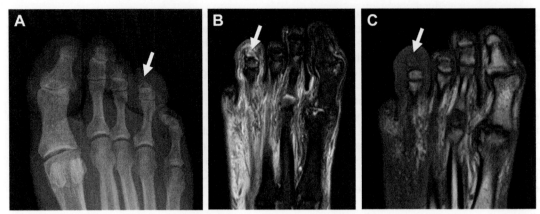

Fig. 8. Osteomyelitis. (*A*) Frontal radiograph demonstrates subtle erosion of the distal tuft of the fourth toe (*arrow*). (*B*) Axial STIR shows edema in the distal phalanx (*arrow*) with surrounding soft tissue swelling. (*C*) Axial T1-weighted MR shows prominent soft tissue swelling of the fourth toe, with confluent intramedullary signal change involving nearly the entire distal phalanx (*arrow*), in keeping with osteomyelitis.

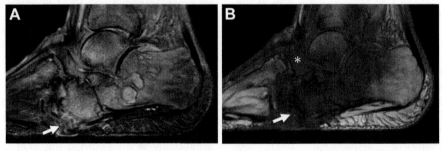

Fig. 9. Charcot arthropathy with superimposed osteomyelitis. (*A*) Coronal STIR MR shows extensive edema throughout the entire hindfoot with partially imaged fragmentation of the TMTs. Note the presence of an ulcer with a sinus tract (*arrow*) tracking directly to the cuboid. (*B*) Sagittal-weighted MR shows erosion of the cuboid at the site of the sinus tract (*arrow*), in keeping with osteomyelitis. It is very difficult to delineate the extent of osteomyelitis on the background of Charcot arthropathy but there is erosion of the navicular (*asterisk*), suggestion extensive osteomyelitis.TMT, tarsometatarsal.

this complexity, the authors thought that focusing on 2 main imaging features can substantially simplify this task. The location, as previously described, the 4 most common sites of diabetic-related osteomyelitis are the fifth metatarsal, first metatarsal, calcaneus, and great toe distal phalanx. The most common location of Charcot arthropathy is the midfoot. That simple distinction will cover the vast majority of cases. However, in cases of altered anatomy due to midfoot collapse or prior surgeries, the separation becomes less reliable (**Fig. 9**). The second important factor to evaluate for is the presence of a sinus tract extending from the ulcer to the infected bone, which has been described as the only imaging finding that is only seen in osteomyelitis.[81] Of note, ulcers may be present in both Charcot arthropathy and osteomyelitis but sinus tracts connecting the ulcer to the bone are only seen in osteomyelitis. All other findings have some degree of overlap so are less useful on a case-by-case basis.

SUMMARY

MR imaging is integral to the evaluation of musculoskeletal trauma and infection. MR is the gold standard for assessment of occult hip and pelvic fractures. MR plays an important role in the evaluation of musculoskeletal infection. In septic arthritis, the hallmark-imaging feature is an effusion with thickened and early enhancing synovium, although septic arthritis may be present even in the absence of effusion. In osteomyelitis, the fluid sensitive sequences provide the highest sensitivity, but the T1-weighted images provide the greatest specificity. In the diabetic foot, both the location of involved bone and the presence of a sinus tract can aid in differentiating osteomyelitis from Charcot arthropathy.

CLINICS CARE POINTS

- For assessment of hip trauma, radiographs are the initial imaging modality. However, if radiographs are negative and there is persistent clinical concern for fracture, then cross-sectional imaging should be performed with CT or MR, with MR preferred if available.

- Septic arthritis is a medical emergency and should be the primary diagnostic consideration in an acute monoarticular arthritis. However, imaging cannot definitively "rule out" septic arthritis and arthrocentesis should be considered depending on clinical context.

DISCLOSURE

The authors have nothing to disclose.

REFERENCES

1. Brown JP, Adachi JD, Schemitsch E, et al. Mortality in older adults following a fragility fracture: real-world retrospective matched-cohort study in Ontario. BMC Musculoskelet Disord 2021;22(1):1–11.
2. Aharonoff GB, Koval KJ, Skovron ML, et al. Hip fractures in the elderly: predictors of one year mortality. J Orthop Trauma 1997;11(3):162–5.
3. Cheung WH, Miclau T, Chow SKH, et al. Fracture healing in osteoporotic bone. Injury 2016;47:S21–6.
4. Beebe MJ, Bauer JM, Mir HR. Treatment of hip dislocations and associated injuries. current state of care. Orthop Clin North Am 2016;47(3):527–49.
5. Mandell JC, Marshall RA, Weaver MJ, et al. Traumatic hip dislocation: what the orthopedic surgeon wants to know. Radiographics 2017;37(7).
6. Barnes R, Brown J, Garden R. Subcapital fractures of the femur. J Bone Jt Surg 1976;58.
7. Ehlinger M, Moser T, Adam P, et al. Early prediction of femoral head avascular necrosis following neck fracture. Orthop Traumatol Surg Res 2011;97(1):79–88.
8. Gautier E, Ganz K, Krügel N, et al. Anatomy of the medial femoral circumflex artery and its surgical implications. J Bone Jt Surg 2000;82(5):679–83. Available at. http://www.ncbi.nlm.nih.gov/pubmed/10963165.
9. Ly TV, Swiontkowski MF. Intracapsular Hip Fractures. In: Browner BD, Jupiter JB, Krettek C, et al, editors. Skeletal trauma: basic science, management, and reconstruction. Fifth Edition. Saunders; 2014. p. 1607–81. Available at. http://www.sciencedirect.com/science/article/pii/B9781455776283000545.
10. Evans PD, Wilson C, Lyons K. Comparison of MRI with bone scanning for suspected hip fracture in elderly patients. J Bone Joint Surg Br 1994;76(1):158–9. Available at. http://www.ncbi.nlm.nih.gov/pubmed/8300666.
11. Dominguez S, Liu P, Roberts C, et al. Prevalence of traumatic hip and pelvic fractures in patients with suspected hip fracture and negative initial standard radiographs - a study of emergency department patients. Acad Emerg Med 2005;12(4):366–9.
12. Rizzo PF, Gould ES, Lyden JP, et al. Diagnosis of occult fractures about the hip. Magnetic resonance imaging compared with bone-scanning. J Bone Joint Surg Am 1993;75(3):395–401. Available at. http://www.ncbi.nlm.nih.gov/pubmed/8444918.
13. Kirby MW, Spritzer C. Radiographic detection of hip and pelvic fractures in the emergency department. Am J Roentgenol 2010;194(4):1054–60.
14. Bogost G a, Lizerbram EK, Crues JV. MR imaging in evaluation of suspected hip fracture: frequency of unsuspected bone and soft-tissue injury. Radiology 1995;197(1):263–7.
15. Verbeeten KM, Hermann KL, Hasselqvist M, et al. The advantages of MRI in the detection of occult hip fractures. Eur Radiol 2005;15(1):165–9.
16. Haj-Mirzaian A, Eng J, Khorasani R, et al. Use of advanced imaging for radiographically occult hip fracture in elderly patients: a systematic review and meta-analysis. Radiology 2020;296(3):521–31.
17. Hossain M, Barwick C, Sinha AK, et al. Is magnetic resonance imaging (MRI) necessary to exclude occult hip fracture? Injury 2007;38(10):1204–8.
18. Peleg K, Rozenfeld M, Radomislensky I, et al. Policy encouraging earlier hip fracture surgery can decrease the long-term mortality of elderly patients. Injury 2014;45(7):1085–90.
19. Kellock TT, Khurana B, Mandell JC. Diagnostic performance of ct for occult proximal femoral fractures: a systematic review and meta-analysis. AJR Am J Roentgenol 2019;213(6):1324–30.
20. Haims AH, Wang A, Yoo BJ, et al. Negative predictive value of CT for occult fractures of the hip and pelvis with imaging follow-up. Emerg Radiol 2021;28(2):259–64.
21. May DA, Purins JL, Smith DK. MR imaging of occult traumatic fractures and muscular injuries of the hip and pelvis in elderly patients. Am J Roentgenol 1996;166(5):1075–8.
22. Pandey R, McNally E, Ali A, et al. The role of MRI in the diagnosis of occult hip fractures. Injury 1998;29(1):61–3. Available at. http://www.ncbi.nlm.nih.gov/pubmed/9659484.
23. Khurana B, Okanobo H, Ossiani M, et al. Abbreviated MRI for patients presenting to the emergency department with hip pain. Am J Roentgenol 2012;198(6):17–9.

24. Davidson A, Silver N, Cohen D, et al. Justifying CT prior to MRI in cases of suspected occult hip fracture. A proposed diagnostic protocol. Injury 2021; 52(6):1429–33.

25. Yun BJ, Myriam Hunink MG, Prabhakar AM, et al. Diagnostic imaging strategies for occult hip fractures: a decision and cost–effectiveness analysis. Acad Emerg Med 2016;23(10):1161–9.

26. Gil H, Tuttle AA, Dean LA, et al. Dedicated MRI in the emergency department to expedite diagnostic management of hip fracture. Emerg Radiol 2020;27(1): 41–4.

27. Ross AB, Chan BY, Yi PH, et al. Diagnostic accuracy of an abbreviated MRI protocol for detecting radiographically occult hip and pelvis fractures in the elderly. Skeletal Radiol 2019;48(1):103–8.

28. Wilson MP, Nobbee D, Murad MH, et al. Diagnostic accuracy of limited mri protocols for detecting radiographically occult hip fractures: a systematic review and meta-analysis. AJR Am J Roentgenol 2020; 215(3):559–67.

29. Mandalia V, Henson JHL. Traumatic bone bruising-a review article. Eur J Radiol 2008;67(1):54–61.

30. Mandell JC, Weaver MJ, Harris MB, et al. Hip fractures: a practical approach to diagnosis and treatment. Curr Radiol Rep 2018;6(7). Available at. http://sfx.hul.harvard.edu/sfx_local?sid=EMBASE&issn=21674825&id=doi:10.1007%2Fs40134-018-0281-9&atitle=Hip+Fractures%3A+A+Practical+Approach+to+Diagnosis+and+Treatment&stitle=Curr.+Radiol.+Rep.&title=Current+Radiology+Reports&volume=6&issue=7&spage=&epage=&aulast=Mandell&aufirst=Jacob+C.&auinit=J.C.&aufull=Mandell+J.C.&coden=&isbn=&pages=–&date=2018&auinit1=J&auinitm=C.

31. Mandell JC, Marshall RA, Banffy MB, et al. Arthroscopy after traumatic hip dislocation: a systematic review of intra-articular findings, correlation with magnetic resonance imaging and computed tomography, treatments, and outcomes. Arthroscopy 2017;1–11. https://doi.org/10.1016/j.arthro.2017.08.295.

32. Richardson P, Young JWR, Porter D. CT detection of cortical fracture of the femoral head associated with posterior hip dislocation. Am J Roentgenol 1990; 155(1):93–4.

33. Ikemura S, Yamamoto T, Motomura G, et al. MRI evaluation of collapsed femoral heads in patients 60 years old or older: Differentiation of subchondral insufficiency fracture from osteonecrosis of the femoral head. Am J Roentgenol 2010;195(1):63–8.

34. Ikemura S, Yamamoto T, Motomura G, et al. The utility of clinical features for distinguishing subchondral insufficiency fracture from osteonecrosis of the femoral head. Arch Orthop Trauma Surg 2013; 133(12):1623–7.

35. Rajan DT, Parker MJ. Does the level of an intracapsular femoral fracture influence fracture healing after internal fixation? a study of 411 patients. Injury 2001; 32(1):53–6.

36. Watson ST, Schaller TM, Tanner SL, et al. Outcomes of low-energy basicervical proximal femoral fractures treated with cephalomedullary fixation. J Bone Joint Surg Am 2016;98(13):1097–102.

37. Lee KH, Kim HM, Kim YS, et al. Isolated fractures of the greater trochanter with occult intertrochanteric extension. Arch Orthop Trauma Surg 2010;130(10): 1275–80.

38. Leslie MP, Baumgaertner MR. Intertrochanteric hip fractures. Fifth Edition. Elsevier Inc.; 2003. https://doi.org/10.1016/B978-1-4557-7628-3.00055-7.

39. Kim S-J, Ahn J, Kim HK, et al. Is magnetic resonance imaging necessary in isolated greater trochanter fracture? A systemic review and pooled analysis. BMC Musculoskelet Disord 2015;16(1): 395.

40. Chung PH, Kang S, Kim JP, et al. Occult intertrochanteric fracture mimicking the fracture of greater trochanter. Hip pelvis 2016;28(2):112–9.

41. Phillips CD, Pope TL, Jones JE, et al. Nontraumatic avulsion of the lesser trochanter: a pathognomonic sign of metastatic disease? Skeletal Radiol 1988; 17(2):106–10. Available at. http://www.ncbi.nlm.nih.gov/pubmed/3363377.

42. Rouvillain J-L, Jawahdou R, Labrada Blanco O, et al. Isolated lesser trochanter fracture in adults: an early indicator of tumor infiltration. Orthop Traumatol Surg Res 2011;97(2):217–20.

43. Sheehan SE, Shyu JY, Weaver MJ, et al. Proximal femoral fractures: what the orthopedic surgeon wants to know. Radiographics 2015;35(5): 1563–84.

44. Sun EX, Mandell JC, Weaver MJ, et al. Clinical utility of a focused hip MRI for assessing suspected hip fracture in the emergency department. Emerg Radiol 2021;28(2):317–25.

45. Mandell JC, Weaver MJ, Khurana B, et al. Computed tomography for occult fractures of the proximal femur, pelvis, and sacrum in clinical practice: single institution, dual-site experience. Emerg Radiol 2018;25(3):265–73.

46. Khurana B, Sheehan SE, Sodickson AD, et al. Pelvic ring fractures: what the orthopedic surgeon wants to know. Radiographics 2014;34(3):1317–33.

47. White LM, Oar DA, Naraghi AM, et al. Gluteus minimus tendon: MR imaging features and patterns of tendon tearing. Skeletal Radiol 2021;50(10): 2013–21.

48. Linklater JM, Hamilton B, Carmichael J, et al. Hamstring injuries: anatomy, imaging, and intervention. Semin Musculoskelet Radiol 2010;14(2): 131–61.

49. Nair AV, Nazar PK, Sekhar R, et al. Morel-Lavallée lesion: a closed degloving injury that requires real attention. Indian J Radiol Imaging 2014;24(3): 288–90.

50. Singh N, Vogelgesang SA. Monoarticular arthritis. Med Clin North Am 2017;101(3):607–13.

51. Goldenberg DL, Reed JI. Bacterial arthritis. N Engl J Med 1985;312(12):764–71.

52. Ross JJ, Saltzman CL, Carling P, et al. Pneumococcal septic arthritis: review of 190 cases. Clin Infect Dis 2003;36(3):319–27.

53. Ohl CA, Forster D. In: Bennett JE, Dolin R, Blaser MJ, editors. Infectious arthritis of native joints. Eighth edition. Elsevier; 2014. https://doi.org/10.1016/B978-0-323-40161-6.00105-4.

54. Keret S, Kaly L, Shouval A, et al. Approach to a patient with monoarticular disease. Autoimmun Rev 2021;20(7):102848.

55. Kaandorp CJ, Van Schaardenburg D, Krijnen P, et al. Risk factors for septic arthritis in patients with joint disease. a prospective study. Arthritis Rheum 1995;38(12):1819–25. Available at. http://www.ncbi.nlm.nih.gov/pubmed/8849354.

56. Kaandorp CJ, Dinant HJ, van de Laar MA, et al. Incidence and sources of native and prosthetic joint infection: a community based prospective survey. Ann Rheum Dis 1997;56(8):470–5. Available at. http://www.ncbi.nlm.nih.gov/pubmed/9306869.

57. Brancós MA, Peris P, Miró JM, et al. Septic arthritis in heroin addicts. Semin Arthritis Rheum 1991;21(2): 81–7.

58. Karchevsky M, Schweitzer ME, Morrison WB, et al. MRI findings of septic arthritis and associated osteomyelitis in adults. Am J Roentgenol 2004;182(1): 119–22.

59. König H, Sieper J, Wolf KJ. Rheumatoid arthritis: evaluation of hypervascular and fibrous pannus with dynamic MR imaging enhanced with Gd-DTPA. Radiology 1990;176(2):473–7.

60. Hayeri MR, Ziai P, Shehata ML, et al. Soft-tissue infections and their imaging mimics: from cellulitis to necrotizing fasciitis. Radiographics 2016;36(6):1888–910.

61. Hyatt BT, Bagg MR. Flexor tenosynovitis. Orthop Clin North Am 2017;48(2):217–27.

62. Chiedozi LC. Pyomyositis. review of 205 cases in 112 patients. Am J Surg 1979;137(2):255–9.

63. Wasserman PL, Way A, Baig S, et al. MRI of myositis and other urgent muscle-related disorders. Emerg Radiol 2021;28(2):409–21.

64. Fugitt JB, Puckett ML, Quigley MM, et al. Necrotizing fasciitis. Radiographics 2004;24(5):1472–6. https://doi.org/10.1148/rg.245035169.

65. Simpfendorfer CS. Radiologic approach to musculoskeletal infections. Infect Dis Clin North Am 2017;31: 299–324.

66. Beaman FD, von Herrmann PF, Kransdorf MJ, et al. ACR appropriateness criteria {®} suspected osteomyelitis, septic arthritis, or soft tissue infection (excluding spine and diabetic foot). J Am Coll Radiol 2017;14(5):S326–37.

67. Capitanio MA, Kirkpatrick JA. Early roentgen observations in acute osteomyelitis. Am J Roentgenol Radium Ther Nucl Med 1970;108(3):488–96. Available at. http://www.ncbi.nlm.nih.gov/pubmed/5415924.

68. Jaramillo D, Treves ST, Kasser JR, et al. Osteomyelitis and septic arthritis in children: appropriate use of imaging to guide treatment. AJR Am J Roentgenol 1995;165(2):399–403.

69. Peltola H, Pääkkönen M. Acute osteomyelitis in children. N Engl J Med 2014;370(4):352–60.

70. Dinh MT, Abad CL, Safdar N. Diagnostic accuracy of the physical examination and imaging tests for osteomyelitis underlying diabetic foot ulcers: meta-analysis. Clin Infect Dis 2008;47(4):519–27.

71. Ledermann HP, Schweitzer ME, Morrison WB. Non-enhancing tissue on MR imaging of pedal infection: characterization of necrotic tissue and associated limitations for diagnosis of osteomyelitis and abscess. AJR Am J Roentgenol 2002;178(1): 215–22.

72. Chang C Di, Wu JS. Imaging of Musculoskeletal Soft Tissue Infection. Semin Roentgenol 2017;52(1): 55–62.

73. Abdel Razek AAK, Samir S. Diagnostic performance of diffusion-weighted MR imaging in differentiation of diabetic osteoarthropathy and osteomyelitis in diabetic foot. Eur J Radiol 2017;89:221–5.

74. Johnson PW, Collins MS, Wenger DE. Diagnostic utility of T1-weighted MRI characteristics in evaluation of osteomyelitis of the foot. AJR Am J Roentgenol 2009;192(1):96–100.

75. Craig JG, Amin MB, Wu K, et al. Osteomyelitis of the diabetic foot: MR imaging-pathologic correlation. Radiology 1997;203(3):849–55.

76. Duryea D, Bernard S, Flemming D, et al. Outcomes in diabetic foot ulcer patients with isolated T2 marrow signal abnormality in the underlying bone: should the diagnosis of "osteitis" be changed to "early osteomyelitis". Skeletal Radiol 2017. https://doi.org/10.1007/s00256-017-2666-x.

77. Collins MS, Schaar MM, Wenger DE, et al. T1-weighted MRI characteristics of pedal osteomyelitis. Am J Roentgenol 2005;185(2):386–93.

78. Skrepnek GH, Mills JL, Armstrong DG. A diabetic emergency one million feet long: disparities and burdens of illness among diabetic foot ulcer cases within emergency departments in the United States, 2006-2010. PLoS One 2015;10(8):1–15.

79. Ramsey SD, Newton K, Blough D, et al. Incidence, outcomes, and cost of foot ulcers in patients with diabetes. Diabetes Care 1999;22(3):382–7.

80. Ledermann HP, Morrison WB, Schweitzer ME. MR image analysis of pedal osteomyelitis: distribution,

patterns of spread, and frequency of associated ulceration and septic arthritis. Radiology 2002;223(7): 747–55.

81. Ahmadi ME, Morrison WB, Carrino JA, et al. Neuropathic arthropathy of the foot with and without superimposed osteomyelitis: mr imaging characteristics. Radiology 2006;238(2):622–31.

82. Berendt AR, Lipsky B. Is this bone infected or not? Differentiating neuro-osteoarthropathy from osteomyelitis in the diabetic foot. Curr Diab Rep 2004;4(6):424–9. Available at. http://www.ncbi.nlm.nih.gov/entrez/query.fcgi?cmd=Retrieve%7B&%7Ddb=PubMed%7B&%7Ddopt=Citation%7B&%7Dlist%7B_%7Duids=15539006.

83. Mandell JC, Khurana B, Smith JT, et al. Osteomyelitis of the lower extremity: pathophysiology, imaging, and classification, with an emphasis on diabetic foot infection. Emerg Radiol 2018;25(2): 175–88.

Imaging Penile and Scrotal Trauma
What the Surgeon Needs to Know

Brian Wells, MD, MS, MPH[a], Laura Avery, MD[b],*

KEYWORDS

• Pelvic • Trauma • MRI • Penile • Scrotal • Testicle

KEY POINTS

- Imaging plays a crucial role in the evaluation of male pelvic trauma.
- MR imaging of the penis is performed in anatomic position with a small field of view and with the protocol focused on triplane T2- and sagittal T1-weighted sequences.
- MR imaging provides excellent anatomic evaluation for injury, often with clear depiction of rupture of the tunica albuginea and hematoma.
- Understanding the normal and abnormal appearance on MR imaging is important to guide patient management, including the need for surgical repair.
- Identification of tunica albuginea or corpus cavernosum rupture requires early surgical exploration and repair.

INTRODUCTION

Male pelvic trauma involving the urethra, penis, and scrotum commonly presents to the emergency department; rapid identification of these traumatic injuries is essential to guide appropriate clinical and surgical management, to prevent long-term comorbidities.[1] Moreover, these injuries can be associated with life-threatening multisystem trauma, which can result in the penile or scrotal lesions being overlooked or deprioritized. Given the fast-paced nature of trauma imaging, as well as the need for timely diagnosis, using various imaging modalities for rapid detection of these injuries with a high degree of certainty is paramount. This article focuses specifically on penile, urethral, and scrotal injuries, with an emphasis on MR imaging evaluation, and uses a case-based approach to educate the reader on imaging techniques, anatomy, and common injury patterns.

NORMAL PENILE ANATOMY AND IMAGING

To best understand the pathologic condition of this region, it is first necessary to understand the normal appearance of the penis on imaging (**Fig. 1**). The normal penile anatomy is composed of 3 bodies of erectile tissue: the corpus cavernosum (left and right) along the dorsal aspect of the penis and the midline corpus spongiosum surrounding the urethra along the ventral surface. Venous sinusoids compose the corpora cavernosa and are the structures that become engorged with blood during erection. The corpora cavernosa are surrounded by a strong fascial sheath called the tunica albuginea ("tunica": a membranous sheath enveloping or lining an organ; "albuginea": tough white fibrous tissue), which creates a septum between them called the intercavernous septum. A tunica albuginea also surrounds the corpus spongiosum. Superficial to the tunica albuginea is Buck fascia, also as known as the deep

a Department of Radiology, Brigham and Women's Hospital, 75 Francis Street, Boston, MA 02115, USA;
b Department of Radiology, Massachusetts General Hospital, 55 Fruit Street, Boston, MA 02114, USA
* Corresponding author.
E-mail address: lavery@mgh.harvard.edu

Magn Reson Imaging Clin N Am 30 (2022) 455–464
https://doi.org/10.1016/j.mric.2022.05.003

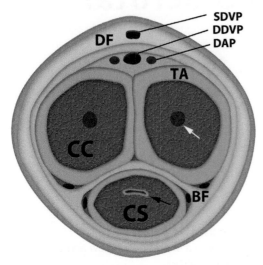

Fig. 1. Penile anatomy. CC, corpus cavernosum; CS, corpus spongiosum; DAP, dorsal artery of the penis; DDVP, deep dorsal vein of the penis; DF, dartos fascia; SDVP, superficial dorsal vein of the penis; TA, tunica albuginea. (*white arrow*) cavernosal artery. (*black arrow*) urethra. (*Courtesy of* Frank M. Corl, MS, Johns Hopkins Medical Institutions, Baltimore, MD) *From:* Avery, L. and Scheinfeld, M. Imaging of Penile and Scrotal Emergencies. RadioGraphics 2013; 33:721–740.

fascia of the penis, and named for the American Civil War plastic surgeon, Gurdon Buck. The crura of the corpora cavernosa attach to the ischial rami proximally.

The vascular anatomy to the penis involves multiple arteries. The arterial supply of the penis is illustrated in **Fig. 2**A, B. The skin of the penis is supplied by the left and right superficial external pudendal arteries arising from the femoral artery. These give rise to dorsolateral and ventrolateral branches, which collateralize across the midline. The ventral skin is supplied by the posterior scrotal artery, which is a superficial branch of the deep internal pudendal artery.[2,3]

The deep structures of the penis are supplied by the right and left internal pudendal arteries from the anterior division of the internal iliac arteries after it gives off a perineal branch.[2,4,5] The internal pudendal artery has 3 branches of arterial flow to the penis: the bulbourethral artery, the dorsal artery, and the deep penile (cavernosal) artery. The bulbourethral artery passes through Buck fascia to supply the bulb of the penis and the penile urethra. The dorsal artery courses along the dorsum of the penis and gives off circumflex branches with the terminus in the glans penis. The deep penile artery arises on each side and enters the corpus cavernosum to give off additional helicine arteries along the penile shaft.[2]

The venous drainage of the penis is divided into the superficial, the intermediate, and the deep. Superficial veins are in the dartos fascia along the dorsolateral surface of the penis and form the superficial dorsal vein, which drains via the superficial external pudendal veins to the great saphenous vein.[2] The intermediate system involves the deep dorsal and circumflex veins deep to Buck fascia. Emissary veins begin within the corpus cavernosa and go through the tunica albuginea to drain into the circumflex or deep dorsal veins. The deep system is via crural and cavernosal veins with crural veins in the midline. Cavernosal veins are consolidations of emissary veins, which form a venous channel to drain to the internal pudendal vein.[2] The venous drainage of the penis is illustrated in **Fig. 2**C.

Attention to the vascular anatomy is important, as vascular injury can result in a myriad of pathologic conditions, such as priapism, torsion, and infarction.

ULTRASOUND AND COMPUTED TOMOGRAPHY CORRELATION WITH NORMAL ANATOMY

Computed tomography (CT) is usually preferred for the evaluation of fractures and hemorrhage/active bleeding and is not usually the first-line imaging modality of choice for scrotal trauma. However, CT is able to depict much of the normal penile anatomy described above, as illustrated in **Fig. 3**. Ultrasound imaging is performed with a high-frequency linear transducer using anatomic positioning.[1] The relatively hypoechoic appearance of the corpus spongiosum contrasts with the homogeneously mixed echogenic appearance of the corpora cavernosa. A region of shadowing is often seen between the corpora cavernosa that extends over the expected location of the urethra. Color and spectral Doppler, as with any other ultrasound, can be used to evaluate the patency and flow in the arteries and veins. The dorsal vein of the penis should be easily compressible with the transducer given its relatively superficial location.[6] Ultrasound correlation of normal penile anatomy is provided in **Fig. 4**.

MR IMAGING CORRELATION OF NORMAL PENILE ANATOMY AND IMAGING PROTOCOL

MR imaging correlation of the normal penile anatomy described above is provided in **Fig. 5**. From a technique perspective, MR imaging is best performed with the penis in the anatomic position, lying on the abdomen. For optimal evaluation, the patient should be placed supine on the

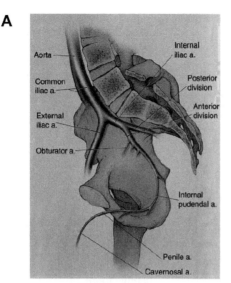

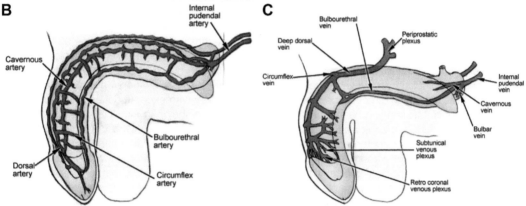

Arterial supply of the penis.　　　　　　　　　　Venous drainage of the penis.

Fig. 2. (*A*) Left parasagittal drawing of the pelvic arterial anatomy. a, artery. (*B, C*) Arterial and venous supply of the penis. The left and right superficial external pudendal arteries arising from the femoral artery provide the blood supply to the skin of the penis. The bulbourethral artery supplies the bulb of the penis and the penile urethra. The dorsal artery gives off circumflex branches and extends to the glans penis. The deep penile artery (cavernosal) artery arises on each side of the corpus cavernosum and gives off helicine arteries. ([*A*] *Courtesy of* Frank M. Corl, MS, Johns Hopkins Medical Institutions, Baltimore, MD) *From*: Pretorius, E., Siegelman, E., Ramchandani, P. et al. MR Imaging of the Penis. RadioGraphics 2001; 21:S283–S299; [*B, C*] *From*: Medscape. Penis Anatomy. https://emedicine.medscape.com/article/1949325-overview#a2.)

imaging table. A towel or other suitable object is placed between the upper thighs to elevate the scrotum. The penis is taped to the anterior abdominal wall in a dorsiflexed position to prevent movement during examination. A multiple phased-array surface coil is placed over the lower abdominopelvic wall and scrotum to optimize image quality.[7]

The MR imaging protocol focuses on a small field of view with triplane high-resolution T2-non–fat-saturated sequences and T1-weighted images in the sagittal and coronal planes. T1-weighted images are ideal for the detection of blood products, as these will by hyperintense on the background of the intermediate signal intensity

of the 3 corpora. T2-weighted images can optimally assess the low-signal tunica albuginea for discontinuity.[1,7] MR.

A review of MR imaging of the penis and scrotum by Parker and colleagues,[7] published in *Radiographics* in 2015, provides a sample protocol used for penile and scrotal MR imaging (**Table 1**).

PENILE INJURIES

The penis is most vulnerable to injury when erect; penile injury may result from either blunt or penetrating mechanisms.[1] Whereas surgical exploration

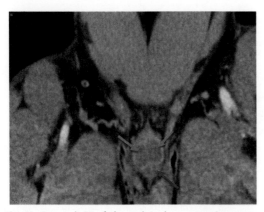

Fig. 3. Coronal CT of the pelvis demonstrating cross-sectional anatomy of the penis. Paired corpora cavernosa superiorly (*blue arrows*) and corpus spongiosum (*red arrow*) inferiorly. *This is an original image.

without initial imaging is typically performed for penetrating trauma, the approach to blunt traumatic injuries is often more nuanced and requires evaluation with imaging. Sonography is often a first-line modality for evaluation, given its wide availability, rapid assessment, and ability to clearly demonstrate patent or injured vascularity. However, ultrasound can be difficult, as it requires direct probe pressure on the injured penis. MR imaging has emerged as a definitive modality assessment, given its ability to clearly delineate anatomic structures and its high sensitivity for detecting subtle traumatic injury. MR imaging and ultrasound-guided clinical decision making can help separate those patients needing surgical intervention from those for whom conservative management is more appropriate.

RUPTURE OF THE TUNICA ALBUGINEA

Less than 1% of all traumas are scrotal traumas, making this a relatively uncommon but still important type of trauma.[8] Most commonly, blunt testicular trauma is seen involving patients between the ages of 10 and 30 years and tends to be sports related. Consequences of blunt force trauma include contusion, hematoma, fracture, or rupture, such as the rupture of the tunica albuginea, as seen in the following case. Note that approximately 50 kg of force is required to rupture a normal tunica albuginea.[9]

Ultrasound has the ability to depict, with high sensitivity, testicular injury as can be seen with altered echogenicity corresponding to injured tissue. Areas of testicular injury, such as infarction, hematocele, fracture, irregular contour, and discontinuity of the tunica albuginea, can be depicted with ultrasound.[1] For example, heterogeneous echotexture combined with loss of normal contour can diagnose testicular rupture. Although useful, there does not need to be depiction of discontinuity of the tunica albuginea. In some studies, ultrasound findings have shown up to 100% sensitivity and 65% to 93.5% specificity.[1,10,11,12] Although it is not typically a first-line modality owing to the imaging time required, MR imaging has additional ability to depict traumatic injury with exceptional anatomic detail.

The case shown in **Fig. 6** involves blunt trauma to a 30-year-old man, who presented with penile swelling and bruising after intercourse. Comparing the pathologic condition shown in **Fig. 6**A, B with the normal appearance of the tunica albuginea (**Fig. 6**C) demonstrates dehiscence of the tunica albuginea. The was confirmed in the operating room (OR), in which the surgeons found "a large opening in the left corpus cavernosum, approximately the size of a dime." No other injury was noted.

Testicular rupture, as evidenced by discontinuity of the tunica albuginea, is an indication for

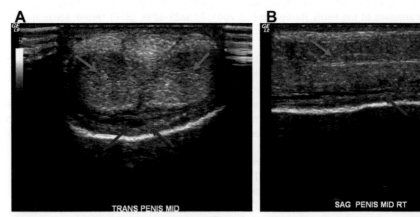

Fig. 4. (*A, B*) Ultrasound images of the penis demonstrating normal anatomy. Paired corpora cavernosa superiorly (*blue arrows*) and corpus spongiosum (*red arrow*) inferiorly. The urethra is highlighted with a yellow arrow. *These are original images. Sag, sagittal; trans, transverse.

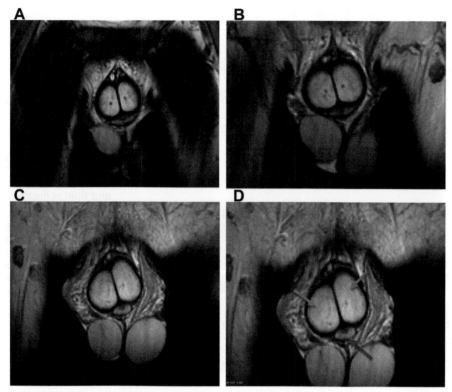

Fig. 5. (*A–D*) Coronal MR images demonstrating normal penile anatomy. Paired corpora cavernosa superiorly (*blue arrows*) and corpus spongiosum (*red arrow*) inferiorly. Note that the signal intensity of the corpora cavernosa on MR imaging may differ from the signal of the corpus spongiosum. The difference is dependent on the rate of blood flow within the cavernous spaces.[4] *Original images.

surgical exploration and repair.[12] Hematocele may also be an indication for exploration.[12,13] Modern treatment algorithms favor exploration in patients with large (>5 cm) or expanding scrotal hematomas, making documentation of scrotal hematoma size, as well as close interval follow-up, important even in patients not initially deemed to be surgical candidates.

Specific imaging findings such as those described above provide a high degree of clinical confidence in the diagnosis and ensure that surgery is only performed on those patients who need it while avoiding unnecessary complications.[6] Complications can include lifelong painful or deviated penile erections related to tunica scar tissue.

SHATTERED TESTICLE

The case illustrated in **Fig. 7** involves a 31-year-old man who was kicked in the groin during karate practice while training. Scrotal ultrasound images (see **Fig. 7**) demonstrated a region of heterogeneous echogenicity within the lower pole of the left testicle consistent with a contusion. In addition, a heterogeneous hypoechoic rind around the left testicle was observed that lacked vascular flow on color Doppler consistent with a hematoma.

Further evaluation with MR imaging (**Fig. 8**) was performed that showed a rim of blood products consistent with hematoma between the tunica vaginalis and tunica albuginea. A focus of heterogeneous signal intensity in the mid and lower pole left testicle was also observed, which was consistent with contusion and hematoma.

The patient was taken to the OR for further evaluation and treatment. On examination in the OR, a large hematoma was found deep to the tunica albuginea. The tunica was then opened with spontaneous passage of the clot. The vast majority of the left testicular tissue appeared necrotic, although the vascular supply and epididymis were intact without injury. The patient was subsequently discharged with outpatient follow-up.

URETHRAL INJURIES

Penile fracture is a rare event and requires emergency diagnosis and intervention. Penile fracture

Table 1
Protocol for penile-scrotal MR imaging

Imaging Sequence and Planes	FOV (mm)	Section Thickness (mm)	Gap (mm)	Matrix Size	Applications
Standard anatomic sequences					
Axial, sagittal, coronal localizer	400	10	5	128 × 256	Prescription of subsequent sequences
Axial, coronal, sagittal T2W FSE	160	4	0.5	256 × 192	Core sequences for anatomic overview, localizing masses, evaluating the integrity of the tunica albuginea, characterizing masses, and fluid collection
Axial T1W SE	340	5	1	256 × 192	Characterizing masses and fluid collections, evaluating the integrity of the tunica albuginea, accessing for deep pelvic disease as well as pelvic and inguinal adenopathy
Additional sequence for trauma					
Axial T1W dual-echo spoiled GRE (in phase and out of phase)	340	4	1	256 × 192	Better characterizing blood products due to T2[a] effects
Sagittal T2W fat-suppressed FSE or STIR	160	4	0.5	256 × 192	Identifying fluid collections and edema

Abbreviations: 3D, three-dimensional; DW, diffusion weighted; FOV, field of view; FSE, fast spin-echo; GRE, gradient-echo; SE, spin-echo; STIR, short inversion time inversion recovery; T1W, T1 weighted; T2W, T2 weighted.

[a] *Modified from*: Parker RA et al, MR Imaging of the Penis and Scrotum. Radiographics. 2015 Jul-Aug;35(4):1033-50. doi: 10.1148/rg.2015140161. Epub 2015 Jun 19. PMID: 26090569.

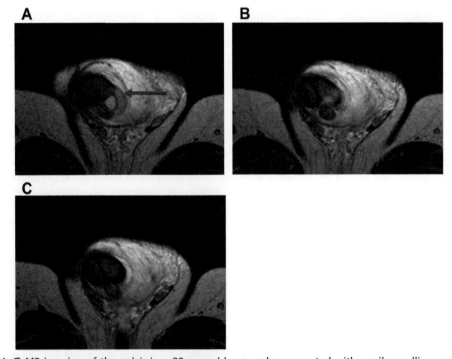

Fig. 6. (*A–C*) MR imaging of the pelvis in a 30-year-old man, who presented with penile swelling and bruising after intercourse. Images showing dehiscence of the tunica albuginea (*A, B: arrow*) compared with the intact tunica imaged at a different level in the same patient (*C*). *Original images.

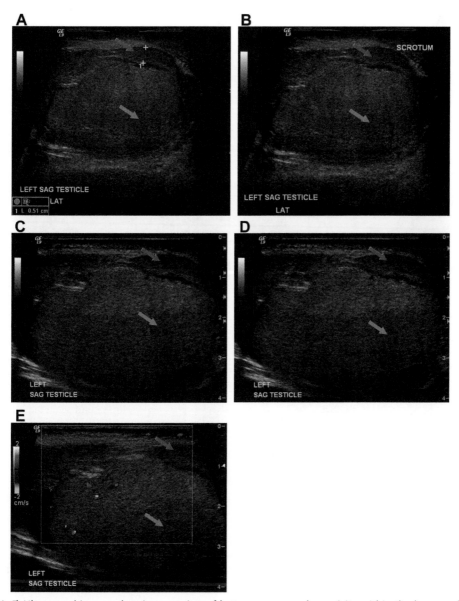

Fig. 7. (*A–E*) Ultrasound images showing a region of heterogeneous echogenicity within the lower pole of the left testicle consistent with a contusion (*blue arrow*). In addition, a heterogeneous hypoechoic rind around the left testicle was observed that lacked vascular flow on color Doppler, consistent with a hematoma (*red arrow*). *Original images.

is defined as a rupture of penile tunica albuginea of the corpora cavernosa or spongiosum, usually caused by trauma to an erect penis, most commonly during sexual intercourse. The urologist needs to know whether the tunica albuginea is ruptured and if the rupture extends to the urethra to determine if an emergent surgical exploration is indicated.[14]

Emergency ultrasound is typically the initial imaging modality. However, this may not be appropriate for all patients, as the penis may be markedly swollen and painful, resulting in a limited, possibly nondiagnostic evaluation. MR imaging of the penis is the best modality to determine the extent of injury.[14]

Fig. 9 illustrates the case of a 47-year-old man, who was brought in by ambulance approximately 1.5 hours after a reported episode of rough sexual intercourse. The patient noted pain in his penis and active bleeding near the meatus, which occurred after feeling his penis "bend" with immediate loss of erection.

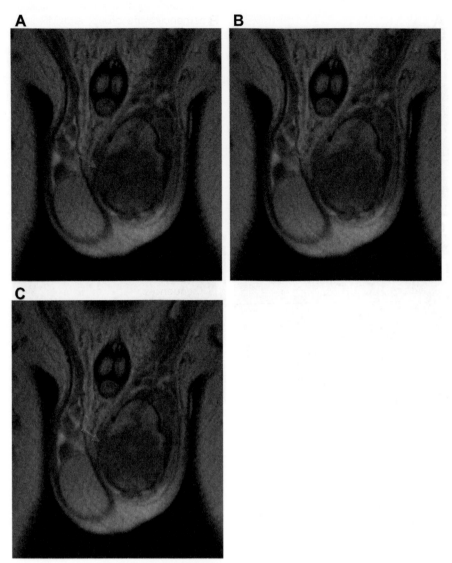

Fig. 8. (*A–C*) Testicular contusion and hematoma, shown as a large area of heterogeneous hypointensity on coronal MR images (*arrows*). Lat, lateral. *Original images.

After evaluation by urology, an MR imaging of the pelvis was obtained through the emergency room. The MR imaging (see **Fig. 9**) demonstrates fluid signal within the distal penile aspect of the corpora spongiosum with extension of the fluid signal into the right corpus cavernosum. There was also apparent dehiscence of the normal low-signal tunica albuginea/Buck fascia along the ventral corpora cavernosum at its junction with corpora spongiosum in the distal penis. The fluid signal was thought to represent urine or blood from a urethral injury.

During this patient's clinical course in the emergency room, a Foley catheter was inserted, and the patient was subsequently discharged from the emergency room observation unit with outpatient urology follow-up.

SEGMENTAL TESTICULAR INFARCT

The case illustrated in **Figs. 10** and **11** involves a 22 year-old man who presented to the emergency room with the chief complaint of right testicular pain for 2 days. A testicular ultrasound was obtained that showed an 11 × 5-mm peripheral wedge-shaped area in the right testis that does not demonstrate any blood flow. Arterial flow was detected within the perfused portions of the right testis. Given that testicular infarct is rare, a contrast-enhanced MR imaging was recommended

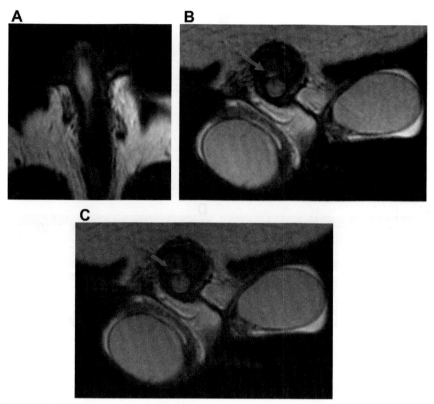

Fig. 9. (A–C) Fluid signal within the distal penile aspect of the corpora spongiosum with extension of the fluid signal into the right corpus cavernosum (arrows). The fluid signal was thought to represent urine or blood from a urethral injury. *These are original case images.

to confirm the diagnosis and to exclude a testicular tumor.

The MR imaging was obtained during the emergency room visit and showed a wedge-shaped perfusion defect in the right testicle with corresponding hyperintensity on T1-weighted images. Postcontrast imaging showed peripheral rim enhancement around this area of abnormality with central hypoenhancement. These findings are consistent with a segmental testicular infarct.

SUMMARY

MR imaging provides excellent soft tissue contrast, spatial resolution, and multiplanar imaging allowing for the evaluation of traumatic injury to the soft tissues and vascular structures of the

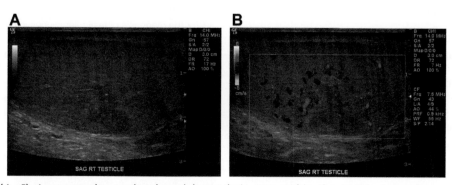

Fig. 10. (A, B) A nonvascular, wedge-shaped hypoechoic area within the testicle (arrows), suggestive of segmental testicular infarction. *Original images.

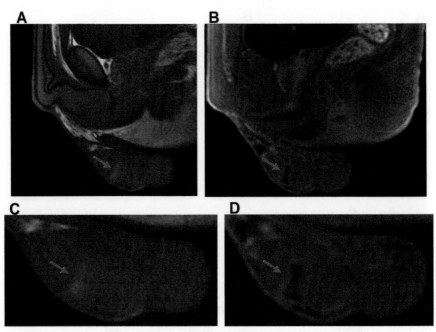

Fig. 11. (*A–D*) A wedge-shaped testicular infarct corresponding to the nonvascular, hypoechoic area on ultrasound (*arrow*). *Original images.

penis and scrotum. Many pathologic conditions can be evaluated with this technique, such as penile fracture, penile masses, arteriogenic impotence, penile prostheses, plaques of Peyronie disease, and periurethral abscesses.[4] Although often a second-line imaging modality after initial evaluation with ultrasound, MR imaging adds high-diagnostic confidence for acute traumatic injuries of the penis and testis, facilitating prompt and appropriate surgical management, while minimizing long-term comorbidities of scrotal trauma.

DISCLOSURE

The authors have nothing to disclose.

REFERENCES

1. Avery L, Scheinfeld M. Imaging of Penile and Scrotal Emergencies. RadioGraphics 2013;33:721–40.
2. Ellsworth P, Gest T. Penile Anatomy. Medscape. Available at: https://emedicine.medscape.com/article/1949325.
3. Bhatt S, Dogra VS. Role of US in Testicular and Scrotal Trauma. Radiographics 2008;28:6.
4. Pretorius E, Siegelman E, Ramchandani P, et al. MR Imaging of the Penis. RadioGraphics 2001;21: S283–99.
5. Evan Siegelman. Body MRI. 1st edition (December 24, 2004).
6. Avery L, Scheinfeld M. Imaging of Male Pelvic Trauma. Radiol Clin North Am 2012;50:1201–17.
7. Parker III R, Menias C, Quazi R. MR Imaging of the Penis and Scrotum. Radiographics 2015;35(4). https://doi.org/10.1148/rg.2015140161.
8. Deurdulian C, Mittelstaedt CA, Chong WK, et al. US of acute scrotal trauma: optimal technique, imaging findings, and management. RadioGraphics 2007; 27(2):357–69.
9. Rao KG. Traumatic rupture of testis. Urology 1982; 20(6):624–5.
10. Guichard G, El Ammari J, Del Coro C, et al. Accuracy of ultrasonography in diagnosis of testicular rupture after blunt scrotal trauma. Urology 2008; 71(1):52–6.
11. Buckley JC, McAninch JW. Use of ultrasonography for the diagnosis of testicular injuries in blunt scrotal trauma. J Urol 2006;175(1):175–8.
12. Buckley JC, McAninch JW. Diagnosis and management of testicular ruptures. Urol Clin North Am 2006; 33(1):111–6, vii.
13. Jeffrey RB, Laing FC, Hricak H, et al. Sonography of testicular trauma. AJR Am J Roentgenol 1983; 141(5):993–5.
14. ha, P., Shah, V. Penile fracture. Reference article, Radiopaedia.org. Available at: https://doi.org/10.53347/rID-26051. Accessed April 27, 2022.

Emergent Magnetic Resonance Angiography for Evaluation of the Thoracoabdominal and Peripheral Vasculature

Daniel R. Ludwig, MD*, Constantine A. Raptis, MD, Sanjeev Bhalla, MD*

KEYWORDS

- Magnetic resonance angiography • Acute aortic syndromes • Aortitis • Aortic aneurysm
- Pulmonary embolism • Peripheral vascular disease

KEY POINTS

- MRA is useful in the evaluation of stable patients who cannot receive IV iodinated contrast such as in the setting of severe allergy, poor IV access, or severe renal insufficiency.
- Non-contrast MRA is sufficient to obtain a diagnostic evaluation in many clinical contexts, although GBCAs are administered whenever possible to improve diagnostic quality and shorten the duration of the exam.
- MRA in plays an important and emerging role in the evaluation of acute aortic syndromes, aortitis, aortic aneurysm, pulmonary embolism, and peripheral vascular disease in the emergency department.

INTRODUCTION

Acute pathology of the thoracoabdominal and peripheral vasculature is often encountered in the emergency department (ED) setting and includes a variety of severe and life-threatening conditions.[1] Computed tomography angiography (CTA) is the first-line modality for imaging of the vasculature in this environment although magnetic resonance angiography (MRA) plays an important and emerging role in the evaluation of carefully selected patients. The goal of this review is to discuss the key strengths and limitations of MRA in the ED, highlighting the role of MRA in the diagnosis of acute aortic syndromes, aortitis, aortic aneurysm, pulmonary embolism (PE), and peripheral vascular disease.

GENERAL IMAGING CONSIDERATIONS

MRA plays an important role in the evaluation of patients who cannot receive intravenous (IV) iodinated contrast, a necessity for performing CTA. History of prior severe allergic-like reaction (ie, anaphylaxis or anaphylactoid-like reactions) to iodinated contrast is a near-absolute contraindication to receiving the same class of contrast media.[2] There is no known cross-reactivity between gadolinium-based contrast agents (GBCAs) and iodinated contrast; thus it is safe to administer the former to patients with a known iodinated contrast allergy.

Additionally, severe renal insufficiency (estimated glomerular filtration rate < 30 mL/min/ 1.73 m^2) and acute kidney injury (AKI) represent

Mallinckrodt Institute of Radiology, Washington University School of Medicine, 510 South Kingshighway Boulevard, Campus Box 8131, Saint Louis, MO 63110, USA
* Corresponding authors.
E-mail addresses: ludwigd@wustl.edu (D.R.L.); sanjeevbhalla@wustl.edu (S.B.)

Magn Reson Imaging Clin N Am 30 (2022) 465–477
https://doi.org/10.1016/j.mric.2022.04.008

relative contraindications to iodinated contrast due to the risk of contrast-induced AKI. Severe renal dysfunction is also a concern with GBCAs, but due to the risk of nephrogenic systemic fibrosis (NSF) rather than contrast-induced AKI as GBCAs are not considered nephrotoxic at doses used for MRA.[3] With regard to NSF, GBCAs (ie, group II agents) can be safely administered to patients with severe renal insufficiency and even with caution in patients with end-stage chronic kidney disease or AKI.[4] In addition, due to the superior contrast resolution of magnetic resonance imaging (MRI), IV contrast is often not required to achieve a diagnostic examination. Furthermore, CTA requires a large bore IV, typically 20 gauge or larger in antecubital fossa or forearm to accommodate a rapid bolus infusion.[5] Contrast-enhanced MRA can be performed in patients with suboptimal IV access due to the lower required infusion rate (ie, 1–2 mL/s vs 4 mL/s for CTA).

MRA has the advantage over CTA of a lack of ionizing radiation. Although rarely a concern in adult patients in the ED setting, ionizing radiation is of specific concern in pediatric and pregnant patients.[6] Another potentially important benefit of MRA is its insensitivity to dense vascular calcifications, which is of particular importance in patients with advanced peripheral vascular disease or diabetes in whom calcifications substantially limit the performance of CTA.[7] Finally, MRA has added value as a problem-solving modality for further characterization of indeterminate findings on CTA most commonly pulsation and flow artifacts. The exam should be tailored to address a specific clinical question and time-resolved imaging may be used in selected circumstances.[8]

There are a number of key considerations that significantly limit the use of MRA in the ED setting. Most importantly, MRA often takes 30 min or longer, rendering it unsuitable for patients who are not hemodynamically stable. By comparison, CTA can be performed in a matter of minutes. In addition, unlike CT scanners, MRI scanners are not commonly found directly in the ED and require a patient to be transported elsewhere in the hospital, often away from critical care resources. MRA also requires a high degree of patient cooperation, often requiring a patient to follow breath-holding instructions and remain motionless for the duration of the exam. There are some patients who also cannot tolerate MR imaging due to severe claustrophobia or have certain nonconditional implanted devices that render the MR environment unsafe.[9] Finally, MRA requires advanced technical experience, robust imaging protocols and often dedicated subspecialist interpretation, which may not be available in certain community practice settings. These factors preclude the use of MRA as a first-line vascular imaging technique. **Table 1** summarizes the key advantages and disadvantages of MRA compared with CTA.

ACUTE AORTIC PATHOLOGY

Acute aortic pathology is commonly encountered in the ED setting and includes a broad spectrum of conditions such as acute aortic syndromes, infectious and noninfectious aortitis, and aortic aneurysm. Imaging plays an important role in confirming the diagnosis, detecting complications, and guiding patient management in the acute setting. CTA is the first-line imaging technique for the diagnosis of aortic pathology although MRA has equivalent diagnostic performance and is the test of choice in hemodynamically stable patients who cannot receive IV iodinated contrast. IV contrast is generally not required for MRA but is administered when possible as it shortens the duration of the exam and increases the diagnostic confidence in the evaluation.[8]

MRA imaging protocols for acute aortic pathology should be kept as brief as possible and tailored to address the specific clinical question. All evaluations include balanced steady-state free-precession (bSSFP) imaging, a robust bright-blood noncontrast MRA imaging technique optimized for luminal evaluation of the thoracoabdominal aorta. In the chest, bSSFP images are acquired with electrocardiographic (EKG)-gating using either a prospective single-shot or retrospective technique. Prospective gating minimizes pulsation artifact, whereas retrospective gating produces cines images that allow for dynamic luminal evaluation. Dark-blood T2-weighted single-shot fast spin echo (SS-FSE) images are another important component of the evaluation and are most useful in the evaluation of the vascular wall. Inversion recovery (IR) imaging is included in the setting of suspected aortitis to depict intramural and periaortic edema. T1-weighted gradient-recalled echo (GRE) imaging highlights blood products within the aortic wall and periaortic soft tissues. Contrast-enhanced MRA, when performed, rapidly creates high contrast-to-background images of the luminal aorta. Noncontrast MRA techniques such as quiescent-interval single-shot (QISS) may be performed when contrast cannot be administered.

Acute Aortic Syndromes

Acute aortic syndromes encompass a spectrum of conditions, which are characterized by disruption of the aortic wall, and include aortic dissection, intramural hematoma (IMH), and penetrating

Table 1
Comparison of magnetic resonance angiography versus computed tomography angiography

	MRA	CTA
Advantages	• Can be performed in patients with contraindications to IV iodinated contrast • Certain GBCAs can be safely administered in severe renal insufficiency and AKI • IV contrast is not required to obtain a diagnostic exam • Superior contrast resolution • Lack of ionizing resolution • Insensitive to dense vascular calcifications • Can be used as a problem-solving tool	• Imaging is significantly faster than MRA • Suitable for hemodynamically unstable patients • CT scanner often found directly in the ED • First-line modality for vascular imaging in the ED • Readily understood by referring MDs
Disadvantages	• Cannot be safely performed in unstable patients • Time intensive • Requires patient cooperation • Not well tolerated in claustrophobic patients • Cannot be performed in patients with certain nonconditional implanted devices • Lack of widespread availability	• Requires IV iodinated contrast to achieve a diagnostic exam • Cannot be performed in patients with severe allergic-like reaction to iodinated contrast or advanced renal insufficiency • Delivers ionizing radiation • Limited in the setting of dense vascular calcification

Abbreviations: AKI, acute kidney injury; CTA, computed tomography angiography; ED, emergency department; GBCA, gadolinium-based contrast agent; IV, Intravenous.

atherosclerotic ulcer (PAU).[10] Aortic dissection results from a tear in the intima and media, resulting in the formation of a medial false lumen in which blood is able to propagate.[11] According to the Stanford classification, dissections can either be type A or type B, according to whether the ascending aorta is involved or spared, respectively. MRA is highly accurate for the diagnosis of aortic dissection, with reported sensitivity and specificity exceeding 95%.[12,13] Notably, noncontrast MRA and contrast-enhanced MRA have comparable diagnostic performance.[14] In patients undergoing MRA from the ED, noncontrast CT should be considered as an initial examination to exclude emergent findings such as aortic rupture or hemopericardium. These findings may call the stability of the patient into question and preclude MRA due to safety concerns.

Aortic dissection is depicted on MRA as a flap within the aortic lumen, the extent of which is easily seen on noncontrast bSSFP images (**Fig. 1**). Contrast-enhanced MRA is generally helpful in assessing the patency of the false lumen, the location of entry and exit tears, and identifying findings of end-organ ischemia. However, contrast-enhanced MRA images are typically not EKG-gated and may harbor pulsation or phase ghosting artifacts, which compromise the evaluation of the aortic root. Careful assessment of EKG-gated bSSFP images, especially retrospectively-gated cine images of the aortic root, is paramount for distinguishing a type A from type B dissection (**Fig. 2**), a distinction that has important management implications. bSSFP cine images are also of value in evaluating for aortic regurgitation or compromise of the left ventricular outflow tract by the dissection. Finally, MRA may also be helpful in characterizing indeterminate findings on CTA such as pulsation or flow-related artifacts, both of which have the potential to mimic a dissection flap.

In IMH, a contained hematoma develops within the aortic wall but does not communicate with the aortic lumen.[15] IMH is usually diagnosed on the basis of noncontrast CT, which classically shows high-attenuation crescentic thickening of the aortic wall.[16] Owing to its superior contrast resolution, the sensitivity of MRA for the diagnosis of IMH approaches 100% and likely exceeds the performance of noncontrast CT due to its ability to portray IMH in the subacute phase, in which the

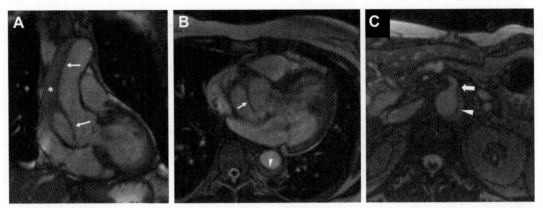

Fig. 1. Type A aortic dissection in a 64-year-old woman presenting with chest pain who underwent evaluation with a noncontrast MRA. Coronal single-shot bSSFP image of the chest (A) and axial single-shot bSSFP images through the chest and upper abdomen (B and C, respectively) show an intimomedial dissection flap involving the ascending aorta, which extends to the aortic root (arrows), in keeping with type A aortic dissection. Note that the majority of the false lumen is thrombosed (asterisk). The dissection extends distally into the abdominal aorta (arrowheads) and involves the origin of the superior mesenteric artery (thick arrow, C).

density of the IMH may approximate that of luminal blood.[17] Dark-blood SS-FSE images often best show the crescentic aortic wall thickening in IMH in contrast to suppressed intraluminal blood (Fig. 3). IMH is usually hyperintense on T1-weighted GRE images due to the internal blood products although the signal intensity is variable based on the acuity of blood products.

Ulcer-like projection (ULP), also known as a focal intimal disruption, is a finger-like outpouching into the IMH that is in communication with the aortic lumen.[18] Importantly, ULP is not readily visible on noncontrast CT. Contrast-enhanced MRA is typically performed in conjunction with noncontrast CT in patients who cannot undergo CTA, as it readily depicts the associated ULP

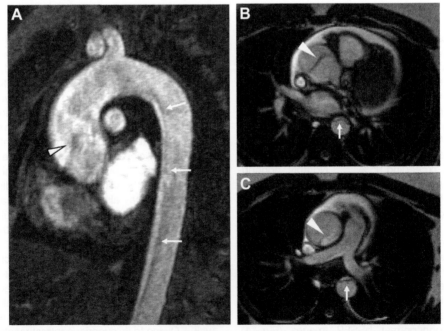

Fig. 2. Type A aortic dissection in a 70-year-old man with chest pain. Contrast-enhanced oblique sagittal MR angiographic image (A) shows a dissection flap within the distal arch and involving the descending thoracic aorta (arrows). There was possible involvement of the ascending aorta, which was difficult to evaluate due to pulsation artifact and turbulent flow (arrowhead). However, retrospectively gated bSSFP images in the diastolic phase of the cardiac cycle (B and C) clearly show the dissection flap extending proximally to the aortic root (arrowheads).

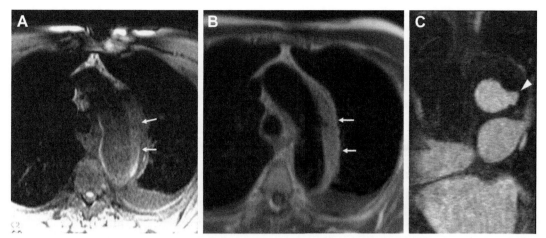

Fig. 3. –Type B intramural hematoma with an ulcer-like projection in an 80-year-old man with chest pain. Axial precontrast T1-weighted volume-interpolated GRE image (*A*) and axial T2-weighted dark-blood single-shot FSE image (*B*) show a crescentic collection within the wall of the aortic arch (*arrows*) with intrinsic T1 and T2 hyperintensity, consistent with an intramural hematoma. Contrast-enhanced MRA image reformatted in the coronal plane (*C*) shows a focal area of contrast opacification within the intramural hematoma (*arrowhead*), which clearly communicates with the aortic lumen and was consistent with an ulcer-like projection.

(see **Fig. 3**). ULP is important to identify, as it is a feature of IMH strongly associated with progression and may direct thoracic endovascular aortic repair.[19] Of note, ULPs should be differentiated from intramural blood pools (IBPs), both of which appear as collections of contrast within the IMH. IBP, unlike ULP, usually has no or occasionally tiny communications (≤3 mm) with the aortic lumen in association with the ostia of small branch arteries and is not associated with IMH progression.[20] In addition to its role in depicting ULPs, MRA may be complementary to noncontrast CT in assessing the proximal extent of an IMH, specifically whether it has a type A or B distribution, as well as determining the age of blood products.

PAU represents an ulceration into the media of the aortic wall, occurring almost exclusively in the setting of atherosclerosis.[21] Although patients with PAU may present with acute chest pain as is common with the other acute aortic syndromes, they are much more often encountered incidentally in asymptomatic patients.[15] PAU is readily depicted on CTA, but may not be apparent on noncontrast CT owing to the difficulty in distinguishing it from adjacent structures. On imaging, a PAU is characterized by a saccular outpouching extending beyond the normal contour of the aorta wall at the site of an intimomedial defect and is generally best appreciated on contrast-enhanced MRA or bSSFP images (**Fig. 4**). PAU should be distinguished from ulcerated atheromatous plaque, the latter of which does not extend beyond the contour of the aortic wall.

Aortitis

Aortitis may be caused by infectious or noninfectious etiologies and is characterized by inflammation involving the aortic wall. Infectious aortitis most commonly occurs as a result of hematogenous seeding of the aorta from an infection elsewhere in the body.[22] Progressive infection often results in the destruction of the aortic wall and the formation of an infectious pseudoaneurysm, which may develop and rapidly enlarge over a period of days to weeks. Infectious aortitis may also occur, albeit infrequently, via the direct extension of an adjacent infection such discitis-osteomyelitis.[23] Imaging findings in infectious aortitis include aortic wall thickening, adjacent soft tissue stranding, reactive lymphadenopathy, and eventual pseudoaneurysm formation, all of which are readily visible on MRA (**Fig. 5**).[24] If IV contrast is administered, a delayed-phase acquisition may be helpful to highlight aortic wall and/or periaortic enhancement. The GRE images should be scrutinized for susceptibility-related signal loss related to intra-aortic or periaortic gas, a finding that may be occult on other sequences and is much better depicted on CT.[25]

Noninfectious aortitis occurs in a variety of conditions, most commonly in the setting of vasculitis (eg, Takayasu and Giant cell), but may be radiation induced or idiopathic.[23] In the setting of immunoglobulin G4-related disease, inflammation may involve periaortic soft tissues (ie, periaortitis) rather than only the aortic wall.[26] The most common imaging manifestation of noninfectious aortitis is

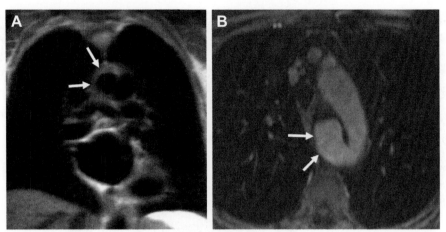

Fig. 4. Penetrating atherosclerotic ulcer in a 72-year-old woman presenting with uncontrolled hypertension and a transient ischemic attack. Coronal T2-weighted dark-blood SS-FSE image (*A*) and contrast-enhanced T1-weighted GRE image (*B*) shows a focal outpouching projecting medially from proximal descending thoracic aorta and extending beyond the expected contour of the aortic wall (*arrows*), consistent with a penetrating atherosclerotic ulcer.

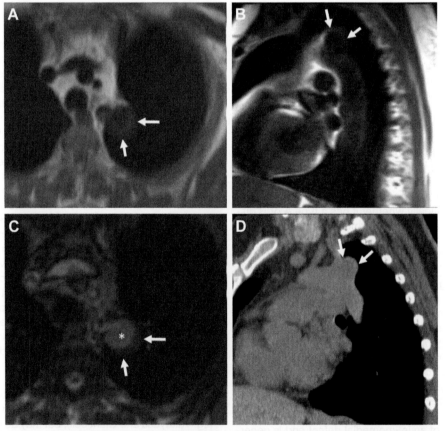

Fig. 5. Infectious pseudoaneurysm in a 46-year-old man with type I diabetes, advanced chronic kidney disease, and lower extremity soft tissue infection. Axial (*A*) and sagittal (*B*) T2-weighted dark-blood SS-FSE images show a saccular pseudoaneurysm projecting superiorly from the distal aortic arch (*arrows*). Axial single-shot bSSFP image (*C*) demonstrates that the pseudoaneurysm is largely patent (*asterisk*). Contemporaneous oblique sagittal non-contrast CT image (*D*) highlights a lack of associated atherosclerosis. The patient was treated with endovascular stenting and chronic suppressive antibiotics.

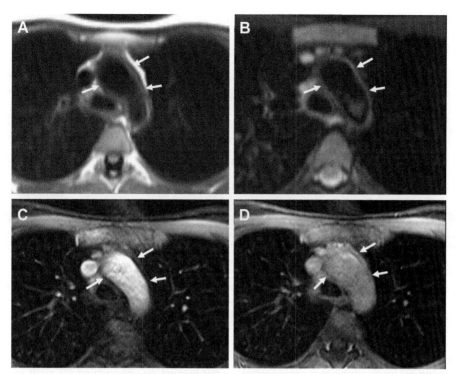

Fig. 6. Takayasu arteritis in a 29-year-old woman. Axial T2-weighted dark-blood SS-FSE image (*A*) and corresponding axial T2-weighted IR image (*B*) show circumferential thickening of the wall of the aortic arch in association with intramural edema (*arrows*), which also involved the proximal great vessels (not shown). Axial contrast-enhanced volume-interpolated GRE images in the arterial phase (*C*) and after a 5-min delay (*D*) show delayed enhancement of the aortic wall (*arrows*), presumed to represent Takayasu arteritis given the patient's age.

concentric wall thickening, with additional imaging findings including narrowing of the vascular lumen and branch vessel occlusion.[27] Rarely, adjacent lymphadenopathy is seen. As in acute aortic syndromes, mural findings are most evident on dark-blood SS-FSE images, whereas luminal findings are easiest to appreciate on contrast-enhanced MRA or bSSFP images (**Fig. 6**). Intramural edema, best depicted on IR (ie, fat-suppressed) T2-weighted images, is usually an indicator of active inflammation. Postcontrast T1-weighted images often show enhancement of the aortic wall, which may occur in the arterial or venous phase in the setting of active aortitis, or often not until a delayed phase in cases of chronic or treated aortitis due to its fibrotic nature. MR can also be helpful in distinguishing aortitis from periaortitis, a distinction that is often challenging on CTA.[28]

Aortic Aneurysm

Aortic aneurysm is defined by segmental dilation of the aorta to a diameter greater than 50% of its normal caliber, typically defined as greater than 4 cm in the ascending aorta and 3 cm in the descending thoracic and abdominal aorta.[29,30] Most aortic aneurysms occur due to atherosclerosis although connective tissue disease and sequela of aortitis of aortic syndromes represent additional causes.[31] Most aneurysms are asymptomatic until they rupture, frequently a lethal occurrence unless the rupture is contained.[32] In the setting of aneurysm instability or chronic contained rupture, patients may present to the ED with nonspecific chest or abdominal pain.[33]

Hematoma adjacent to an aortic aneurysm is diagnostic of rupture, which can confidently be diagnosed on CT and MRA.[34] If chronic and contained, a draped configuration of the aneurysm may be evident, in which the posterior wall follows the contour of the adjacent vertebral body or retroperitoneal musculature.[35] Additionally, findings of aneurysm instability have been well-documented using noncontrast CT and CTA and include a high-attenuating crescent on noncontrast images, changing thrombus morphology, discontinuous or tangential calcification in the aortic wall, focal eccentric contour bulge, and mild periaortic stranding.[36] MRA readily depicts many of these

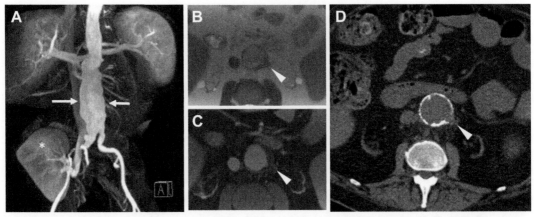

Fig. 7. Abdominal aortic aneurysm with findings of instability in a 70-year-old man with prior kidney transplantation. MIP image derived from a contrast-enhanced MRA acquisition (*A*) shows an infrarenal abdominal aortic aneurysm, which measured approximately 5.5 cm (*arrows*) in a patient with a transplanted kidney in the right iliac fossa (*asterisk*). Axial T2-weighted SS-FSE (*B*) and contrast-enhanced volumetric-interpolated GRE (*C*) shows a small focal outpouching arising from the right posterolateral aspect of the abdominal aorta (*arrowheads*), suspicious for aneurysm instability. Subsequent noncontrast axial CT image (*D*) confirmed this finding (*arrowhead*) and highlighted the discontinuity in the otherwise continuous peripheral intimal calcifications.

findings of aneurysm instability (**Figs. 7** and **8**). Notably, calcifications are rarely visible on MRA, limiting assessment for discontinuous or tangential calcification. Furthermore, there is no reported MRA equivalent for the high-attenuating crescent. Mural thrombus within an aneurysm often has intrinsic T1 hyperintensity, which should not be interpreted as a feature of aneurysm instability unless there is a prior study to document an interval change.

As with acute aortic syndromes, patients with a known or suspected aortic aneurysm who cannot undergo CTA should be initially evaluated with noncontrast CT to identify findings of instability

or rupture. MRA is complementary to noncontrast CT and may portray findings of instability that are not evident on noncontrast CT such as changing thrombus morphology. Additionally, MRA is often helpful in characterizing the location of the aneurysm relative to the visceral arteries for surgical planning or showing the coexistence of aorto-iliac occlusive disease.

PULMONARY EMBOLISM

PE is a frequent clinical concern in the ED setting and is almost exclusively evaluated by CT pulmonary angiography or ventilation/perfusion

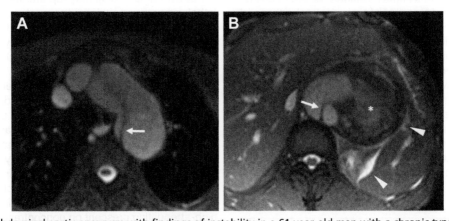

Fig. 8. Abdominal aortic aneurysm with findings of instability in a 61-year-old man with a chronic type B dissection and back pain. Axial single-shot bSSFP images through the chest and abdomen (*A* and *B*, respectively) show a type B aortic dissection (*arrows*) with a large suprarenal abdominal aortic aneurysm arising from the false lumen (*asterisk*). Moderate periaortic and retroperitoneal fat stranding (*arrowheads*) was indicative of aneurysm instability.

scintigraphy. Pulmonary MRA may be useful in carefully selected patients, such as when other examinations are contraindicated, there is a desire to minimize radiation exposure in the pregnant or pediatric patient, or IV access is suboptimal. As with other indications, MRA cannot be performed in patients who are clinically unstable.

MRA has a high diagnostic accuracy for the detection of PE. Indeed, a 2015 meta-analysis on the performance of MRA for detection of PE reported a sensitivity of 84% and specificity of 97%, after the exclusion of studies that were technically inadequate (approximately 20%).[37] Technical inadequacy is an important limitation of MRA, with the most common causes including suboptimal pulmonary arterial opacification and respiratory motion. More recent studies report a higher rate of technical adequacy (>95%), likely owing to advances in scanner technology, widespread use of accelerated imaging techniques, and motion-insensitive acquisitions.[38] Dynamic contrast-enhanced (DCE) sequences with high temporal resolution using compressed sensing (eg, GRASP-VIBE [Golden-angle RAdial Sparse Parallel Volume-Interpolated 3D GRE]), for instance, allow for a free-breathing acquisition in patients unable to hold their breath.[39] IV contrast is generally necessary for the evaluation of the pulmonary vessels; however, in patients who cannot receive GBCA, ferumoxytol (superparamagnetic iron oxide particle) may represent a valid alternative.[40] Furthermore, noncontrast MRA techniques such as bSSFP may be sufficient for diagnosing PE within the central and lobar pulmonary arteries.[40,41]

MRA imaging protocols for pulmonary embolism are designed to maximize the likelihood of a diagnostic evaluation. Multiple phases of contrast are obtained, the first timed for optimal pulmonary arterial opacification, to help ensure at least one phase is free of respiratory motion or in case the first phase is acquired too early. In the setting of suboptimal breath holding, an additional radial *k*-space acquisition may be added to minimize respiratory artifact. In a patient who cannot perform breath holds, DCE with compressed sensing (eg, GRASP-VIBE) may be performed in lieu of standard MRA sequences although this technique is only available on newer scanners. Otherwise, respiratory gating can be used with standard MRA sequences to account for respiratory motion. On MRA images, PE is visible as a nonenhancing filling defect within the pulmonary arterial tree (**Fig. 9**). Maximum intensity projection (MIP) images are generated after subtraction of the precontrast MRA image, which may improve the visibility of subtle findings.[8] A comprehensive protocol incorporating multiple different types of acquisitions (ie, bSSFP, GRE, etc.) improves the overall diagnostic performance of the evaluation.[42]

PERIPHERAL MAGNETIC RESONANCE ANGIOGRAPHY

Peripheral arterial disease (PAD) encompasses a spectrum of conditions including atherosclerosis and embolic disease, which can result in stenosis or occlusion of the arteries of the lower extremities. Patients often present to the ED with symptoms of claudication, or in advanced cases, rest pain, critical limb ischemia, nonhealing wounds, and infection.[43] Doppler ultrasound may be performed as an initial imaging test but

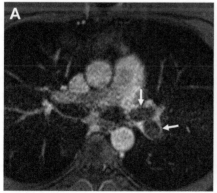
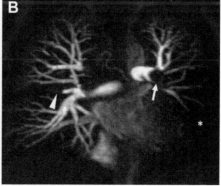

Fig. 9. Pulmonary embolism in a 38-year-old woman with chest pain and shortness of breath. Axial contrast-enhanced volumetric-interpolated GRE image (*A*) shows multiple filling defects within the left main pulmonary artery, consistent with acute pulmonary embolism (*arrows*). Coronal MIP MRA image (*B*) again shows the embolism within the left main pulmonary artery (*arrow*) and oligemia in the left lower lobe (*asterisk*). An additional pulmonary embolism in the superior segment of the right lower lobe is also evident (*arrowhead*).

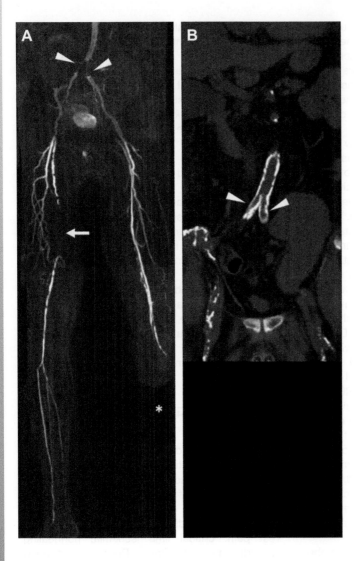

Fig. 10. Chronic occlusion of the right superficial femoral artery in a 62-year-old man with prior renal transplantation and left below-the-knee amputation who presented with right lower extremity pain at rest. Contrast-enhanced MRA MIP image of abdominal aorta, iliac arteries, and lower extremities (*A*) shows long segment occlusion of the right superficial femoral artery (*arrow*) with distal reconstitution via branches of the profundal femoris. Elsewhere there was multifocal stenosis with diminutive three-vessel runoff to the right foot. Susceptibility-related loss within both common iliac arteries (*arrowheads*) was related to the presence of indwelling stents, as seen on prior noncontrast coronal CT image (*B, arrowheads*). Note the changes from prior left below-the-knee amputation (*asterisk*).

does not comprehensively depict the anatomy of the affected arterial territory.[44] Both CTA and MRA of the aortic-iliac-femoral vasculature with lower extremity runoff are highly accurate in the assessment and staging of PAD (>95%) and have essentially replaced catheter angiography in the diagnostic setting.[45,46] CTA is often preferred in the ED setting due owing to its broader availability and rapid acquisition speeds, whereas MRA is essentially reserved for patients who cannot receive IV iodinated contrast.[47] As mentioned above, the insensitivity of MRA to dense vascular calcifications is an important advantage over CTA. However, susceptibility artifact from metallic stents, clips, and prostheses may mimic stenosis and limit the evaluation of the adjacent vessel (**Fig. 10**).

Contrast-enhanced MRA is used whenever possible, as it results in images of higher

diagnostic quality compared with noncontrast MRA. Nonetheless, noncontrast MRA techniques such as QISS provide an evaluation with comparable diagnostic performance to contrast-enhanced MRA, albeit at the expense of a longer evaluation.[48] In contrast-enhanced MRA, time-resolved imaging using k-space sharing techniques (eg, time-resolved imaging with stochastic trajectories) may be performed to eliminate the risk of mistiming the contrast bolus and introducing venous contamination, which is of greatest concern when evaluating the vessels of the calf.[49,50] Differences in blood flow between the limbs in the setting of PAD may further impair bolus timing in the calf station using traditional continuous-table-movement MRA. We perform time-resolved imaging of the calf using one-fifth of the contrast dose, followed by continuous-table-movement MRA imaging of the abdominal aorta and

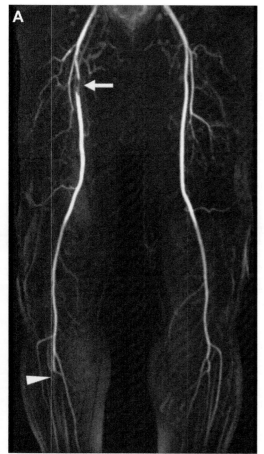

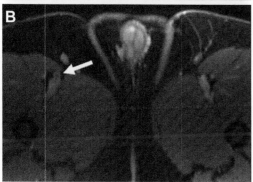

Fig. 11. Right superficial femoral artery (SFA) embolism in a 41-year-old man with cardiogenic embolic disease. Contrast-enhanced MRA MIP image of the lower extremities (*A*) shows a nonocclusive thrombus within the right superficial femoral artery (*arrow*). There was also embolic occlusion of the proximal right peroneal artery (*arrowhead*). The right SFA thrombus was confirmed on contrast-enhanced axial volumetric-interpolated GRE image (*B, arrow*).

iliofemoral arteries using the remainder of the contrast dose. Postcontrast MRA images are postprocessed by mask subtraction to create thick-slice MIP images, which highlight the

positive vascular findings and are useful for the referring clinician who may be unfamiliar with MRA (see **Fig. 10; Fig. 11**). All findings on the MIP images should be confirmed on the source dataset to ensure the finding is not related to a postprocessing artifact.

SUMMARY

Thoracoabdominal and peripheral vasculature pathology includes a broad spectrum of conditions that are commonly encountered in the ED setting. CTA is most commonly preferred for the evaluation of these patients owing to its widespread availability, rapid speed of acquisition, and applicability in hemodynamically unstable patients. MRA plays an important role in the evaluation of stable patients who cannot receive IV iodinated contrast such as in the setting of severe allergy, poor IV access or severe renal insufficiency. In the setting of acute aortic pathology, noncontrast CT is often complementary to MRA and is performed before MRA to exclude emergent findings such as aortic rupture, which may call the stability of the patient into question. Noncontrast MRA is sufficient to obtain a diagnostic evaluation in most clinical settings. However, GBCAs are administered whenever possible, as they generally improve diagnostic quality and shorten the duration of the exam. As such, MRA in plays an important and emerging role in the evaluation of acute aortic syndromes, aortitis, aortic aneurysm, pulmonary embolism, and peripheral vascular disease in the emergency setting.

CLINICS CARE POINTS

- MRA is useful in the evaluation of stable patients who cannot receive IV iodinated contrast such as in the setting of severe allergy, poor IV access, or severe renal insufficiency.

- Non-contrast MRA is sufficient to obtain a diagnostic evaluation in many clinical contexts, although GBCAs are administered whenever possible to improve diagnostic quality and shorten the duration of the exam.

- MRA in plays an important and emerging role in the evaluation of acute aortic syndromes, aortitis, aortic aneurysm, pulmonary embolism, and peripheral vascular disease in the emergency department.

DISCLOSURE OF CONFLICTS OF INTEREST

The authors have no relevant relationships to disclose.

REFERENCES

1. Clough RE, Nienaber CA. Management of acute aortic syndrome. Nat Rev Cardiol 2015;12(2): 103–14.
2. American College of Radiology, Committee on Drugs and Contrast Media. ACR manual on contrast media v2021. 2021. Available at: https://www.acr.org/Clinical-Resources/Contrast-Manual. Accessed September 10, 2021.
3. Fraum TJ, Ludwig DR, Bashir MR, et al. Gadolinium-based contrast agents: a comprehensive risk assessment. J Magn Reson Imaging JMRI 2017; 46(2):338–53.
4. Weinreb JC, Rodby RA, Yee J, et al. Use of intravenous gadolinium-based contrast media in patients with kidney disease: consensus statements from the american college of radiology and the national kidney foundation. Radiology 2021;298(1):28–35.
5. American College of Radiology. ACR–NASCI–SIR–SPR practice parameter for the performance and interpretation of body computed tomography angiography (CTA) 2017. Available at: https://www.acr.org/-/media/acr/files/practice-parameters/body-cta.pdfCited. Accessed September 10, 2021.
6. Brenner DJ, Elliston CD, Hall EJ, et al. Estimated risks of radiation-induced fatal cancer from pediatric CT. Am J Roentgenol 2001;176(2):289–96.
7. Pollak AW, Norton PT, Kramer CM. Multimodality imaging of lower extremity peripheral arterial disease. Circ Cardiovasc Imaging 2012;5(6):797–807.
8. Ludwig DR, Shetty AS, Broncano J, et al. Magnetic resonance angiography of the thoracic vasculature: technique and applications. J Magn Reson Imaging JMRI 2020;52(2):325–47.
9. Greenberg TD, Hoff MN, Gilk TB, et al. ACR guidance document on MR safe practices: updates and critical information 2019. J Magn Reson Imaging 2020;51(2):331–8.
10. Corvera JS. Acute aortic syndrome. Ann Cardiothorac Surg 2016;5(3):188–93.
11. McMahon MA, Squirrell CA. Multidetector CT of aortic dissection: a pictorial review. RadioGraphics 2010;30(2):445–60.
12. Sommer T, Fehske W, Holzknecht N, et al. Aortic dissection: a comparative study of diagnosis with spiral CT, multiplanar transesophageal echocardiography, and MR imaging. Radiology 1996;199(2):347–52.
13. Prince MR, Narasimham DL, Jacoby WT, et al. Three-dimensional gadolinium-enhanced MR angiography of the thoracic aorta. Am J Roentgenol 1996;166(6):1387–97.
14. Krishnam MS, Tomasian A, Malik S, et al. Three-dimensional imaging of pulmonary veins by a novel steady-state free-precession magnetic resonance angiography technique without the use of intravenous contrast agent: initial experience. Invest Radiol 2009;44(8):447–53.
15. Bonaca MP. Descending aortic dissection, penetrating aortic ulcer, and intramural hematoma (Acute and Chronic) including kommerell's diverticulum. In: Dieter RS, Dieter RA Jr, Dieter RA, editors. Diseases of the aorta. Cham, Switzerland: Springer; 2019. p. 149–60.
16. Chao CP, Walker TG, Kalva SP. Natural history and CT appearances of aortic intramural hematoma. Radiographics 2009;29(3):791–804.
17. Goldstein SA, Evangelista A, Abbara S, et al. Multimodality Imaging of diseases of the thoracic aorta in adults: from the american society of echocardiography and the european association of cardiovascular imaging: endorsed by the society of cardiovascular computed tomography and society for cardiovascular magnetic resonance. J Am Soc Echocardiogr 2015;28(2):119–82.
18. Moral S, Cuéllar H, Avegliano G, et al. Clinical implications of focal intimal disruption in patients with Type B intramural hematoma. J Am Coll Cardiol 2017;69(1):28–39.
19. Takeshi K, Shuichiro K, Atsushi Y, et al. Impact of new development of ulcer-like projection on clinical outcomes in patients with Type B aortic dissection with closed and thrombosed false lumen. Circulation 2010;122(11_suppl_1):S74–80.
20. Wu M-T, Wang Y-C, Huang Y-L, et al. Intramural blood pools accompanying aortic intramural hematoma: CT appearance and natural course. Radiology 2011;258(3):705–13.
21. Chow SC, Wong RH, Underwood MJ. Acute aortic syndrome: current understandings. In: Tintoiu I, Elefteriades J, Ursulescu A, et al, editors. New approaches to aortic diseases from valve to abdominal bifurcation. Elsevier; 2018. p. 479–89.
22. Gornik Heather L, Creager Mark A. Aortitis. Circulation 2008;117(23):3039–51.
23. Restrepo CS, Ocazionez D, Suri R, et al. Aortitis: imaging spectrum of the infectious and inflammatory conditions of the aorta. RadioGraphics 2011;31(2): 435–51.
24. Macedo TA, Stanson AW, Oderich GS, et al. Infected aortic aneurysms: imaging findings. Radiology 2004;231(1):250–7.
25. Yu HS, Gupta A, Soto JA, et al. Emergency abdominal MRI: current uses and trends. Br J Radiol 2016; 89(1061):20150804.
26. Lian L, Wang C, Tian J-L. IgG4-related retroperitoneal fibrosis: a newly described disease. Int J Rheum Dis 2016;19(11):1049–55.

27. Töpel I, Zorger N, Steinbauer M. Inflammatory diseases of the aorta: Part 1: non-infectious aortitis. Gefasschirurgie 2016;21(Suppl 2):80–6.

28. Mitnick H, Jacobowitz G, Krinsky G, et al. Periaortitis: gadolinium-enhanced magnetic resonance imaging and response to therapy in four patients. Ann Vasc Surg 2004;18(1):100–7.

29. Sakalihasan N, Limet R, Defawe OD. Abdominal aortic aneurysm. Lancet Lond Engl 2005; 365(9470):1577–89.

30. Mao SS, Ahmadi N, Shah B, et al. Normal thoracic aorta diameter on cardiac computed tomography in healthy asymptomatic adult; impact of age and gender. Acad Radiol 2008;15(7):827–34.

31. Gunn TM, Gupta VA, Nadig V, et al. Ascending aortic aneurysm. In: Dieter RS, Dieter RA Jr, Deiter RA, editors. Diseases of the aorta. Springer; 2019. p. 161–73.

32. Newman JD, Motiwala A, Turin A, et al. Abdominal aortic aneurysms. In: Deiter RS, Deiter RA Jr, Deiter RA, editors. Diseases of the aorta. Springer; 2019. p. 199–216.

33. Curtis W, Yano M. Acute non-traumatic disease of the abdominal aorta. Abdom Radiol NY 2018; 43(5):1067–83.

34. Siegel CL, Cohan RH, Korobkin M, et al. Abdominal aortic aneurysm morphology: CT features in patients with ruptured and nonruptured aneurysms. AJR Am J Roentgenol 1994;163(5):1123–9.

35. Halliday KE, al-Kutoubi A. Draped aorta: CT sign of contained leak of aortic aneurysms. Radiology 1996;199(1):41–3.

36. Bhalla S, Menias CO, Heiken JP. CT of acute abdominal aortic disorders. Radiol Clin North Am 2003; 41(6):1153–69.

37. Zhou M, Hu Y, Long X, et al. Diagnostic performance of magnetic resonance imaging for acute pulmonary embolism: a systematic review and meta-analysis. J Thromb Haemost 2015;13(9):1623–34.

38. Schiebler ML, Nagle SK, François CJ, et al. Effectiveness of MR angiography for the primary diagnosis of acute pulmonary embolism: Clinical outcomes at 3 months and 1 year. J Magn Reson Imaging 2013;38(4):914–25.

39. Chen L, Liu D, Zhang J, et al. Free-breathing dynamic contrast-enhanced mri for assessment of pulmonary lesions using golden-angle radial sparse parallel imaging. J Magn Reson Imaging JMRI 2018;48(2):459–68.

40. Benson DG, Schiebler ML, Repplinger MD, et al. Contrast-enhanced pulmonary MRA for the primary diagnosis of pulmonary embolism: current state of the art and future directions. Br J Radiol 2017; 90(1074):20160901.

41. Kaya F, Ufuk F, Karabulut N. Diagnostic performance of contrast-enhanced and unenhanced combined pulmonary artery MRI and magnetic resonance venography techniques in the diagnosis of venous thromboembolism. Br J Radiol 2019; 92(1095):20180695.

42. Kalb B, Sharma P, Tigges S, et al. MR imaging of pulmonary embolism: diagnostic accuracy of contrast-enhanced 3D MR pulmonary angiography, contrast-enhanced low-flip angle 3D GRE, and nonenhanced free-induction FISP sequences. Radiology 2012;263(1):271–8.

43. Hirsch AT, Haskal ZJ, Hertzer NR, et al. ACC/AHA 2005 guidelines for the management of patients with peripheral arterial disease (lower extremity, renal, mesenteric, and abdominal aortic): a collaborative report from the American Association for Vascular Surgery/Society for Vascular Surgery, Society for Cardiovascular Angiography and Interventions, Society for Vascular Medicine and Biology, Society of Interventional Radiology, and the ACC/AHA Task Force on Practice Guidelines (Writing Committee to Develop Guidelines for the Management of Patients With Peripheral Arterial Disease). J Am Coll Cardiol 2006;47(6):e1–192.

44. Sibley RC, Reis SP, MacFarlane JJ, et al. Noninvasive physiologic vascular studies: a guide to diagnosing peripheral arterial disease. RadioGraphics 2017;37(1):346–57.

45. Menke J, Larsen J. Meta-analysis: Accuracy of contrast-enhanced magnetic resonance angiography for assessing steno-occlusions in peripheral arterial disease. Ann Intern Med 2010;v153(5): 325–34.

46. Napoli A, Anzidei M, Zaccagna F, et al. Peripheral arterial occlusive disease: diagnostic performance and effect on therapeutic management of 64-section CT angiography. Radiology 2011;261(3):976–86.

47. Ahmed O, Hanley M, Bennett SJ, et al. ACR appropriateness criteria® vascular claudication—assessment for revascularization. J Am Coll Radiol 2017; 14(5, Supplement):S372–9.

48. Saini A, Wallace A, Albadawi H, et al. Quiescent-interval single-shot magnetic resonance angiography. Diagnostics 2018;8(4).

49. Sandhu GS, Rezaee RP, Jesberger J, et al. Time-resolved MR angiography of the legs at 3 T using a low dose of gadolinium: initial experience and contrast dynamics. Am J Roentgenol 2012;198(3): 686–91.

50. Hansmann J, Michaely HJ, Morelli JN, et al. Impact of time-resolved MRA on diagnostic accuracy in patients with symptomatic peripheral artery disease of the calf station. Am J Roentgenol 2013;201(6): 1368–75.

Use of MR in Pancreaticobiliary Emergencies

Hailey Chang, MD[a],*, David D.B. Bates, MD[b], Avneesh Gupta, MD[a],
Christina A. LeBedis, MD[a]

KEYWORDS

- Emergency MR imaging • Pancreatitis • Cholecystitis • Biliary obstruction • Cholangitis • Bile leak
- MRCP • MR cholangiopancreatography

KEY POINTS

- MR plays a role in the evaluation of a number of acute pancreaticobiliary conditions, including cholecystitis, pancreatitis, biliary obstruction, pancreatic trauma, and bile leak.
- Several MR imaging features may be used to assist in the diagnosis and classification of pancreatic and biliary emergencies, including specific complications.
- Several imaging artifacts and pitfalls exist in the MR imaging of pancreaticobiliary emergencies that can mimic pathology.
- Abbreviated MR protocols are increasingly being used in the emergency setting to decrease imaging acquisition times while maintaining diagnostic accuracy.

INTRODUCTION

Acute abdominal symptoms are a common cause of emergency department (ED) visits in the United States. Per the National Hospital Ambulatory Medical Care Survey (NHAMCS), the US Department of Health and Human Services reported 11 million ED visits for noninjury abdominal pain in 2018.[1] Disorders of the biliary system and pancreas constitute a large portion of these conditions, with approximately 270,000 admissions for acute pancreatitis[2] and more than 700,000 emergent cholecystectomies performed annually in the United States.[3] Cross-sectional imaging has become an invaluable tool in the clinicians' armamentarium to aid in the diagnosis and triage of patients presenting with acute abdominal conditions.

Technological advances in multidetector and dual-energy computed tomography (CT) over the past several years, particularly involving the increased speed of acquisition and reduced radiation dose, have made them the workhorses of emergency abdominal imaging. The widespread utility of CT in abdominal emergencies is well established.

Despite its secondary role to CT, certain clinical scenarios may require evaluation with MR imaging. MR cholangiopancreatography (MRCP), first described in 1991 by Wallner and colleagues,[4] has become an essential tool for imaging the pancreas and biliary system. Heavily T2-weighted MRCP images enable rapid, noninvasive evaluation of the biliary tree and localization of pathology. In addition, MR may provide relevant information in patients being evaluated for pancreatic or biliary trauma, bile leaks, acute cholecystitis, biliary obstruction, or pancreatitis. When compared with CT, MR also offers the distinct advantage of avoiding ionizing radiation.

Funding sources: Dr H. Chang: Nil. Dr D.D.B. Bates: Nil. Dr A. Gupta: Nil. Dr C.A. LeBedis: Nil.
[a] Department of Radiology, Boston Medical Center, 820 Harrison Avenue, FGH Building 3rd Floor, Boston, MA 02118, USA; [b] Department of Radiology, Cornell University, Memorial Sloan Kettering Cancer Center, 1275 York Avenue, New York, NY 10065, USA
* Corresponding author.
E-mail address: hailey.chang@bmc.org

NORMAL ANATOMY AND IMAGING TECHNIQUE

The pancreas is a retroperitoneal organ that arises from the endodermal lining of the duodenum. It is formed by fusion of the dorsal and ventral pancreatic buds.[5] The main pancreatic duct (of Wirsung) drains the body of the pancreas, whereas in some the accessory pancreatic duct of Santorini drains into the minor papilla.[5] Certain congenital anomalies can occur that may be relevant in acute abdominal conditions later in life, as discussed later.

The 3 components of a portal triad are the hepatic artery, portal vein, and bile duct. The left and right hepatic ducts join shortly after the porta hepatis to form the common hepatic duct. The common hepatic duct joins the cystic duct to form the common bile duct, which runs in parallel to the pancreatic duct until they merge to form the hepatopancreatic ampulla of Vater.[6] Variant ductal anatomy may have implications in diagnosis and clinical management and will be addressed later in the discussion on choledocholithiasis.

IMAGING PROTOCOLS

At our institution, abdominal MR with MRCP sequences using phased-array surface body or torso coils are standardized (**Table 1**), but certain modifications may be implemented to address a specific clinical question. The contrast agent of choice at our institution is Gadoteridol (ProHance; Bracco Imaging, Milan, Italy). In select cases where detection of a ductal leak is required, gadoxetate disodium (Eovist; Bayer Healthcare Pharmaceuticals, Berlin, Germany) may be used, with additional delayed hepatocellular phase images acquired 10 to 20 minutes after the injection of contrast. Currently, the use of hepatobiliary contrast agents to detect bile leak is off-label. If a hepatocyte specific agent such as gadoxetate disodium (Eovist) is administered, MRCP and other T2-weighted sequences must be acquired before contrast administration to prevent T2 shortening in the biliary tree, as discussed in the following section.

In addition to the aforementioned, MRCP sequences are typically performed when evaluating for pancreaticobiliary pathology. If desired, a negative oral contrast agent may be given immediately before imaging to reduce or eliminate the background signal of the proximal gastrointestinal tract. Before its discontinuation, an oral suspension of ferumoxsil (Gastromark, AMAG pharmaceuticals, Lexington, Massachusetts) was routinely administered in our department. Oral administration of pineapple juice or blueberry juice may achieve a similar effect. MRCP is typically acquired with both 2-dimensional (2D) and 3D techniques in our department. 2D MRCP technique is performed using a heavily T2-weighted fat-suppressed single-shot turbo spinecho with 40-mm slice thickness. Six breath-hold or respiratory-triggered images are acquired in the coronal oblique plane at various angles centered about the head of the pancreas. 2D MRCP images have the advantage of rapid acquisition and are therefore relatively resistant to motion artifact. 3D MRCP images are acquired in the coronal plane using a 3D TSE technique using 1.6-mm slice thickness. Although acquisition time is significantly longer than the 2D technique, 3D MRCP imaging allows high-resolution imaging of the biliary tree, improved signal-to-noise ratio, and the ability to perform multiplanar reconstructions. MIP reformats are acquired in the coronal oblique plane, and additional multiplanar reconstructions may be performed for additional information, including the distinction between choledocholithiasis and air in the duct, as discussed later.

A growing trend among institutions is the implementation of abbreviated MR (A-MR) protocols for pancreaticobiliary imaging. These protocols aim to answer focused clinical questions using fewer, more targeted sequences to decrease imaging acquisition and interpretation times while maintaining diagnostic accuracy.

One main application for A-MR protocols in the ED is the use of abbreviated magnetic resonance cholangiopancreatography (A-MRCP) for the detection of choledocholithiasis and biliary obstruction. A retrospective study by Tso and colleagues[7] demonstrated that A-MRCP protocols with 4 noncontrast sequences, as opposed to the standard 8 sequences with gadolinium, cut imaging acquisition time in half without compromising diagnostic accuracy. The A-MRCP protocol consisted of coronal fast spin echo, axial gradient echo with fat saturation, and 2D and 3D MRCP sequences.

A-MR sequences also play a role in routine surveillance and follow-up imaging. They are meant to be used following the acquisition of a reference baseline that includes the A-MR sequences as well as standard contrast-enhanced, diffusion-weighted, and chemical shift sequences. A-MR protocols were first proposed by Macari and colleagues[8] who demonstrated that use of gadolinium-based contrast agents only altered clinical recommendations in a minority of cases, a finding that was subsequently supported by other retrospective and prospective studies.[9,10]

Table 1
Standard 3 T magnetic resonance abdomen protocol with intravenous contrast

Parameter	T1-Weighted In- and Out-of-Phase	T2-Weighted SPIR	T2-Weighted Single-Shot TSE	Diffusion (b = 0, 600 s/mm²)	MR Cholangiopancreatography	T1-Weighted 3D GRE SPIR (THRIVE)
FOV mm	400	400	400	400	300	400
Technique	GRE	Fast SE	Fast SE	Diffusion	Fast SE for 2D, 3D TSE for 3D	GRE
Scanning Mode	Multisection, dual echo	Multisection 2D	Multisection, 2D	Multisection, 2D	Multisection, 2D or 3D	3D
TR (ms)	180	2000	∞	3.6	8000	3.6
TE (ms)	2.3 (out-of-phase)/4.6 (in-phase) a1.1 (out-of-phase)/2.3 (in-phase) on 3T	80	80	1.8	800	1.7
Section Thickness (mm)	5	5	5	7	40 for 2D, 1.6 for 3D	4
Flip Angle	90	90	90	60	90	15
SENSE Acceleration Factor	1.8	2	2	2	2	1.7
Respiration Control	Breath-holding	Respiratory triggering[a]	Respiratory triggering[a]	Respiratory triggering[a]	Respiratory triggering[a]	Breath-holding

Abbreviations: GRE, gradient-recalled echo; SP, spin echo; SPIR, selective partial inversion recovery; TSE, turbo spin echo.
[a] May perform with breath-hold technique as tolerated by patient.

Delaney and colleagues[11] further demonstrated the safety of A-MR protocols when used for routine surveillance of nonmalignant lesions. An A-MR protocol proposed by Pedrosa[12] consists of coronal and axial single-shot fast spin echo T2-weighted, 2D MRCP and 3D MRCP, and 3D T1-weighted spoiled gradient echo sequences.

IMAGING FINDINGS AND PATHOLOGY
Pancreatic Trauma

Although MR acquisition times have decreased with advances in technology, CT remains the imaging modality of choice in the setting of blunt and penetrating abdominal trauma due to its speed, availability, and high spatial resolution. However, select patients with blunt pancreaticobiliary injury on CT may benefit from additional MR imaging.[13]

Pancreatic injury in the setting of abdominal trauma is relatively uncommon with reported incidences ranging from 3% to 12%, approximately 37% of which are due to blunt abdominal injury.[14] However, the associated mortality for blunt pancreatic trauma is considerable and may be as high as 30% to 50%, largely secondary to concomitant injuries.[13] Factors associated with poor outcomes include a delay in the time to definitive diagnosis, high-grade injury, and disruption of the main pancreatic duct (MPD).[15] Elevated serum amylase may be present, but the clinical presentation of pancreatic injury is variable and nonspecific.[16] Blunt pancreatic injuries occur more commonly in the body of the gland, accounting for two-thirds of cases, and are typically caused by a crushing impact against the vertebral column. Because the main cause for morbidity and mortality is disruption of the main pancreatic duct, assessment for ductal injuries is critical. Deep lacerations (involving greater than 50% of the thickness of the pancreas) are predictive of ductal disruption and may be detected using T1-weighted postcontrast and T2-weighted sequences. Direct injury to the duct may be visible using T2-weighted sequences, including MRCP images (Fig. 1).

Pancreatic lacerations, defined as irregular linear, low attenuation regions in the pancreatic parenchyma on CT,[17] may be either superficial (when involving < 50% of the parenchymal thickness) or deep (>50% of the parenchymal thickness).[18] The sensitivity of MDCT for pancreatic injury is limited, ranging from 47% to 60%.[13] A deep pancreatic laceration is traditionally considered indirect evidence of a main pancreatic duct injury, and further evaluation with endoscopic retrograde cholangiopancreatography (ERCP)

may be warranted if duct integrity is questionable on MR.

Because of the invasive nature of ERCP and its associated complications, particularly in unstable trauma patients, MRCP offers a noninvasive alternative to evaluate the extent of pancreatic injury and MPD involvement. A recent single-center prospective study by Panda and colleagues[13] compared MDCT and MRCP in patients with blunt abdominal trauma using laparotomy as the gold standard. The study found that both MDCT and MRCP performed well in the evaluation of pancreatic injury and suggested that the combination of these modalities increased diagnostic confidence and allowed for more accurate evaluation of MPD involvement.[13] Thus, when pancreatic laceration is suspected, particularly deep lacerations, further evaluation of the MPD with MRCP (if feasible) may be appropriate. Alternatively, an ERCP should be performed.

Bile Leak

Bile leaks may occur after blunt or penetrating hepatic injury or surgical intervention and can present a diagnostic challenge. The lack of specific symptoms may result in a delay in diagnosis. Some of the more common symptoms associated with bile leak include abdominal discomfort, anorexia, and lethargy. Left undiagnosed and untreated bile leaks can progress to bilomas and bile peritonitis. Eventually, superimposed infection of the intraperitoneal fluid can result in peritonitis and sepsis, often requiring surgical intervention.[19]

Traditionally, hepatobiliary scintigraphy has been used to diagnose bile leaks. However, poor anatomic detail and low spatial resolution limit the ability of scintigraphy to precisely localize the source of a bile leak.[19] The addition of single-photon emission computed tomography images may improve the sensitivity and specificity for the detection of leaks, but with the disadvantage of increased exposure to ionizing radiation.

With the advent of gadolinium-based hepatobiliary contrast agents such as gadoxetate disodium (Eovist; Bayer Healthcare Pharmaceuticals, Berlin, Germany), which has 50% renal excretion and 50% hepatic excretion, MRCP may now play a role in the evaluation of patients with suspected bile leaks.[20] Its use for this purpose is currently off-label, but a 2013 study by Kantarci and colleagues[21] demonstrated improved detection and localization of bile leaks with Eovist when compared with traditional MRCP. The additional acquisition of delayed phase images following Eovist administration further increased the

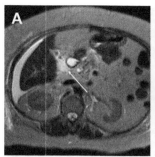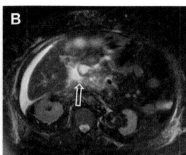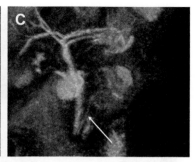

Fig. 1. Pancreatic contusion. A 58-year-old unrestrained driver in an MVC, with stranding around the duodenum and pancreas on MDCT. (A) Axial T2-weighted image demonstrating edema in the fat around the neck of the pancreas (*arrow*) and ascites, which becomes more evident on (B) T2-weighted fat suppressed image (*open arrow*). (C) 2D MRCP demonstrates an intact pancreatic duct (*arrow*). (*From* Bates, D., LeBedis, C., Soto, J. and Gupta, A., 2016. Use of Magnetic Resonance in Pancreaticobiliary Emergencies. Magnetic Resonance Imaging Clinics of North America, 24(2), pp.433-448.)

sensitivity of detecting and localizing active bile leaks[22] (**Fig. 2**).

Gadolinium-based hepatobiliary contrast agents result in T1 shortening of excreted bile, rendering it hyperintense on T1-weighted images. Biliary excretion may begin as early as 10 minutes after intravenous contrast administration, and fat-saturated T1-weighted images to assess for bile leak may be acquired at 20 minutes.[19] Key imaging findings include extraluminal accumulation of contrast in the liver parenchyma, around the liver or free spillage into the peritoneal cavity. Secondary signs of bile leak parallel those seen in other imaging modalities, including a collapsed gallbladder, pericholecystic or perihepatic fluid collections, and ascites.[19]

Acute Cholecystitis

Acute cholecystitis is one of the most common surgical emergencies, with a prevalence of approximately 5%.[23] In approximately 90% to 95% of cases, acute cholecystitis is due to gallstone impaction in the neck of the gallbladder or cystic duct.[24] Cholelithiasis is present in approximately 10% of the population, with a higher prevalence seen in middle-aged and elderly women.[25] As a result of the obstruction, bile stasis, ischemia, and development of systemic infection can occur.[26] As cystic duct obstruction leads to increased intraluminal pressure and the gallbladder wall is weakened by ischemia, subsequent gallbladder perforation can result.

Diagnostic imaging plays a central role in the Tokyo Guidelines, which seek to improve the diagnostic sensitivity and specificity for acute cholecystitis and acute cholangitis.[27,28] A number of imaging modalities are used to assist in the diagnosis of acute cholecystitis, primarily including ultrasound (US), but CT and MR imaging may be helpful in select cases. Since its introduction in 1991,[4] MRCP has been an invaluable tool to evaluate the biliary tree.

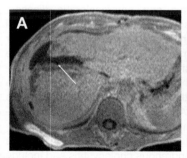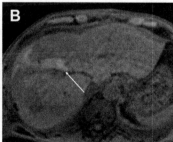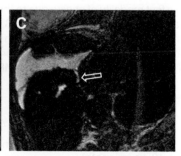

Fig. 2. Hepatic duct laceration. A 63-year-old man after blunt abdominal trauma with grade V liver laceration. (A) Precontrast and (B) postcontrast T1-weighted fat-suppressed images acquired at 20 minutes after the injection of gadoxetate disodium demonstrate a deep laceration in the right lobe of the liver (*arrows*). Note accumulation of excreted T1 hyperintense bile at the site of laceration (B), indicating active biliary leakage. (C) 3D MRCP image demonstrates direct continuity of the fluid collection with the right hepatic duct, indicating the site of ductal injury (*open arrow*) (**Fig. 3**). (*From* Bates, D., LeBedis, C., Soto, J. and Gupta, A., 2016. Use of Magnetic Resonance in Pancreaticobiliary Emergencies. Magnetic Resonance Imaging Clinics of North America, 24(2), pp.433-448.)

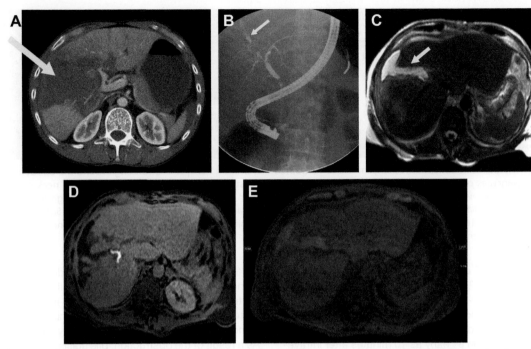

Fig. 3. Hepatic laceration with bile leak. A 46-year-old man after motor vehicle collision. (*A*) Contrast-enhanced CT abdomen and pelvis in the portal venous phase demonstrates a large hepatic laceration (*yellow arrow*). (*B*) ERCP demonstrates contrast extravasation in the region of the laceration consistent with bile leak and contrast extravasation at site of hepatic laceration (*yellow arrow*). (*C*) Axial T2-weighted image demonstrates fluid at the laceration site and fluid at site of hepatic laceration (*yellow arrow.*). Axial postcontrast T1-weighted fat-suppressed image demonstrates a biliary tree branch at the base of the laceration (*D*) with extravasation of contrast into the laceration on delayed phase image performed 12 hours later (*E*).

Imaging features of acute cholecystitis are common to US, CT, and MR imaging (**Box 1**) and include cholelithiasis, gallbladder distention to a diameter greater than 4 cm or length greater than 10 cm, gallbladder wall thickening, pericholecystic fluid, and perihepatic fluid (the so-called C-sign). CT and MR imaging may also show hyperenhancement of the adjacent liver on postcontrast arterial phase images.[24] Although not routinely the first modality of choice due to the speed, accuracy, and low cost of abdominal US, MR imaging is more sensitive for the detection of gallstones affected in the gallbladder neck or cystic duct.[24] The sensitivity and specificity of MR for detection

of cholecystitis when any one of these imaging features is present on MR have been reported at 88% and 89%, respectively[29] (**Fig. 4**).

Certain forms of cholecystitis also demonstrate unique imaging features and may be readily classified on MR imaging. Emphysematous cholecystitis is a distinct entity and has a different pathogenesis than typical acute calculous cholecystitis. It is more commonly seen in patients with underlying diabetes mellitus and atherosclerotic disease. Small vessel ischemia results in gallbladder wall inflammation and necrosis, allowing gas to enter the gallbladder wall. Although US and CT are extremely sensitive for detection of air in the gallbladder wall, this finding may also be detectable by MR. Air in the gallbladder wall will appear as signal voids.[24] Air may also be visible as susceptibility artifact on gradient echo imaging. Other imaging features of emphysematous cholecystitis overlap with gangrenous cholecystitis and include irregular wall thickening or asymmetric heterogeneous hyperintense signal in the gallbladder wall on T2-weighted images[27] (**Fig. 5**).

In addition to demonstrating diagnostic features of acute cholecystitis, MR is an invaluable tool to identify its most common complications, including

---

Box 1
Imaging features of acute cholecystitis

- Gallbladder distention > 4 cm in diameter (or 10 cm in length)
- Gallbladder wall thickening > 3 mm
- Pericholecystic fluid
- Perihepatic fluid (the "C-sign")
- Hyperenhancement of the adjacent liver

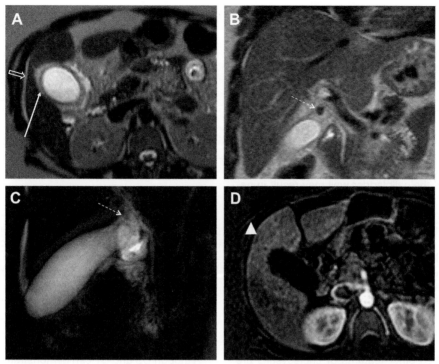

Fig. 4. Acute cholecystitis. A 42-year-old woman with right upper quadrant pain. (*A*) Axial T2-weighted image demonstrates gallbladder wall thickening (*arrow*) and distention, with trace perihepatic ascites (*open arrow*). (*B*) Coronal T2-weighted and (*C*) radial MRCP images demonstrate a T2 hypointense stone (*dashed arrow*) lodged in the cystic duct. (*D*) Arterial phase postcontrast imaging demonstrates relative hyperenhancement of the adjacent liver parenchyma (*arrowhead*), indicative of inflammation. (*From* Bates, D., LeBedis, C., Soto, J. and Gupta, A., 2016. Use of Magnetic Resonance in Pancreaticobiliary Emergencies. Magnetic Resonance Imaging Clinics of North America, 24(2), pp.433-448.)

empyema, perforation, gangrenous cholecystitis, and gallbladder empyema.[24]

Gallbladder empyema refers to filling of the inflamed and distended gallbladder with purulent material. In typical acute cholecystitis, the gallbladder is usually distended with T2-hyperintense bile. In the setting of empyema, the inflamed gallbladder fills with pus, which appears as layering-dependent, hypointense, inhomogeneous material on heavily T2-weighted sequences.[24]

Perforation may be diagnosed when there is discontinuity of the gallbladder wall in the setting of acute cholecystitis. MR may aid in the

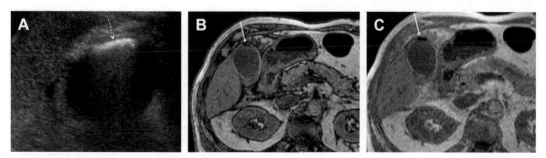

Fig. 5. Emphysematous cholecystitis. A 69-year-old man with abdominal pain. (*A*) Abdominal US demonstrates a linear echogenic area in the antidependent aspect of the gallbladder wall (*dashed arrow*), with dirty shadowing posteriorly, consistent with air. (*B*) Out-of-phase and (*C*) in-phase phase T1 gradient echo images demonstrate patchy decreased T1 signal with prolonged TE (*arrows*, in-phase imaging), consistent with air in the gallbladder wall. (*From* Bates, D., LeBedis, C., Soto, J. and Gupta, A., 2016. Use of Magnetic Resonance in Pancreaticobiliary Emergencies. Magnetic Resonance Imaging Clinics of North America, 24(2), pp.433-448.)

visualization of wall disruption when it is unclear on US or CT, particularly on T1-weighted post-gadolinium and T2-weighted fat-suppressed images. Although subacute perforation with abscess formation in the gallbladder wall is the most common form, free perforation into the peritoneal cavity and the development of enterocholecystic fistulas may also be seen[24] (**Fig. 6**).

Gangrenous cholecystitis is a complication that occurs when cholecystitis has become advanced. As with other complications, US and CT findings tend to be specific, but relatively insensitive. Ischemia of the gallbladder wall may result in necrosis and sloughing of the mucosa. Key findings suggesting microabscesses or gallbladder wall necrosis include heterogeneous areas of hyperintensity on fat-suppressed T1- and T2-weighted images. Heterogeneous or disrupted wall or mucosal enhancement on postcontrast T1-weighted fat-suppressed images may also be suggestive[24] (**Fig. 8**).

Hemorrhagic cholecystitis may be diagnosed on CT by the presence of hyperattenuating blood in the setting of cholecystitis but can be confirmed on MR. When other features of cholecystitis are present on imaging, hemorrhage may be seen in the gallbladder lumen or wall as T1 hyperintense signal as a result of the T1-shortening effects of methemoglobin.[24]

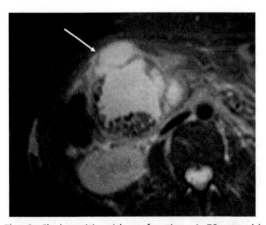

Fig. 6. Cholecystitis with perforation. A 59-year-old man presenting with right upper quadrant pain and cholecystitis. Axial fat-suppressed T2-weighted image demonstrates discontinuity of the anterior gallbladder wall (*arrow*), with loculated fluid collections consistent with gallbladder perforation. This finding was not well seen on US (**Fig. 7**). (*From* Bates, D., LeBedis, C., Soto, J. and Gupta, A., 2016. Use of Magnetic Resonance in Pancreaticobiliary Emergencies. Magnetic Resonance Imaging Clinics of North America, 24(2), pp.433-448.)

Dual-energy CT has shown promise for improved detection and characterization of acute cholecystitis. In a study by Huda and colleagues,[30] dual-energy CT demonstrated improved sensitivity for detection of numerous imaging findings of acute cholecystitis, including gallbladder fossa hyperemia, gangrene, heterogeneous gallbladder wall enhancement, and acute cholecystitis. In addition, an iodine density measurement of 0.5 mg/mL or lower in a visibly hypoenhancing region of the gallbladder wall was 95.7% specific for diagnosis of gangrenous cholecystitis.

Biliary Obstruction

Obstruction of the biliary tree may result in intrahepatic biliary ductal dilation, with associated increase in pressure. In addition to obstructive jaundice, the increased pressure in the biliary tree can result in hepaticovenous reflux of bacteria.[24] The resultant acute cholangitis and biliary sepsis can be life-threatening, and emergent intervention may be required with either percutaneous or endoscopic drainage.

Although US and CT can demonstrate the presence of biliary obstruction, the exact cause is often most clearly identified by MRCP. Choledocholithiasis, iatrogenic stricture, and malignant obstruction may all contribute to biliary obstruction and can be differentiated on MR.

As mentioned earlier in the discussion of cholecystitis, choledocholithiasis is common in western populations. When gallstones migrate through the cystic duct and into the common bile duct, choledocholithiasis occurs and can result in acute biliary obstruction. Identifying gallstones in the common bile duct can help guide therapeutic options. Because choledocholithiasis and cholecystitis may occur together, dilation of the common bile duct greater than 8 mm should raise suspicion for choledocholithiasis when imaging features of cholecystitis are present. Because CT may not detect choledocholithiasis, MRCP may be performed in cases where it is suspected[28] (**Fig. 9**).

In addition to demonstrating a high sensitivity and specificity for detecting choledocholithiasis,[28] excluding the presence of gallstones in the biliary tree may prevent an unnecessary ERCP, an invasive procedure that is associated with complications such as pancreatitis. On heavily T2-weighted MRCP images, gallstones appear as rounded signal voids within the bile duct, with a meniscus both above and below. Cholesterol stones will generally be both T1 and T2 hypointense, but pigmented stones may show variable T1 signal that can be hyperintense. The distinction is significant, as pigmented stones are susceptible

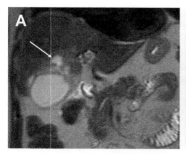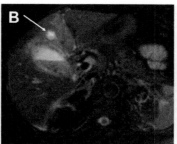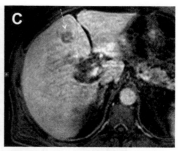

Fig. 7. Cholecystitis with perforation and liver abscess formation. A 70-year-old man with cholelithiasis and abdominal pain. (*A*) Coronal T2-weighted and (*B*) axial fat-suppressed T2-weighted images show a hyperintense fluid collection in the hepatic parenchyma adjacent to an inflamed gallbladder (*arrows*). (*C*) Axial T1-weighted postcontrast imaging during equilibrium phase demonstrates mild peripheral enhancement around the collection, consistent with intrahepatic abscess (*dashed arrow*). (*From* Bates, D., LeBedis, C., Soto, J. and Gupta, A., 2016. Use of Magnetic Resonance in Pancreaticobiliary Emergencies. Magnetic Resonance Imaging Clinics of North America, 24(2), pp.433-448.)

to fragmentation via endoscopic lithotripsy, whereas cholesterol stones are not.[25] Rarely, a gallstone may become affected in the cystic duct and cause extrinsic compression of the common hepatic duct, resulting in intrahepatic biliary duct obstruction (Mirizzi syndrome). This unique condition is named after Pablo Luis Mirizzi, the Argentinian surgeon who first described it (**Fig. 10**).

Several congenital anomalies of the biliary tree have been described that may have an impact on diagnosis and treatment of patients with choledocholithiasis.[31] Low medial insertion of the cystic duct is one such anomaly and may be diagnosed when the cystic duct inserts at or near the hepatopancreatic ampulla. In this setting, superimposition of the cystic duct on the distal bile duct may appear to represent a stone in the distal bile duct on ERCP. Mirizzi syndrome may also occur due to a low cystic duct insertion. In addition, ERCP may be more technically difficult in patients with this anomaly, and the gastroenterologist should be alerted to its presence before endoscopy.[31]

A second but rare cause of acute biliary obstruction worth noting is inadvertent occlusion of the cystic duct during surgery; this may occur during liver transplant, hepatic resection, or cholecystectomy. The rate of iatrogenic bile duct injury remains relatively low, with reported rates of 1.0% for laparoscopic and 0.5% for open cholecystectomy.[32] However, given the large volume of cholecystectomies performed each year, as high as 700,000 per year in the United States, even a low rate of 0.5% to 1.0% can result in a substantial incidence of iatrogenic bile duct injuries.[25] It is associated with significant need for reintervention, increased hospital cost, and decreased quality of life for the patient.[33]

Malignant biliary obstruction does not occur acutely in the same manner as choledocholithiasis or iatrogenic biliary stricture, but patients may

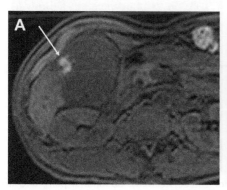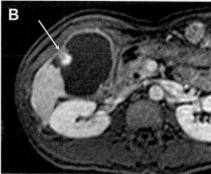

Fig. 8. Hemorrhagic cholecystitis. Axial fat-suppressed T1-weighted precontrast (*A*) and postcontrast (*B*) images show an area of focal T1 hyperintensity in the gallbladder fundus (*arrows*). Pathology showed cholecystitis with an area of focal hemorrhage corresponding to the imaging findings. (*From* Bates, D., LeBedis, C., Soto, J. and Gupta, A., 2016. Use of Magnetic Resonance in Pancreaticobiliary Emergencies. Magnetic Resonance Imaging Clinics of North America, 24(2), pp.433-448.)

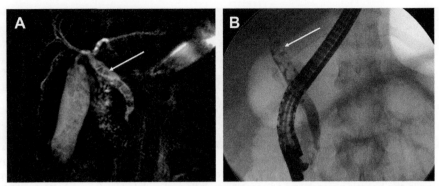

Fig. 9. Choledocholithiasis. A 25-year-old woman with right upper quadrant pain and cholelithiasis on US. (*A*) MRCP demonstrates choledocholithiasis and dilation of the common bile duct to 11 mm (*arrow*). (*B*) ERCP was performed with stone retrieval (*arrow*). (*From* Bates, D., LeBedis, C., Soto, J. and Gupta, A., 2016. Use of Magnetic Resonance in Pancreaticobiliary Emergencies. Magnetic Resonance Imaging Clinics of North America, 24(2), pp.433-448.)

present emergently with obstructive jaundice and complicating cholangitis, as the growing tumor occludes the biliary tree. Cholangiocarcinoma, gallbladder carcinoma, ampullary tumors, or pancreatic adenocarcinoma may all result in obstruction of the biliary tree once they have progressed. Identifying the level of obstruction will help guide therapeutic options, whether via percutaneous biliary decompression, endoscopic stent placement, or surgical resection.[34]

Lastly, acute ("ascending") cholangitis represents a feared complication of biliary obstruction and is diagnosed clinically by the presence of right upper quadrant pain, jaundice, and fever.[29] In one study, the most common imaging finding in patients with cholangitis was cholestasis, characterized by dilation of the intrahepatic bile ducts. Biliary sludge, periductal edema (increased T2

signal), and ascites/retroperitoneal fluid are additional findings associated with acute cholangitis. Pus within the biliary tree may be identified as intraductal hypointense signal on heavily T2-weighted images.[24] (**Box 2, Fig. 11**).

Care must be taken to avoid mistaking certain imaging findings for biliary obstruction. Potential pitfalls that may cause apparent filling defects in the bile ducts and mimic stones include impression from the right hepatic artery, intraductal air, signal voids from flow of bile through the bile ducts, and metal artifact from surgical clips or stents. Impression from the right hepatic artery will appear as an extrinsic signal void in the common hepatic duct on MRCP images, but this pitfall may be avoided by recognizing the characteristic location of this artifact and by identifying the right hepatic artery on T2-and T1-weighted post-

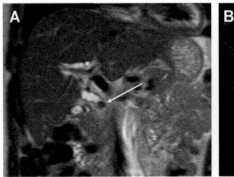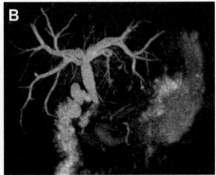

Fig. 10. Mirizzi syndrome. A 59-year-old man with prior cholecystectomy, abdominal pain, and intrahepatic biliary ductal (IHBD) dilation seen on US. (*A*) Coronal T2-weighted image demonstrates a retained hypointense stone (*arrow*) in the remnant cystic duct, causing mass effect on the common hepatic duct. (*B*) MIP projection of 3D MRCP demonstrates intra- and extrahepatic biliary ductal dilation. (*From* Bates, D., LeBedis, C., Soto, J. and Gupta, A., 2016. Use of Magnetic Resonance in Pancreaticobiliary Emergencies. Magnetic Resonance Imaging Clinics of North America, 24(2), pp.433-448.)

gadolinium sequences. Intraductal air will appear as rounded signal voids within the bile ducts, but unlike gallstones, air will be antidependent on axial images. Axial reformatted images of 3D MRCP data may be particularly valuable to determine if such rounded filling defects are dependent or antidependent. Flowing bile can create a central signal void in the bile duct. This pitfall may be avoided by noting the characteristic central location of the signal void, which usually is not reproducible on repeat sequences. Susceptibility artifact from metal clips or stents may create artificial signal voids, particularly on gradient echo sequences (**Figs. 12–16**).

Pancreatitis

Acute pancreatitis is a common cause of acute abdominal pain in the western hemisphere, and the incidence has increased in recent decades.[35] Acute pancreatitis accounts for one-quarter of a million hospital admissions each year in the United States. Choledocholithiasis and alcohol use are the leading causes of acute pancreatitis, but no inciting factor is identified in as many as one-third of cases.[36] The clinical course of acute pancreatitis is variable. Mild pancreatitis typically follows a self-limited course and requires only supportive care with low associated morbidity and mortality. In its severe acute form, necrotizing pancreatitis can be life-threatening, with morbidity and mortality as high as 36% to 50%.[37]

In response to considerable variability and confusion regarding the classification and terminology of acute pancreatitis in the medical literature, the Atlanta classification was developed[38] and most recently updated in 2012.[39]

The 2012 revised Atlanta classification states that acute pancreatitis may be diagnosed when 2 of the following 3 criteria are met: elevated lipase 3 times the upper limit of normal, characteristic abdominal pain, or radiologic findings that suggest pancreatic inflammation. The report suggests that when acute pancreatitis is suspected based on characteristic abdominal pain, but serum lipase is less than 3 times the upper limit of normal, cross-sectional imaging is indicated to establish the diagnosis.

Acute pancreatitis is divided into early and late phases, and the severity is classified as mild, moderate, or severe. The early phase of acute pancreatitis typically lasts up to one week and is the result of systemic response to local pancreatic inflammation. During the early phase, the presence and duration of organ failure determines the severity. In mild acute pancreatitis, there is no associated organ failure or systemic complication. Moderate pancreatitis occurs when transient organ failure (<48 hours) is present and may be associated with local or systemic complications such as exacerbation of preexisting cardiac or pulmonary disease. Severe acute pancreatitis is diagnosed

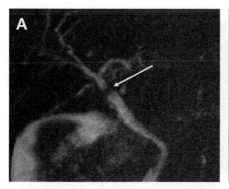
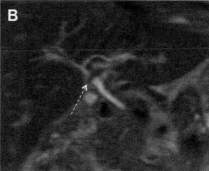

Fig. 11. Hepatic artery impression mimicking a ductal stone. (*A*) 2D MRCP shows an apparent filling defect in the proximal common hepatic duct (*arrow*). (*B*) Coronal T2-weighted image demonstrates flow void from the right hepatic artery (*dashed arrow*) corresponding to the artifact on MRCP images. (*From* Bates, D., LeBedis, C., Soto, J. and Gupta, A., 2016. Use of Magnetic Resonance in Pancreaticobiliary Emergencies. Magnetic Resonance Imaging Clinics of North America, 24(2), pp.433-448.)

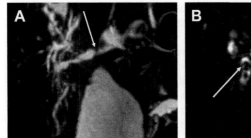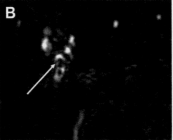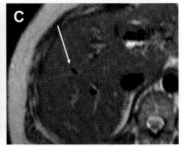

Fig. 12. Air in the cystic duct mimicking a stone. (*A*) 3D and (*B*) 2D MRCP show antidependent signal void consistent with air (*arrows*). (*C*) Axial T2-weighted image shows antidependent signal void in the bile ducts, consistent with pneumobilia. (*From* Bates, D., LeBedis, C., Soto, J. and Gupta, A., 2016. Use of Magnetic Resonance in Pancreaticobiliary Emergencies. Magnetic Resonance Imaging Clinics of North America, 24(2), pp.433-448.)

when organ failure, either single or multiple, persists beyond 48 hours.[37]

The late phase of acute pancreatitis occurs after the first week of presentation and only in moderate and severe cases. Local complications include the development of pancreatic or peripancreatic fluid collections, vascular complications (thrombosis or pseudoaneurysm), or gastric outlet obstruction.[37] Cross-sectional imaging, with either CT or MR, plays an essential role in the characterization of local complications in acute pancreatitis and has significant implications in management. Dual-energy CT has shown to improve sensitivity for detection of acute pancreatitis. In a study by Martin and colleagues,[40] an iodine density threshold of 2.1 mg/mL and less was 96% sensitive and 77% specific for detection of acute pancreatitis, and dual-energy CT was significantly more sensitive for detection of pancreatitis than conventional CT images.

Although CT is generally the preferred modality due to widespread availability and rapid acquisition, MR may be desirable for a variety of reasons. Detection of cholelithiasis or choledocholithiasis, characterization of nonliquefied collections, or a contraindication to iodinated CT contrast may make MR the modality of choice in certain clinical situations. Familiarity with the MR imaging appearance of acute pancreatitis, its causes, and complications is essential.

When first evaluating a patient with acute pancreatitis, the distinction must first be made between interstitial edematous pancreatitis (IEP) and necrotizing pancreatitis. IEP will appear as diffuse or local pancreatic enlargement with homogenous or slightly heterogeneous enhancement. T2 hyperintense signal may also be seen in the surrounding fat, indicating inflammation and edema. Pancreatic necrosis is present when an area of the pancreas does not enhance on postcontrast imaging. Nonliquefied components in the collection (hemorrhage, fat, or necrotic fat) should also be classified as necrotizing pancreatitis and not IEP.[41] The presence of ascites in acute pancreatitis is highly associated with pancreatic necrosis.[42] If the presence or absence of necrosis is indeterminate, and repeat imaging may be performed 5 to 7 days later (**Figs. 17–20**).

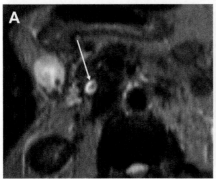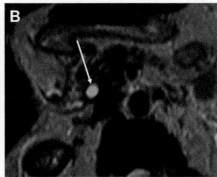

Fig. 13. (*A*) Axial T2-weighted image shows a central signal void in the CBD due to flow of bile (*arrow*), which does not persist upon repeat imaging (*B, arrow*). (*From* Bates, D., LeBedis, C., Soto, J. and Gupta, A., 2016. Use of Magnetic Resonance in Pancreaticobiliary Emergencies. Magnetic Resonance Imaging Clinics of North America, 24(2), pp.433-448.)

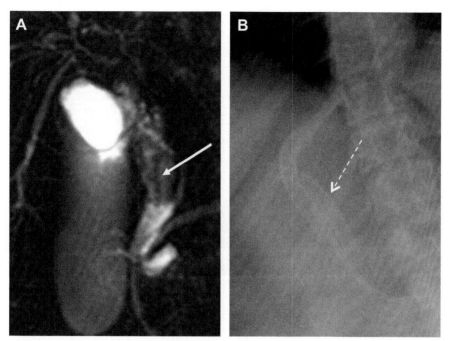

Fig. 14. Apparent filling defect in the bile duct on 2D MRCP (*A, arrow*) is due to metallic artifact from a biliary stent (*B, dashed arrow*). (*From* Bates, D., LeBedis, C., Soto, J. and Gupta, A., 2016. Use of Magnetic Resonance in Pancreaticobiliary Emergencies. Magnetic Resonance Imaging Clinics of North America, 24(2), pp.433-448.)

Four types of fluid collections are described in the new classification, stratified by the presence or absence of necrosis and duration. A peripancreatic fluid collection that is present during the first 4 weeks of IEP that does not contain a solid component is described as an acute peripancreatic fluid collection (APFC). A fluid collection present within the parenchyma of the pancreas should not be described as an APFC and should be considered necrosis.[41] When the fluid collection persists beyond 4 weeks in IEP, it is termed a pancreatic pseudocyst. To qualify as a pancreatic pseudocyst, the collection must be entirely fluid and must have a well-defined wall.[37] Pancreatic pseudocysts may communicate with the pancreatic duct via a side branch or the main pancreatic duct. MRCP may demonstrate the communication, indicating a pseudocyst may be amenable to transpapillary drainage.[41,43]

Within the category of necrotizing pancreatitis, 3 subtypes are described: pancreatic parenchymal necrosis alone, peripancreatic necrosis alone, and combined pancreatic parenchymal necrosis with peripancreatic necrosis. The combined form is most common (75%–80%), with peripancreatic necrosis typically seen in the retroperitoneum and lesser sac.[41] Once necrotizing pancreatitis has been diagnosed, a peripancreatic fluid collection should be termed an acute necrotic collection

in the first 4 weeks and may contain variable amounts of solid components. After 4 weeks, once a capsule has developed, the collection should be termed walled-off necrosis (WON) and not a pseudocyst[41] (**Figs. 21–23, Table 2**)

Treatment of the collections associated with acute pancreatitis is variable. It should be noted that any of the 4 types of collection may be either sterile or infected. An APFC does not generally require intervention and often resolves spontaneously on its own. Likewise, pseudocysts generally do not require intervention, unless the patient is symptomatic from local mass effect or superimposed infection is suspected. If infection is suspected, percutaneous drainage of the pseudocyst is often sufficient, and most patients do not require additional surgical intervention following drainage.[44] In contrast, patients with WON require debridement via percutaneous catheter drainage or surgery to remove all of the nonliquid components.[41]

In addition to collections, potential vascular complications should be identified in patients with acute pancreatitis. Venous complications are relatively common and typically involve thrombosis of the splenic or portal vein. Venous thrombosis is more common in necrotizing pancreatitis, with some investigators reporting an incidence as high as 45%.[45] Arterial complications

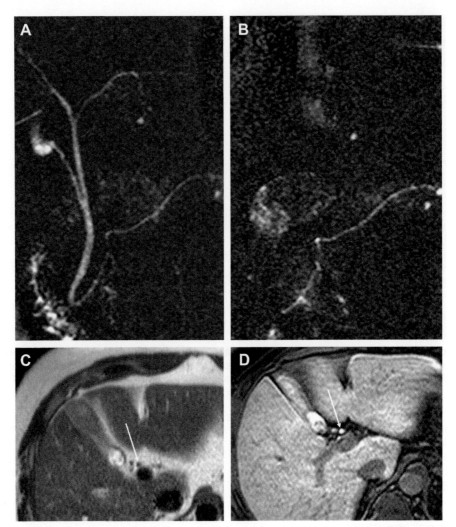

Fig. 15. (*A*) MRCP acquired before and (*B*) several minutes after the administration of hepatobiliary contrast. Signal in the biliary tree is obscured on delayed postcontrast images due to the T2-shortening effect of excreted contrast in the bile ducts. (*C*) Axial T2-weighted image acquired several minutes after the administration of gadoxetate disodium shows corresponding hypointense signal in the bile duct (*arrow*). (*D*) T1-weighted fat-suppressed image acquired 10 minutes postcontrast demonstrates hyperintense signal in the duct (*arrow*), indicating biliary excretion of contrast. (*From* Bates, D., LeBedis, C., Soto, J. and Gupta, A., 2016. Use of Magnetic Resonance in Pancreaticobiliary Emergencies. Magnetic Resonance Imaging Clinics of North America, 24(2), pp.433-448.)

in acute pancreatitis are far less common, with the main complications being pseudoaneurysm formation and acute hemorrhage. The left gastric, splenic, gastroduodenal, superior mesenteric, and hepatic arteries are most commonly involved.[45] Identification of pseudoaneurysm formation is crucial, and timely intervention must be performed to prevent life-threatening hemorrhage (**Fig. 24**).

The identification of hemorrhagic pancreatitis is another distinct advantage of MR imaging. The presence of T1 hyperintense methemoglobin is easily recognized to aid in this diagnosis. Hemorrhage in the pancreatic bed is typically thought to be the result of erosion of a vessel, and prompt surgical intervention may be required to prevent potentially fatal consequences.[28]

A final complication of acute necrotizing pancreatitis is disrupted duct syndrome, a condition in which the main pancreatic duct is interrupted along its course. Because of its noninvasive nature, MRCP is preferred over ERCP to evaluate for pancreatic duct disruption. On imaging, the presence of an intrapancreatic fluid collection

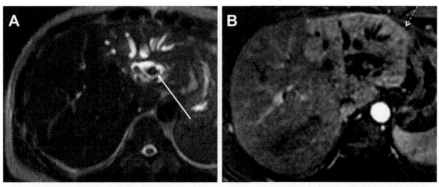

Fig. 16. Acute pyogenic cholangitis. A 26-year-old man with severe epigastric pain, leukocytosis, and IHBD dilation on abdominal US. (A) Axial T2-weighted image demonstrates IHBD dilation isolated to the left lobe of the liver, with rounded hypointense filling defects in the bile ducts consistent with stones (*arrow*). The liver parenchyma in the left lobe is asymmetrically T2 hyperintense. (B) T1-weighted postcontrast imaging demonstrates early enhancement of the left lobe of the liver (*dashed arrow*). (*From* Bates, D., LeBedis, C., Soto, J. and Gupta, A., 2016. Use of Magnetic Resonance in Pancreaticobiliary Emergencies. Magnetic Resonance Imaging Clinics of North America, 24(2), pp.433-448.)

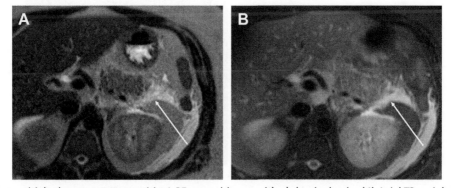

Fig. 17. Interstitial edematous pancreatitis. A 25-year-old man with abdominal pain. (A) Axial T2-weighted image through the upper abdomen demonstrates an enlarged pancreas with edema and fluid in the surrounding fat (*arrow*). The degree of inflammation is more readily apparent on (B) axial fat-suppressed T2-weighted image through the same location, with adjacent acute peripancreatic fluid collection (*arrow*, APFC). APFC, acute peripancreatic fluid collection. (*From* Bates, D., LeBedis, C., Soto, J. and Gupta, A., 2016. Use of Magnetic Resonance in Pancreaticobiliary Emergencies. Magnetic Resonance Imaging Clinics of North America, 24(2), pp.433-448.)

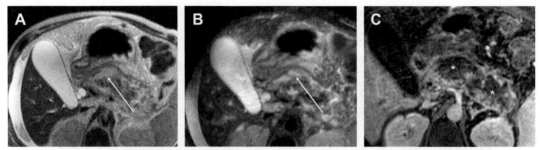

Fig. 18. Necrotizing pancreatitis. A 51-year-old man with pancreatitis. (*A*) Axial T2-weighted and (*B*) fat-suppressed T2-weighted images through the upper abdomen demonstrate ascites and significant edema in the region of the pancreas and an adjacent acute necrotic collection (*arrow*, ANC). (*C*) Postcontrast fat-suppressed T1-weighted image acquired during the portal venous phase shows hypoenhancement of nearly the entire pancreatic body and tail (*asterisk*), consistent with necrotizing pancreatitis. ANC, acute necrotic collection. (*From* Bates, D., LeBedis, C., Soto, J. and Gupta, A., 2016. Use of Magnetic Resonance in Pancreaticobiliary Emergencies. Magnetic Resonance Imaging Clinics of North America, 24(2), pp.433-448.)

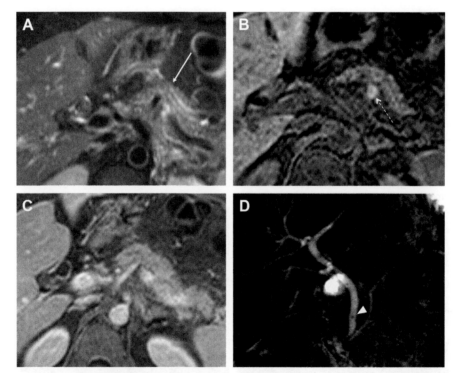

Fig. 19. Pancreatitis with hemorrhage. A 52-year-old man with pancreatitis. (*A*) Axial fat-suppressed T2-weighted image shows an edematous pancreas with surrounding inflammation (*arrow*). (*B*) Precontrast fat-suppressed T1-weighted image shows a hyperintense focus along the superior, posterior aspect of the pancreas consistent with hemorrhage (*dashed arrow*). (*C*) Postcontrast fat-suppressed T1-weighted image demonstrates homogenous enhancement without evidence of necrosis. (*D*) 2D MRCP images show a small stone in the distal CBD (*arrowhead*). (*From* Bates, D., LeBedis, C., Soto, J. and Gupta, A., 2016. Use of Magnetic Resonance in Pancreaticobiliary Emergencies. Magnetic Resonance Imaging Clinics of North America, 24(2), pp.433-448.)

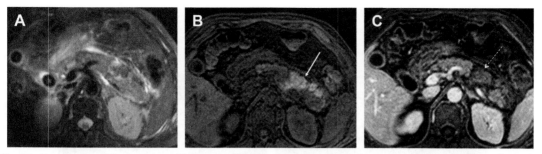

Fig. 20. Pancreatitis with necrosis and hemorrhage. A 43-year-old man admitted with abdominal pain and pancreatitis on CT. (*A*) Axial fat-suppressed T2-weighted image demonstrates extensive inflammation in the pancreatic bed and enlargement of the gland. (*B*) Precontrast fat-suppressed T1-weighted image shows a large area of T1 hyperintensity in the body and tail of the pancreas consistent with hemorrhage (*arrow*). (*C*) Postcontrast fat-suppressed T1-weighted image shows hypoenhancement in the area of hemorrhage (*dashed arrow*), indicating concurrent necrosis. (*From* Bates, D., LeBedis, C., Soto, J. and Gupta, A., 2016. Use of Magnetic Resonance in Pancreaticobiliary Emergencies. Magnetic Resonance Imaging Clinics of North America, 24(2), pp.433-448.)

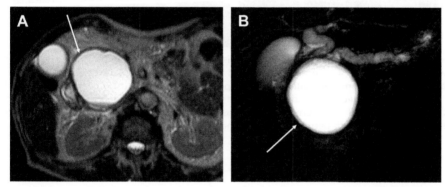

Fig. 21. Pancreatic pseudocyst. A 67-year-old man with acute on chronic pancreatitis. (*A*) Axial T2-weighted image demonstrates a T2 hyperintense fluid collection adjacent to the head of the pancreas (*arrow*). (*B*) 2D MRCP image demonstrates the pseudocyst (*arrow*). (*From* Bates, D., LeBedis, C., Soto, J. and Gupta, A., 2016. Use of Magnetic Resonance in Pancreaticobiliary Emergencies. Magnetic Resonance Imaging Clinics of North America, 24(2), pp.433-448.)

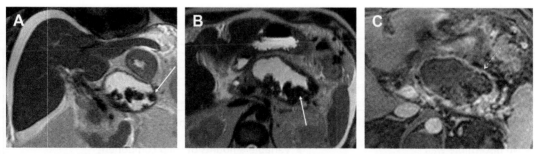

Fig. 22. Walled-off necrosis. A 45-year-old man with history of pancreatitis and abdominal pain. (*A*) Coronal and (*B*) axial T2-weighted images demonstrate a T2 hyperintense fluid collection in the body of the pancreas with hypointense internal debris (*arrows*). (*C*) Postcontrast fat-suppressed T1-weighted image acquired during equilibrium demonstrates peripheral enhancement and a clearly defined capsule (*dashed arrow*). (*From* Bates, D., LeBedis, C., Soto, J. and Gupta, A., 2016. Use of Magnetic Resonance in Pancreaticobiliary Emergencies. Magnetic Resonance Imaging Clinics of North America, 24(2), pp.433-448.)

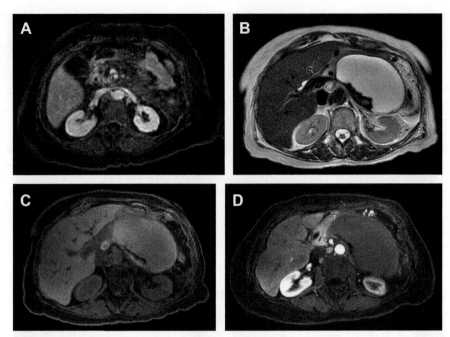

Fig. 23. Necrotizing pancreatitis with walled-off necrosis. 76 year-old female with history of gallstone pancreatitis. (a) Axial post-contrast fat suppressed T1-weighted image demonstrates lack of enhancement throughout the pancreatic body and tail consistent with necrotizing pancreatitis (*arrows*). (b) Repeat MRI 8 months later demonstrates a T2 hyperintense fluid collection with hypointense internal necrotic debris in the pancreatic body and tail (*arrows*). Axial T1-weighted fat suppressed precontrast (c) and post contrast arterial phase (d) images demonstrate a well-defined capsule with peripheral enhancement (*arrows*).

Table 2
Fluid collections in pancreatitis

Interstitial Edematous Pancreatitis (IEP)	Necrotizing Pancreatitis
Acute Peripancreatic Fluid Collection: • < 4 weeks • No discernible wall • No solid component	Acute Necrotic Collection: • < 4 weeks • Variable amounts of solid component • Any fluid collection *within* the pancreatic parenchyma
Pancreatic Pseudocyst • 4 weeks • Well defined wall • No solid component	Walled-Off Necrosis: • 4 weeks • Variable amounts of solid component • Any fluid collection *within* the pancreatic parenchyma

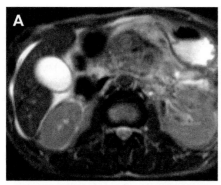
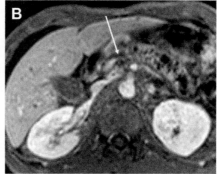

Fig. 24. Pancreatitis with splenic vein and SMV thrombosis. A 58-year-old man with pancreatitis. (*A*) Axial T2-weighted image demonstrates ascites, pancreatic edema, and surrounding fluid. (*B*) Axial fat-suppressed T1-weighted postcontrast image acquired in the equilibrium phase shows abrupt tapering of the portal vein (*arrow*) at the expected confluence of the splenic and superior mesenteric veins, which were not visualized. The splenic vein and SMV were patent on abdominal CT performed 3 months prior, suggesting thrombosis. SMV, superior mesenteric vein. (*From* Bates, D., LeBedis, C., Soto, J. and Gupta, A., 2016. Use of Magnetic Resonance in Pancreaticobiliary Emergencies. Magnetic Resonance Imaging Clinics of North America, 24(2), pp.433-448.)

along the expected course of the duct suggests ductal disruption,[46] a finding that increases the risk of pancreatic fistula formation and that often requires surgical treatment.[47]

SUMMARY

Evaluation of patients with acute abdominal conditions is common in diagnostic radiology, and a multimodality approach to imaging is often required. Although CT is the main workhorse of emergency abdominal imaging, additional information gathered from modalities such as US, MR, and nuclear medicine can be of the utmost value. In the evaluation of patients with pancreaticobiliary trauma, suspected bile leak, cholecystitis, biliary obstruction, and pancreatitis, MR is invaluable. Familiarity with the optimal imaging protocols, imaging appearance of pathology and mimics, established guidelines, and therapeutic implications is key to the accurate diagnosis and management of these patients.

DISCLOSURE

Conflicts of interest: Dr H. Chang: Nil. Dr D.D.B. Bates: Nil. Dr A. Gupta: Nil. Dr C.A. LeBedis: Nil.

REFERENCES

1. US Department of Health and Human Services. National Hospital Ambulatory Medical Care Survey: 2018 emergency department summary tables. Natl Hosp Ambul Med Care Surv 2018;13.
2. Peery AF, Dellon ES, Lund J, et al. Burden of gastrointestinal disease in the United States: 2012 update. Gastroenterology 2012;143(5):1179.
3. Knab LM, Boller AM, Mahvi DM. Cholecystitis. Surg Clin North Am 2014;94(2):455–70. Available at: https://pubmed.ncbi.nlm.nih.gov/24679431/.
4. Wallner BK, Schumacher KA, Weidenmaier W, et al. Dilated biliary tract: evaluation with MR cholangiography with a T2-weighted contrast-enhanced fast sequence. Radiology 1991;181(3):805–8. Available at. https://pubmed.ncbi.nlm.nih.gov/1947101/.
5. Sadler TW. Langman's medical embryology. 12th edition. Philadelphia: Wolters Kluwer Health/Lippincott Williams & Wilkins; 2012. Available at. https://www.ncbi.nlm.nih.gov/nlmcatalog/101562744.
6. Moore KL, Dalley AF II, Agur AMR. Clinically oriented anatomy. Clinical Anatomy. 7th edition. Baltimore: Lippincott Williams & Wilkins; 2014.
7. Tso DK, Almeida RR, Prabhakar AM, et al. Accuracy and timeliness of an abbreviated emergency department MRCP protocol for choledocholithiasis. Emerg Radiol 2019;26(4):427–32. Available at. https://pubmed.ncbi.nlm.nih.gov/31030393/.
8. Macari M, Lee T, Kim S, et al. Is gadolinium necessary for mri follow-up evaluation of cystic lesions in the pancreas? Preliminary results. AJR Am J Roentgenol 2012;192(1):159–64. Available at: www.ajronline.org.
9. Nougaret S, Reinhold C, Chong J, et al. Incidental pancreatic cysts: natural history and diagnostic accuracy of a limited serial pancreatic cyst MRI protocol. Eur Radiol 2014;24(5):1020–9. Available at. https://pubmed.ncbi.nlm.nih.gov/24569848/.
10. Pozzi-Mucelli RM, Rinta-Kiikka I, Wünsche K, et al. Pancreatic MRI for the surveillance of cystic neoplasms: comparison of a short with a comprehensive imaging protocol. Eur Radiol 2016;27(1):41–50. Available at. https://link.springer.com/article/10.1007/s00330-016-4377-4.

11. Delaney FT, Fenlon HM, Cronin CG. An abbreviated MRI protocol for surveillance of cystic pancreatic lesions. Abdom Radiol 2021;46(7):3253–9. https://doi.org/10.1007/s00261-021-02987-z. Available at.

12. Pedrosa I. A 10-min MRI protocol for follow up incidental cystic pancreatic lesions. In: Oak Brook I, editor. Radiological society of north America scientific assembly and annual meeting program. Dallas (TX): Radiological Society of North America; 2017. Available at. https://archive.rsna.org/2017/17001338.html.

13. Panda A, Kumar A, Gamanagatti S, et al. Evaluation of diagnostic utility of multidetector computed tomography and magnetic resonance imaging in blunt pancreatic trauma: a prospective study. Acta Radiol 2015;56(4):387–96. Available at. https://pubmed.ncbi.nlm.nih.gov/24760286/.

14. Dave S, Toy FK, London S. Pancreatic trauma. Surg Liver Bile Ducts Pancreas Child Third Ed 2021;13: 329–37. Available at. https://www.ncbi.nlm.nih.gov/books/NBK459365/.

15. Ayoob AR, Lee JT, Herr K, et al. Pancreatic trauma: Imaging review and management update. Radiographics 2021;41(1):58–74. Available at. https://pubs.rsna.org/doi/abs/10.1148/rg.2021200077.

16. Bradley EL, Young PR, Chang MC, et al. Diagnosis and initial management of blunt pancreatic trauma: guidelines from a multiinstitutional review. Ann Surg 1998;27(6):861–9. Available at. https://pubmed.ncbi.nlm.nih.gov/9637549/.

17. Rekhi S, Anderson SW, Rhea JT, et al. Imaging of blunt pancreatic trauma. Emerg Radiol 2010;17(1): 13–9. Available at. https://pubmed.ncbi.nlm.nih.gov/19396480/.

18. Wong YC, Wang LJ, Lin BC, et al. CT grading of blunt pancreatic injuries: prediction of ductal disruption and surgical correlation. J Comput Assist Tomogr 1997;21(2):246–50. Available at. https://pubmed.ncbi.nlm.nih.gov/9071293/.

19. Melamud K, LeBedis CA, Anderson SW, et al. Biliary imaging: multimodality approach to imaging of biliary injuries and their complications. Radiographics 2014;34(3):613–23. Available at. https://pubmed.ncbi.nlm.nih.gov/24819784/.

20. LeBedis C, Luna A, Soto JA. Use of magnetic resonance imaging contrast agents in the liver and biliary tract. Magn Reson Imaging Clin N Am 2012; 20(4):715–37. Available at. https://pubmed.ncbi.nlm.nih.gov/23088947/.

21. Kantarci M, Pirimoglu B, Karabulut N, et al. Noninvasive detection of biliary leaks using Gd-EOB-DTPA-enhanced MR cholangiography: comparison with T2-weighted MR cholangiography. Eur Radiol 2013;23(10):2713–22. Available at. https://pubmed.ncbi.nlm.nih.gov/23695221/.

22. Cieszanowski A, Stadnik A, Lezak A, et al. Detection of active bile leak with Gd-EOB-DTPA enhanced MR cholangiography: Comparison of 20–25 min delayed and 60–180 min delayed images. Eur J Radiol 2013; 82(12):2176–82. Available at. http://www.ejradiology.com/article/S0720048X13004208/fulltext.

23. Kiewiet JJS, Leeuwenburgh MMN, Bipat S, et al. A systematic review and meta-analysis of diagnostic performance of imaging in acute cholecystitis. Radiology 2012;264(3):708–20. Available at. https://pubmed.ncbi.nlm.nih.gov/22798223/.

24. Watanabe Y, Nagayama M, Okumura A, et al. MR imaging of acute biliary disorders. Radiographics 2007;27(2):477–95. Available at. https://pubmed.ncbi.nlm.nih.gov/17374864/.

25. Yam BL, Siegelman ES. MR imaging of the biliary system. Radiol Clin North Am 2014;52(4):725–55. Available at. https://pubmed.ncbi.nlm.nih.gov/24889169/.

26. O'Connor OJ, Maher MM. Imaging of cholecystitis. AJR Am J Roentgenol 2011;196(4):369–71. Available at. https://pubmed.ncbi.nlm.nih.gov/21427298/.

27. Adusumilli S, Siegelman ES. MR imaging of the gallbladder. Magn Reson Imaging Clin N Am 2002; 10(1):165–84. Available at. https://pubmed.ncbi.nlm.nih.gov/11998573/.

28. Tkacz JN, Anderson SA, Soto J. Mr imaging in gastrointestinal emergencies. Radiographics 2009; 29(6):1767–80. Available at. https://pubs.rsna.org/doi/abs/10.1148/rg.296095509.

29. Hakansson K, Leander P, Ekberg O, et al. MR imaging in clinically suspected acute cholecystitis. A comparison with ultrasonography. Acta Radiol 2000; 41(4):322–8. Available at. https://pubmed.ncbi.nlm.nih.gov/10937751/.

30. Huda F, LeBedis CA, Qureshi MM, et al. Acute cholecystitis: diagnostic value of dual-energy CT-derived iodine map and low-keV virtual monoenergetic images. Abdom Radiol (NY) 2021;46(11): 5125–33. Available at. https://pubmed.ncbi.nlm.nih.gov/34223959/.

31. Turner MA, Fulcher AS. The cystic duct: normal anatomy and disease processes. Radiographics 2001;21(1):3–22. Available at. https://pubmed.ncbi.nlm.nih.gov/11158640/.

32. Mungai F, Berti V, Colagrande S. Bile leak after elective laparoscopic cholecystectomy: Role of MR imaging. J Radiol Case Rep 2013;7(1):25.

33. Buddingh KT, Nieuwenhuijs VB, Van Buuren L, et al. Intraoperative assessment of biliary anatomy for prevention of bile duct injury: a review of current and future patient safety interventions. Surg Endosc 2011;25(8):2449–61. Available at. https://www.researchgate.net/publication/51046522_Intraoperative_assessment_of_biliary_anatomy_for_prevention_of_bile_duct_injury_A_review_of_current_and_future_patient_safety_interventions.

34. Soto JA, Alvarez O, Lopera JE, et al. Biliary obstruction: findings at MR cholangiography and

cross-sectional MR imaging. Radiographics 2000; 20(2):353–66. Available at. https://pubmed.ncbi. nlm.nih.gov/10715336/.

35. Goldacre MJ, Roberts SE. Hospital admission for acute pancreatitis in an English population, 1963-98: database study of incidence and mortality. BMJ 2004;328(7454):1466–9. Available at. https:// pubmed.ncbi.nlm.nih.gov/15205290/.

36. Murphy KP, O'Connor OJ, Maher MM. Updated imaging nomenclature for acute pancreatitis. AJR Am J Roentgenol 2014;203(5):W464–9. Available at. https://pubmed.ncbi.nlm.nih.gov/25341160/.

37. Banks PA, Bollen TL, Dervenis C, et al. Classification of acute pancreatitis 2012: revision of the Atlanta classification and definitions by international consensus. Gut 2013;62(1):102–11. Available at. https://pubmed.ncbi.nlm.nih.gov/23100216/.

38. Bradley EL. A clinically based classification system for acute pancreatitis. Summary of the International Symposium on Acute Pancreatitis, Atlanta, Ga, September 11 through 13, 1992. Arch Surg 1993; 128(5):586–90. Available at. https://pubmed.ncbi. nlm.nih.gov/8489394/.

39. Foster BR, Jensen KK, Bakis G, et al. Revised Atlanta classification for acute pancreatitis: a pictorial essay. Radiographics 2016;36(3):675–87. Available at. https:// pubs.rsna.org/doi/abs/10.1148/rg.2016150097.

40. Martin SS, Trapp F, Wichmann JL, et al. Dual-energy CT in early acute pancreatitis: improved detection using iodine quantification. Eur Radiol 2019;29(5): 2226–32. Available at. https://pubmed.ncbi.nlm.nih. gov/30488112/.

41. Thoeni RF. The revised Atlanta classification of acute pancreatitis: its importance for the radiologist and its effect on treatment. Radiology 2012;262(3):751–64. Available at. https://pubmed.ncbi.nlm.nih.gov/ 22357880/.

42. Yang E, Nguyen NH, Kwong WT. Abdominal free fluid in acute pancreatitis predicts necrotizing pancreatitis and organ failure. Ann Gastroenterol 2021;34(6):872.

43. Aghdassi AA, Mayerle J, Kraft M, et al. Pancreatic pseudocysts- when and how to treat? HPB (Oxford) 2006;8(6):432–41. Available at. https://pubmed. ncbi.nlm.nih.gov/18333098/.

44. Keshavarz P, Azrumelashvili T, Yazdanpanah F, et al. Percutaneous catheter drainage of pancreatic associated pathologies: a systematic review and meta-analysis. Eur J Radiol 2021;144:109978.

45. Mendelson RM, Anderson J, Marshall M, et al. Vascular complications of pancreatitis. ANZ J Surg 2005;75(12):1073–9. Available at. https://pubmed. ncbi.nlm.nih.gov/16398814/.

46. Manikkavasakar S, AlObaidy M, Busireddy KK, et al. Magnetic resonance imaging of pancreatitis: An update. World J Gastroenterol 2014;20(40):14760.

47. Sandrasegaran K, Tann M, Jennings SG, et al. Disconnection of the pancreatic duct: an important but overlooked complication of severe acute pancreatitis. Radiographics 2007;27(5):1389–400. Available at. https://pubmed.ncbi.nlm.nih.gov/ 17848698/.

Magnetic Resonance Imaging in Gastrointestinal and Genitourinary Emergencies

Khyati Bidani, MD[a], Ramandeep Singh, MD[b], Garima Chandra, MD[a],
Rubal Rai, MD[a], Ajay Kumar Singh, MD[b],*

KEYWORDS

• MRI • Emergency department • Abdominal pain • Radiation exposure

KEY POINTS

- Owing to concerns of computed tomography (CT) radiation exposure, magnetic resonance imaging (MRI) applications in acute settings are increasing.
- Among the patients presenting in the emergency department, a significant proportion is present with abdominopelvic complaints.
- Magnetic resonance imaging offers better soft-tissue contrast and diagnostic interpretation critical for the early interpretation and management of acute abdominal pathologies.

INTRODUCTION

The ever-rising volume of patients in emergency departments has necessitated the requirement of rapid and efficient diagnostic techniques. While the role of ultrasound and computed tomography (CT) scans is relatively well established, clinical applications of magnetic resonance imaging (MRI) in emergency settings are being increasingly validated.

Among the patients presenting in the emergency department, a significant proportion present with abdominopelvic complaints. Acute abdominal pain is one of the most common symptoms (accounting for 5%–10% of all ED visits)[1,2] and encompasses a wide range of possible differential diagnoses. Early detection with imaging and timely intervention can significantly decrease morbidity and mortality, especially in conditions such as acute pancreatitis or ovarian torsion.

CT and ultrasound (US) imaging is routinely used in emergency settings to aid prompt diagnosis and appropriate patient care. Both these modalities have the advantage of being quick and easily accessible. While CT allows for accurate assessment of the whole abdomen for a wide range of gastrointestinal conditions within a shorter scan time, its usage carries the risk of exposing patients to ionizing radiation. Per published data, a single scan can contribute to up to 10 times the natural radiation exposure in 1 year.[3] Additionally, the diagnostic ability of a CT scan is limited in situations such as coexisting chronic renal failure or allergy to intravenous (IV) iodinated contrast media. Alternative modalities such as ultrasound could be used in such scenarios; however, operator dependency, inability to image in the presence of significant bowel gas, and patients with higher body mass index (BMI), limit its significance.

MRI is being increasingly considered as an alternative and sometimes primary diagnostic modality in specific emergency settings owing to its exceptional soft-tissue resolution, nonusage of ionizing

[a] Department of Radiology, Massachusetts General Hospital, 55 Fruit Street, Boston, MA 02114, USA;
[b] Department of Emergency Radiology, Massachusetts General Hospital, 55 Fruit Street, Boston, MA 02114, USA
* Corresponding author. Massachusetts General Hospital, 55 Fruit Street, Boston, MA 02114.
E-mail address: asingh1@mgh.harvard.edu

Magn Reson Imaging Clin N Am 30 (2022) 501–513
https://doi.org/10.1016/j.mric.2022.03.005
1064-9689/22/© 2022 Elsevier Inc. All rights reserved.

radiation and iodinated contrast media, nonoperator dependency, and higher reproducibility. In several instances, MRI can be used as a critical imaging tool for equivocal CT findings. Despite its several imaging advantages, MRI acquisition is relatively time-consuming, bears higher cost and patient cooperation which could be of clinical challenge in an acute emergency. American College of Radiology currently recommends the usage of MRI in acute abdominal emergencies involving pregnant and pediatric patient groups.[4,5]

MAGNETIC RESONANCE IMAGING PROTOCOLS

In acute settings, designing and execution of MRI protocols allows high-quality imaging at an expense of minimum diagnostic time interval.[6] Unlike CT imaging whereby the usage of IV contrast media is often imperative, the use of fluid-sensitive sequences such as single-shot T2-weighted imaging can obviate MRI-based contrast media in several pathologies. Such avoidance of IV contrast in clinical situations whereby diagnostic accuracy remains unaffected, reduces the table time and improves patient experience, as quick diagnosis is directly linked to efficient patient management.

MRI techniques valuable in emergency settings include T2-weighted fluid sensitive sequences; precontrast, and when applicable, postcontrast T1-weighted sequences; and diffusion-weighted sequences. MRI protocols should be tailored to the patient's clinical condition with free-breathing protocols preferable over breath-hold protocols for patients unable to hold their breath for optimal imaging.

T2-weighted imaging (T2WI) techniques are fluid sensitive and thus allow for the detection of free fluid or tissue edema. Routinely used T2-weighted techniques include coronal short inversion time recovery sequence (STIR) and axial single-shot T2-weighted sequence (fast spin-echo or half-Fourier RARE). STIR images can be acquired in multiple planes (axial, coronal, and sagittal) for abdomen and pelvis to identify areas with high signal intensity corresponding to regions of free fluid. Image acquisition and generation with STIR sequences can be performed in about 3 minutes of imaging time.[7,8] Axial and coronal single-shot T2-weighted sequences have lesser degree of motion artifacts and very short acquisition times (approximately 1 second per section).[9] Similar to STIR imaging, these images show high signal in the region of free fluid and allow tissue characterization for assessment of pathologies.[9,10] Additional advantage of T2WI is that it

can be performed with free breathing and can be used in intubated patients or those who cannot perform breath-holding for the study.

T1-weighted imaging (T1WI) uses gradient echo-based sequences and provides higher anatomic detail, and tissue differentiation for the detection of blood products and protein deposits, unlike T2WI which is helpful for identifying inflammatory pathologies. T1WI can be acquired with and without fat-saturation, the latter suppressing the fat signal and retaining other tissue signals. Examples of fat-suppressed three-dimensional volumetric T1-weighted sequences include VIBE, LAVA, and THRIVE. Dual-echo GRE T1-weighted sequences used obtains both out-of-phase followed by in-phase images in the same acquisition and allow for the characterization of lipid content and magnetic artifacts. T1WI can be performed both with and without the administration of gadolinium-based IV contrast media. An example of gadolinium-based contrast media includes gadobenate dimeglumine which can be injected at a rate of 2 mL/s for high-resolution postcontrast dynamic images.[5,11] Certain example situations whereby the use of gadolinium-based IV contrast is shown to be beneficial include bile leak, inflammatory bowel wall thickening, and intraabdominal abscesses.[5–7] As mentioned earlier, it leads to the improved depiction of bowel wall defects, abscesses, and perfusion defects. The absolute contraindication to the usage of gadolinium-based IV contrast includes pregnancy and significant renal dysfunction (especially when the glomerular filtration rate is < 30 mL min-1 1.73 m-2[5]). T1WI is motion sensitive, imaging requires a breath-hold for about 15 to 20 seconds.[9,11,12] T1WI can be affected by susceptibility artifacts from materials such as iron, calcium, air. One of the methods to address this limitation is by using shorter echo times.[9]

Diffusion-weighted imaging (DWI) allows for the measurement of diffusion restriction of water molecules in various tissues. Normally, water molecules can freely diffuse in random directions but pathologic events interfering with cellular organization or permeability may restrict this free diffusion. DWI is a spin-echo-based sequence with longer echo times (due to strong and opposite diffusion gradients) that allows for T2-weighting on these images. Tissues with fluid restriction appear bright on DWI but dark on apparent diffusion coefficient (ADC) map. ADC maps are needed to distinguish the increased signal intensity of the tissue due to fluid restriction from the possible T2 shine-through effect. DWI technique can be used for the evaluation of cellular tumors, abscesses/cysts, and lymph nodes with increasing applications in the near future.[7,13]

In our single institutional experience, administration of rectal saline improves the diagnostic ability of MRI for equivocal cases of acute appendicitis. Following rectal saline administration, a fluid distended appendix seems hyperintense on noncontrast T2WI and can be demonstrated on both axial and coronal planes. In cases with wall thickening or appendicolith at the appendix base, there is absence of appendiceal luminal filling on postrectal saline administered T2W sequence and paired nonsaline and saline administered image can help differentiate the presence of acute appendicitis.

CLINICAL APPLICATIONS
Acute Appendicitis

Globally, acute appendicitis is one of the most common causes of acute abdomen and is the most common indication for surgery in children and pregnant patients (excluding the obstetric causes).[14,15] In the United States, around 300,000 appendectomies are performed annually.[15] For accurate diagnosis, a combination of clinical symptoms, physical examination, laboratory findings, and imaging is important. Typical clinical features of acute appendicitis include right lower quadrant pain, fever, nausea, and vomiting. Laboratory evidence of both white blood cell (WBC) count of greater than 10,000 mm-3 and C-reactive protein (CRP) level greater than 8 improves the diagnostic accuracy.[16] However, these findings are nonspecific and often not demonstrated in a pregnant patient. One of the features in pregnancy, for example, leukocytosis could be physiologic.

Per ACR appropriateness criteria, the imaging modality of choice for acute appendicitis in adults includes CT scan of abdomen and pelvis with the administration of IV contrast.[17] CT abdomen and pelvis without iv contrast and US are also considered appropriate. The sensitivity and specificity of CT range between 85.7% to 100% and 94.8% to 100%, respectively, and that of US range between 21% to 95.7% and 71.4% to 97.9%, respectively.[17] While CT is not suitable for the patients in whom exposure to ionizing radiation is of major concern, such as pregnant and pediatric populations, US is not an ideal investigation for obese or overweight patients.[18,19] An exception to this is graded compression US is the modality of choice in pregnant patients, even though the gravid uterus displacing the appendix upwards may interfere with proper examination.

MRI is a second-line investigation for pregnant patients and is preferred over CT in cases with equivocal or nondiagnostic US results.[9] MRI has reported sensitivity of 97% to 100% and specificity of 92% to 93.6% for the diagnosis of acute appendicitis.[20,21] The goals of MRI include the localization and visualization of the inflamed appendiceal wall as well as the presence of any peri-appendiceal fluid collection. Localization can be challenging in pregnant patients due to the displacement of the appendix by the gravid uterus. The inflamed appendiceal wall has a diameter of $\geq$ 7 mm and wall thickness of $\geq$ 2 mm and shows hypointense signal on T1WI and hyperintense signal on T2WI, relative to the skeletal muscle.[5] Coronal STIR and axial single-shot T2WI are sensitive for the detection of the inflamed appendix. In nonpregnant patients, fat-suppressed T1WI can be acquired before and after the administration of gadolinium-based contrast medium. The presence of peri appendiceal fluid signal usually indicates abscess formation and can also be demonstrated on postcontrast images (**Fig. 1**). MRI is useful in demonstrating direct signs of appendicitis such as thickened fluid-filled dilated appendix (see **Fig. 1**), wall thickening and enhancement, and indirect signs such as T2 hyperintense peri appendiceal stranding and enhancement, overlying peritoneal thickening, and enlarged mesenteric lymph nodes. Appendicolith may be demonstrated as T1 and T2 hypointense focus within the appendix lumen (**Fig. 2**). In suspected clinical cases with perforated appendicitis, a T2 hyperintense collection with peripheral wall enhancement in the right iliac fossa or pelvis favors ruptured appendix (**Fig. 3**). Additionally, DWI can be used for the characterization of the abscess and phlegmon with affected areas exhibiting restricted diffusion compared with normal and can be compared with ADC mapping. If none of the above-mentioned findings are evident on imaging, owing to higher soft-tissue details, MRI can assist in yielding an alternative diagnosis.

ACUTE PANCREATITIS

Acute pancreatitis is not an uncommon etiology encountered in emergency settings. The 2 most common etiologies of acute pancreatitis are gallstones and alcohol consumption. The clinical manifestations include severe and constant epigastric pain often radiating to the back, with associated nausea and vomiting. Laboratory findings include elevated serum levels of amylase and lipase. A combination of clinical and laboratory findings can clinch the primary diagnosis in most of the cases. Imaging is reserved for circumstances whereby the diagnosis cannot be made with certainty, visualize any potential complications, or if the patient's clinical condition fails to improve even after 72 hours of receiving appropriate management.[22]

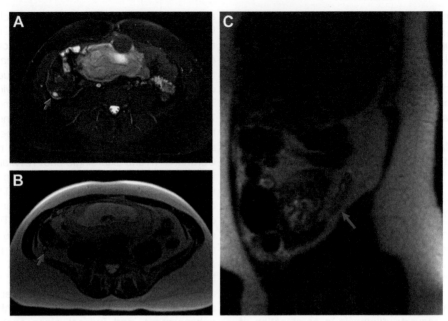

Fig. 1. MRI images (*A, B*) of an adult pregnant female presenting to the emergency department with acute right lower quadrant pain, nausea, and vomiting. Axial T2W fat-suppressed (*A*) and non–fat-suppressed SSFSE (*B*) images show dilated fluid-filled appendix (*red arrows*). Sagittal SSFSE image (*C*) shows tubular appendix with thickened wall.

Both contrast-enhanced CT and MRI are found to be equally effective for the initial assessment of acute pancreatitis.[23] However, MR cholangio-pancreatography (MRCP) is superior to contrast-enhanced CT for the anatomic depiction of the pancreatic duct and necrosis/collections. MRI and MRCP are useful for the detection of potential complications of pancreatitis such as pseudocyst formation and hemorrhagic pancreatitis. MRI is

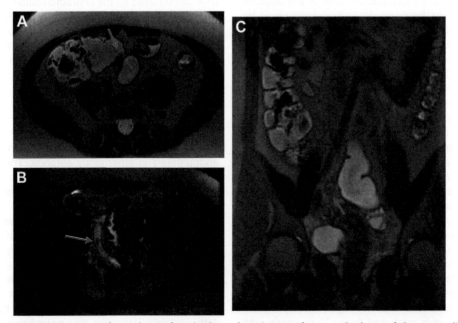

Fig. 2. Axial SSFSE (*A*) image of a pediatric female shows hypointense focus at the base of the appendix consistent with appendicolith (*red arrow*). The appendix is diffusely distended with fluid appearing hyperintense on axial fat-suppressed T2WI (*B*) with additional appendicolith (*red arrow*) also demonstrated on coronal SSFSE image (*C*).

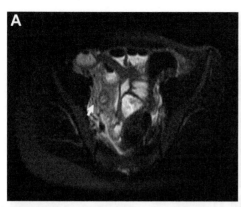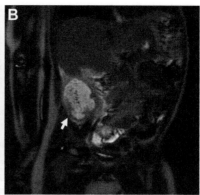

Fig. 3. Axial T2W fat-suppressed image (*A*) of a young female shows hyperintense dilated fluid-filled appendix with peri-appendiceal fluid and phlegmon (*white arrows*). Coronal fat-suppressed T2WI (*B*) showing a ruptured appendix with abscess in the right iliac fossa (*white arrows*).

also preferred over CT in situations whereby contrast cannot be administered.[24]

Normal pancreas seems hypointense on T2WI and hyperintense on fat-suppressed T1WI due to the presence of acinar proteins.[5,25] Axial fat-suppressed single-shot T2WI readily depicts the presence of edema, pancreatic or peripancreatic fluid collection, and any solid necrotic debris (**Fig. 4**). The inflammation is often extensive with elevated T2 signal intensity frequently observed beyond the pancreas into the adjacent peripancreatic soft tissues and even retroperitoneum. Hemorrhagic collections as seen in hemorrhagic pancreatitis or the presence of blood products within the pseudocyst demonstrate high signal intensity on fat-suppressed T1WI (**Fig. 5**).

BILIARY DISORDERS

Frequently encountered biliary disorders in emergency settings include cholelithiasis, acute cholecystitis, and choledocholithiasis commonly presenting as right upper quadrant abdominal pain. As per ACR appropriateness criteria, in acute settings, US is considered the imaging modality of choice for the evaluation of suspected biliary pathologies.[26,27] Right upper quadrant US allows for the evaluation of gall bladder, intrahepatic and extrahepatic bile ducts, and liver. When US findings are negative, or equivocal but clinical suspicion is still high, alternative imaging modalities can be utilized. MRI abdomen with MRCP, CT abdomen with iv contrast, and radionuclide imaging of gall bladder are the recommended second-line imaging modalities.[26] However, it is important to note that CT and radionuclide scans expose patients to ionizing radiation. CT scan additionally provides lower soft-tissue resolution than MRI.

Cholelithiasis is one of the commonest health problems in the United States with a prevalence of approximately 10% to 20%.[28] Only 1% to 4% of these patients are symptomatic and the rest are largely asymptomatic.[29] When symptomatic, biliary colic is the most presented symptom.[29] The US is extremely sensitive and specific for the diagnosis of uncomplicated gallstone disease making the utilization of other imaging techniques very rare. The possible complications of cholelithiasis include acute cholecystitis, choledocholithiasis, cholangitis, acute pancreatitis, and gallstone ileus.

Acute cholecystitis is the inflammation of the gall bladder. It most commonly occurs due to the obstruction of the cystic duct by a calculus. Acalculous etiologies account for 5% to 10% of the cases.[30] Clinical manifestations include right upper quadrant pain, fever, and usually a positive sonographic Murphy's sign. US remains the primary modality for acute cholecystitis. US findings consistent with the diagnosis are the presence of distended gallbladder with transverse diameter > 5 cm, thickened gallbladder wall (>3 mm), and pericholecystic fluid.[12] These findings can also be demonstrated adequately on MRI sequences such as fat-suppressed T2WI with high signal in gallbladder wall edema and pericholecystic fluid (see **Fig. 3**). Postcontrast T1-weighted sequences can show abnormal enhancement of thickened gallbladder wall. The absence of gallbladder wall enhancement can suggest gangrenous cholecystitis, a serious complication of acute cholecystitis usually seen in immunocompromised patients.

Choledocholithiasis typically results from the migration of gallstone(s) from the gallbladder to the common bile duct (CBD), potentially resulting in biliary obstruction. Primary CBD calculi are a rare occurrence. Mirizzi syndrome is caused by

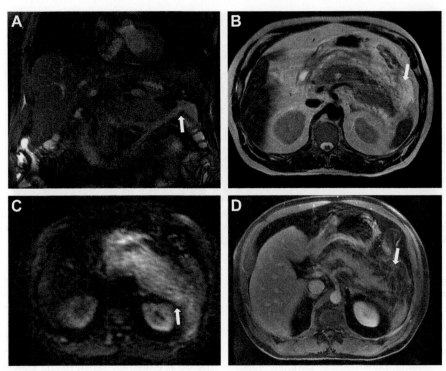

Fig. 4. Coronal T2 fat-suppressed (*A*) and axial T2 non–fat-suppressed (*B*) images show peripancreatic hyperintensity (white arrow) consistent with edema and fluid suggestive of acute edematous pancreatitis. Pancreas is diffusely edematous and restricts diffusion on axial DWI (*C*) image. Postcontrast T1 fat-suppressed (*D*) image shows enhancing septae (white arrow) within the peripancreatic region.

the external impression of CBD by impacted gallstones within the neck or Hartmann pouch of gallbladder. About 3% to 22% of all the cholecystectomies performed each year document the evidence of choledocholithiasis.[31,32] Unlike for the detection of cholelithiasis and acute cholecystitis, US reports relatively low sensitivity and specificity for the diagnosis of choledocholithiasis due to the presence of bowel gas. US and CT are limited in diagnosis of choledocholithiasis, suspected when CBD diameter ≥ 8 mm. MRCP demonstrates a sensitivity of 97% to 99% and specificity of 95% to 99% for the diagnostic evaluation of biliary duct abnormalities.[12] Heavily T2-weighted images of MRCP demonstrate biliary stones as filling defects (**Fig. 6**). Postcontrast T1-weighted images might provide further information on the degree of obstruction. However, the diagnostic accuracy of T2 MRCP and contrast-enhanced T1 images is comparable for the diagnosis of choledocholithiasis.[31,33] MRCP is also useful for the diagnosis of complications of biliary disorders such as Mirizzi syndrome and gangrenous cholecystitis.

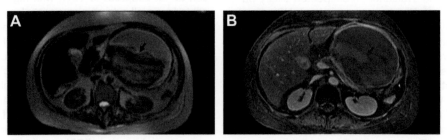

Fig. 5. Axial T2 WI image (*A*) of an adult female demonstrating well defined T2 hyperintense cyst with internal hemorrhage (*black arrow*) anterior to the pancreatic body and tail with evidence of peripheral enhancement (*blue arrow*) on postgadolinium T1WI (*B*).

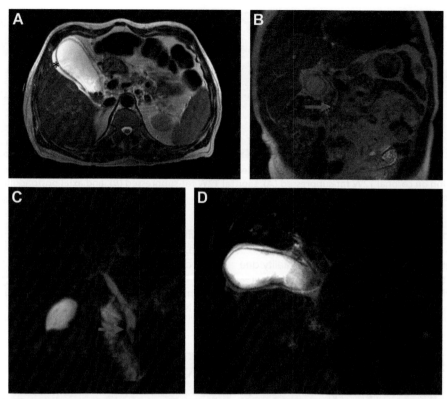

Fig. 6. Axial T2W MRI image (*A*) of an adult female presenting to emergency department with acute right upper quadrant pain, nausea, and vomiting showing T2 hypointense foci (*red arrow*) within the gallbladder lumen representing cholelithiasis with gallbladder wall edema (*asterisk*) consistent with acute cholecystitis. Coronal T2WI non–fat-suppressed (*B*) and MRCP image (*C*) showing evidence of stone in distal CBD (*blue arrow*). T2 hyperintense edema (*D*) within the gall bladder wall consistent with acute cholecystitis.

BOWEL DISORDERS

Crohn's disease is a chronic granulomatous inflammatory bowel disease with the second-highest prevalence in North America.[34] The incidence and prevalence of Crohn's disease are also on the rise globally.[34] The most frequently affected age group is 15 to 30 years old although few cases have also been reported in pediatric population.[7,35] The inflammatory process can essentially involve any part of the gastrointestinal tract from mouth to anus; however, it most typically involves the small bowel. Erosions, strictures, sinuses, fistulas are common associated findings.

Barium studies and MR enterography are common investigations that can be used early in the disease process. Limitations of barium studies include the inability to determine the extent of the disease and the inability to differentiate active disease from quiescent disease. MR enterography, on the other hand, can provide information on disease activity and bowel motility.

CT and MRI despite not being the ideal investigations for the establishment of early diagnosis,

are still valuable for the characterization of pathologic changes occurring over time, identification of extraintestinal manifestations, and guiding patient management. The sensitivity of both CT and MRI is greater than 95% with adequate bowel distension using intraluminal contrast.[36] T2WI can demonstrate bowel wall thickening, intramural inflammation, and mesenteric edema (**Fig. 7**). Differential diagnosis in colonic involvement of Crohn's disease could be clostridium difficile colitis frequently from prolonged hospitalization or antibiotics use (**Fig. 8**). The differential bowel wall enhancement on postcontrast T1WI can demonstrate fibrosis of the bowel wall, abscesses, sinuses, and fistulas. Whereas fibrosed/strictured bowel wall shows decreased contrast enhancement, abscesses display thickened circumferential peripheral enhancement, and sinuses/fistulas show enhancing linear tracts between adjacent structures (**Fig. 9**). Indeed, it is noteworthy that MRI with contrast is the imaging modality of choice for the detection/characterization of potential peri-anal and other bowel fistulous tracts, owing

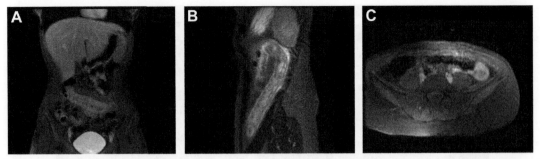

Fig. 7. An adult male patient with Crohn's disease demonstrating diffuse wall thickening of the descending and sigmoid colon on coronal T2W fat-suppressed (*A*), sagittal T2W fat-suppressed (*B*), and axial postgadolinium T1W fat-suppressed (*C*) images.

to its more sensitive evaluation of soft-tissue structures than CT.[37]

Although CT scan is the preferred modality due to shorter scan time, MRI sensitivity is 86% to 94% and specificity is 88% to 92% for acute diverticulitis.[38] Similar findings on MRI have been reported as with CT which include the presence of diverticula, bowel wall thickening, pericolic stranding, and complications such as peri-colonic abscess (see **Fig. 6**). Additionally, MRI can help identify alternative diagnoses whereby required. However, MRI is limited in its ability to percutaneously drain

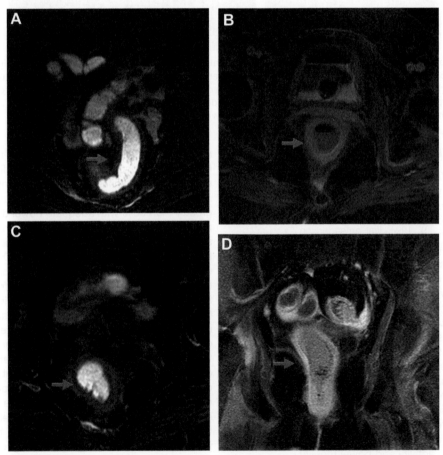

Fig. 8. Axial T2W fat-suppressed images (*A*, *B*) of an elderly female with clostridium difficile colitis following prolonged use of antibiotics show diffuse wall thickening of the rectosigmoid colon (red arrow) with evidence of enhancement on axial (*C*) and coronal (*D*) fat-suppressed postcontrast T1W image.

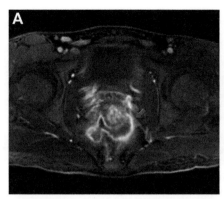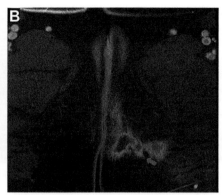

Fig. 9. Axial postgadoliniumT1 weighted fat-suppressed image (*A, B*) showing perianal abscess (*red arrow*) in the left ischiorectal fossa extending superiority into the perirectal region in a patient of Crohn's disease. The perianal fistula track is located at 5 o clock position on the left side.

abdominal abscesses and such applications could be further explored.

GYNECOLOGIC EMERGENCIES

OVARIAN TORSION: Ovarian torsion presents with acute onset lower abdominal or pelvic pain due to the twisting of the ovary over its supporting ligaments. Without prompt treatment, the ovary loses its vascular supply resulting in hemorrhagic infarction. Torsion is most typically associated with benign neoplasms such as mature cystic teratoma (**Fig. 10**). Enlarged corpus luteal cysts, malignant tumors, or developmental anomalies are other possible etiologies.[7] According to ACR appropriateness criteria, US is the recommended first-line imaging modality for the evaluation of adnexal lesions.[39] MR Imaging is considered second-line for cases with negative or inconclusive US findings. The presence of an enlarged ovary with thickened walls, edematous stroma, absence of contrast enhancement, evidence of hemorrhagic collections can be visualized with MRI sequences.[9] Incidence of ovarian torsion is increased with the presence of ovarian/adnexal masses. In a reproductive age female, certain cystic ovarian pathologies such as corpus luteal cyst, endometrioma, teratoma which could predispose to torsion can be diagnosed with MRI. A corpus luteum cyst is visualized as T1 hypointense and T2 hyperintense thin-walled cystic adnexal lesion without any solid component. An endometrioma can show fluid levels within the thin wall cyst corresponding to various stages of hemorrhage and seen as "T2 shading" on T2WI (**Fig. 11**). Mature cystic teratoma classically

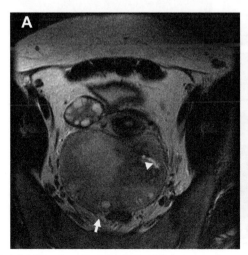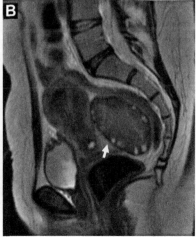

Fig. 10. Axial (*A*) and sagittal (*B*) T2W MRI images of a reproductive age female with ovarian torsion demonstrating bulky and centrally heterogeneous left ovary r(white arrow) epresenting hemorrhage with peripherally arranged follicles. The vascular pedicle can be seen on the left side (arrow head).

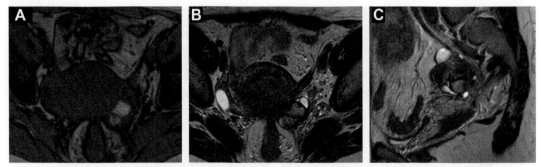

Fig. 11. T1W axial (*A*) and T2W axial (*B*) and sagittal (*C*) images of a reproductive age female show T1 hyperintense and T2 hyperintense cysts in the left adnexa with evidence of T2 shading consistent with endometriomas.

includes all 3 germ layers and shows fluid, fat and solid component (**Fig. 12**).

TUBO-OVARIAN ABSCESS: Tubo-ovarian abscesses result as a complication of pelvic inflammatory disease (PID). Sexually active young females are most susceptible to PID and thereby to tubo-ovarian abscesses. The signs and symptoms are nonspecific and include pelvic pain, vaginal discharge, abnormal vaginal bleeding.[40] MRI is considered superior to US for the

demonstration of the changes consistent with PID.[9] Tubo-ovarian abscess is visualized as complex adnexal cyst/mass with fluid-filled thick-walled fallopian tubes and abscess walls demonstrated well on T2WI and postcontrast T1WI (**Fig. 13**).

DEGENERATING FIBROIDS: Fibroids are benign tumors arising from the myometrium of the uterus and are most common in reproductive-age women. Fibroids are often

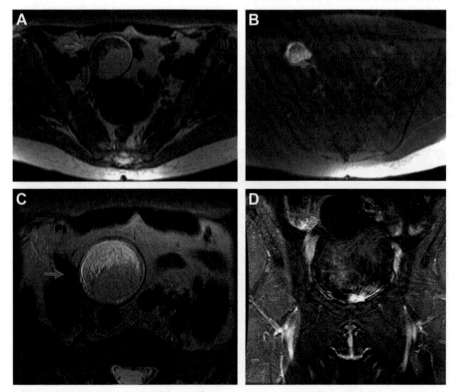

Fig. 12. Axial T1W (*A*) and coronal T2W (*B*) non–fat-suppressed images of an adult female show hyperintense right ovarian cystic mass (red *arrow*) with signal suppression on T1W fat-suppressed (*C*) images. Postcontrast T1W fat-suppressed images show no enhancing solid component within the lesion (red arrow) suggesting ovarian dermoid.

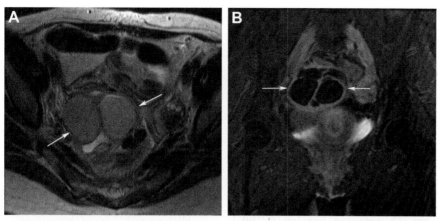

Fig. 13. Axial T2 non fat suppressed image (*A*) of an adult female with right tubo-ovarian abscess shows a complex T2 hyperintense cystic mass within the right adnexa (*white arrows*). Peripheral enhancement is noted on axial post gadolinium T1W fat suppressed images (*B*).

multiple, and based on their location, can be classified as submucosal, intramural, or subserosal. Fibroids can be asymptomatic or can present with lower abdominal pain, abnormal uterine bleeding, or pressure symptoms. Large fibroids eventually undergo degeneration due to an inadequate supply of blood or nutrients. Degenerating fibroids present with acute abdominal pain. MRI is sensitive for the detection of fibroid and related complications. The hyperintense signal in the

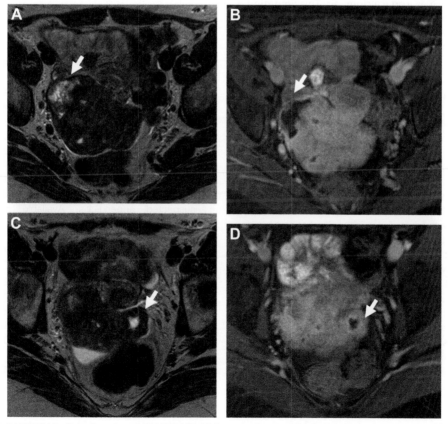

Fig. 14. Axial T2W (*A, C*) and postcontrast T1W (*B, D*) images show multiple heterogenous uterine fibroids with evidence of cystic degeneration appearing as areas of T2 hyperintensity and T1 hypointensity (*white arrow*).

fibroids on T1WI and T2WI could represent areas of hemorrhage, while hyperintense signal only on T2WI could indicate the presence of edema **(Fig. 14)**. Degenerating fibroids demonstrate comparatively less and heterogenous contrast enhancement compared with solid fibroids.[9]

CLINICS CARE POINTS

- MRI protocols can be tailored to the clinical presentation of the patient and suspected pathology; however, T2 weighted imaging (T2WI) and T1 weighted imaging (T1WI) with contrast are the most diagnostically useful sequences in an emergency radiology setting.

- In an acute setting use of gadolinium-based IV contrast is particularly beneficial in situations such as bile leak, inflammatory bowel wall thickening, and intraabdominal abscesses.

- T1WI is motion sensitive, requires a breath-hold for about 15 to 20 seconds and can be affected by susceptibility artifacts from materials such as iron, calcium, air. This limitation can be addressed by using shorted echo times.

DISCLOSURE

The authors have nothing to disclose.

REFERENCES

1. Laméris W, van Randen A, Van Es HW, et al. Imaging strategies for detection of urgent conditions in patients with acute abdominal pain: diagnostic accuracy study. BMJ 2009;338.
2. Bhuiya FA, Pitts SR, McCaig LF. Emergency department visits for chest pain and abdominal pain: United States, 1999-2008. NCHS Data Brief 2010; 43:1–8.
3. Aldrich JE, Bilawich AM, Mayo JR. Radiation doses to patients receiving computed tomography examinations in British Columbia. Can Assoc Radiol J 2006;57:79–85.
4. Ditkofsky NG, Singh A, Avery L, et al. The role of emergency MRI in the setting of acute abdominal pain. Emerg Radiol 2014;21(6):615–24.
5. Yu HS, Gupta A, Soto JA, et al. Emergency abdominal MRI: current uses and trends. Br J Radiol 2016; 89(1061):20150804.
6. Heverhagen JT, Ishaque N, Zielke A, et al. Feasibility of MRI in the diagnosis of acute diverticulitis: initial results. MAGMA 2001;12:4–9.
7. Heverhagen JT, Klose KJ. MR imaging for acute lower abdominal and pelvic pain. Radiographics 2009;29(6):1781–96.
8. Pedrosa I, Zeikus EA, Levine D, et al. MR imaging of acute right lower quadrant pain in pregnant and nonpregnant patients. RadioGraphics 2007;27: 721–43.
9. Singh A, Danrad R, Hahn PF, et al. MR imaging of the acute abdomen and pelvis: acute appendicitis and beyond. RadioGraphics 2007;27:1419–31.
10. Patel SJ, Reede DL, Katz DS, et al. Imaging the pregnant patient for non-obstetric conditions: algorithms and radiation dose considerations. RadioGraphics 2007;27:1705–22.
11. SemelkaRC, Balci NC, Op de Beeck B, et al. Evaluation of a 10-minute comprehensive MR imaging examination of the upper abdomen. Radiology 1999; 211(1):189–95.
12. Tkacz JN, Anderson SA, Soto J. MR imaging in gastrointestinal emergencies. Radiographics 2009; 29(6):1767–80.
13. Bouman DE, Wiarda BM. Diffusion-weighted imaging of acute abdominal and pelvic pain [abstr]. In: Radiological Society of North America scientific assembly and annual meeting program. Oak Brook, Ill: Radiological Society of North America; 2008. p. 845.
14. Glass CC, Rangel SJ. Overview and diagnosis of acute appendicitis in children. Semin Pediatr Surg 2016;25(No. 4):198–203. WB Saunders.
15. Snyder MJ, Guthrie M, Cagle SD. Acute appendicitis: efficient diagnosis and management. Am Fam Physician 2018;98(1):25–33.
16. Cole MA, Maldonado N. Evidence-based management of suspected appendicitis in the emergency department. Emerg Med Pract 2011;13(10):1–29.
17. Smith MP, Katz DS, Rosen MP, et al. ACR appropriateness criteria®—right lower quadrant pain—suspected appendicitis. Available at: https://acsearch.acr.org/docs/69357/Narrative. Accessed October 2015.
18. Kotagal M, Richards MK, Flum DR, et al. Use and accuracy of diagnostic imaging in the evaluation of pediatric appendicitis. J Pediatr Surg 2015;50(4): 642–6.
19. Schuh S, Man C, Cheng A, et al. Predictors of non-diagnostic ultra-sound scanning in children with suspected appendicitis. J Pediatr 2011;158(1): 112–8.
20. NittaN, Takahashi M, Furukawa A, et al. MR imaging of the normal appendix and acute appendicitis. J Magn Reson Imaging 2005;21(2):156–65.
21. IncesuL, Coskun A, Selcuk MB, et al. Acute appendicitis: MR imaging and sonographic correlation. AJR Am J Roentgenol 1997;168(3):669–74.

22. James TW, Crockett SD. Management of acute pancreatitis in the first 72 hours. Curr Opin Gastroenterol 2018;34(5):330.

23. Štimac D, Miletic D, Radic M, et al. The role of non-enhanced magnetic resonance imaging in the early assessment of acute pancreatitis. Official J Am Coll Gastroenterol ACG 2007;102(5):997–1004.

24. Wongwaisayawan S, Kaewlai R, Dattwyler M, et al. Magnetic resonance of pelvic and gastrointestinal emergencies. Magn Reson Imaging Clin 2016;24(2):419–31.

25. Miller FH, Keppke AL, Dalal K, et al. MRI of pancreatitis and its complications: part 1, acute pancreatitis. Am J Roentgenol 2004;183(6):1637–44.

26. American College of Radiology. ACR appropriateness criteria: right upper quadrant pain. 2013. Available at: https://acsearch.acr.org/docs/69474/Narrative/. Accessed January 26, 2018.

27. Joshi G, Crawford KA, Hanna TN, et al. US of right upper quadrant pain in the emergency department: diagnosing beyond gallbladder and biliary disease. Radiographics 2018;38(3):766–93.

28. Pak M, Lindseth G. Risk factors for cholelithiasis. Gastroenterol Nurs 2016;39(4):297–309.

29. Sanders G, Kingsnorth AN. Gallstones. Bmj 2007; 335(7614):295–9.

30. Meacock LM, Sellars ME, Sidhu PS. Evaluation of gallbladder and biliary duct disease using microbubble contrast-enhanced ultrasound. Br J Radiol 2010;83(991):615–27.

31. Gurusamy KS, Giljaca V, Takwoingi Y, et al. Ultrasound versus liver function tests for diagnosis of common bile duct stones. Cochrane Database Syst Rev 2015;(2).

32. Molvar C, Glaenzer B. Choledocholithiasis: Evaluation, Treatment, and Outcomes. Semin Intervent Radiol 2016 Dec;33(4):268–76. https://doi.org/10.1055/s-0036-1592329.

33. Choi IY, Yeom SK, Cha SH, et al. Diagnosis of biliary stone disease: T1-weighted magnetic resonance cholangiography with Gd-EOB-DTPA versus T2-weighted magnetic resonance cholangiography. Clin Imaging 2014;38(2):164–9.

34. Molodecky NA, Soon S, Rabi DM, et al. Increasing incidence and prevalence of the inflammatory bowel diseases with time, based on systematic review. Gastroenterology 2012;142(1):46–54.

35. Ali S, Tamboli CP. Advances in epidemiology and diagnosis of inflammatory bowel diseases. Curr Gastroenterol Rep 2008;10:576–84.

36. Furukawa A, Saotome T, Yamasaki M, et al. Cross-sectional imaging in Crohn disease. Radiographics 2004;24(3):689–702.

37. Buchanan GN, Halligan S, Bartram CI, et al. Clinical examination, endosonography, and MR imaging in preoperative assessment of fistula in ano: comparison with outcome-based reference standard. Radiology 2004;233(3):674–81.

38. Destigter KK, Keating DP. Imaging update: acute colonic diverticulitis. Clin Colon Rectal Surg 2009; 22(3):147–55. https://doi.org/10.1055/s-0029-1236158.

39. https://acsearch.acr.org/docs/69503/Narrative/ (Accessed 31 March 2022.).

40. Sweet RL. Pelvic inflammatory disease: current concepts of diagnosis and management. Curr Infect Dis Rep 2012;14(2):194–203.

Magnetic Resonance Imaging of Acute Abdominal Pain in the Pregnant Patient

Abigail D. Stanley, BM[a],*, Miltiadis Tembelis, MD[b], Michael N. Patlas, MD, FRCPC[c], Mariam Moshiri, MD[d], Margarita V. Revzin, MD, MS[e], Douglas S. Katz, MD[b]

KEYWORDS

• MR imaging • Pregnancy • Acute abdomen • Abdominal pain • Appendicitis

KEY POINTS

- Evaluating the pregnant patient with acute abdominal pain can be difficult due to alterations in normal physiology, the inherent limited capability of ultrasound, particularly during pregnancy, and the need to limit radiation exposure.
- MR imaging can be used to accurately diagnose most abdominal and pelvic pathologies in the pregnant patient without posing a risk to the mother or to the fetus.
- All radiologists should have current information regarding performing and interpreting MR imaging of the pregnant patient.

INTRODUCTION
Discussion of Problem/Clinical Presentation

Compared with nonpregnant patients, pregnant patients who present with acute abdominal pain can be difficult to evaluate and accurately diagnose both clinically and radiologically due to the physiologic changes that occur during pregnancy and the challenges of choosing the imaging modalities that are safest for the mother and the fetus. This article aims to review some common as well as uncommon causes of nonobstetric abdominal pain in pregnancy and discusses various imaging options for the evaluation of pregnant patients with acute abdominal abnormalities, including the utility and risks associated with each imaging modality. Pathologies discussed in this article include some of the more common gastrointestinal, hepatobiliary, genitourinary, and gynecologic causes of abdominal pain occurring in pregnancy, as well as traumatic injuries.

NORMAL ANATOMY AND IMAGING TECHNIQUE
Discussion of Important Anatomic Considerations

When interpreting cross-sectional imaging in a pregnant patient including abdominal and pelvic MRI, pregnancy-related alterations in anatomy and physiology must be considered. Some of the changes become noticeable within the first few weeks of pregnancy, and may not subside until a few weeks post partum.[1,2] The most obvious of these is the displacement of anatomic structures by the gravid uterus, which becomes

---

[a] NYIT College of Osteopathic Medicine, Old Westbury, 101 Northern Boulvard, Glen Head, NY 11545, USA; [b] Department of Radiology, NYU Langone Hospital, 222 Station Plaza North, Suite 501, Mineola, NY 11501, USA; [c] Department of Radiology, McMaster University, Hamilton General Hospital, 237 Barton Street, East Hamilton, ON L8L 2X2, Canada; [d] Department of Radiology, Vanderbilt University Medical Center, 1161-21st Avenue, South Medical Center North CCC-117, Nashville, TN 37232, USA; [e] Department of Radiology and Biomedical Imaging, Yale University, 330 Cedar Street, New Haven, CT 06520, USA
* Corresponding author.
E-mail address: astanley@nyit.edu

Magn Reson Imaging Clin N Am 30 (2022) 515–532
https://doi.org/10.1016/j.mric.2022.04.010

progressively larger as the pregnancy progresses, complicating interpretations of findings as well as adding difficulty to the accurate identification of structures. The uterus can reach volumes of up to 5L just before delivery when these changes are the most apparent. Additionally, adnexal vessels enlarge, making accurate identification and evaluation of the adjacent bowel, particularly the appendix, whether normal or abnormal, more challenging. Along with the mass effect from the gravid uterus, hormonal changes can also induce alterations in anatomy as well as affect laboratory data. Data points such as leukocytosis, which would normally support a specific radiological diagnosis, are no longer as helpful as this is a natural response to pregnancy itself.[2] In addition, symptoms that would be more alarming in nonpregnant patients can frequently be seen as normal consequences of pregnancy, particularly nausea, vomiting, and pelvic pain.

Some relative common anatomic considerations are listed below[1-3]:

- Cephalad displacement of the appendix
- Displacement of the intra-abdominal aorta into the thorax
- Dilation of the urinary tract
- Temporary esophageal varices
- Colonic compression
- Decreased lower esophageal sphincter tone
- Decreased gastrointestinal motility leading to constipation
- Compression of inferior vena cava and common iliac veins

Imaging Protocols

When imaging pregnant patients, nonionizing modalities are strongly preferred if possible due to concerns for both fetal and maternal safety. The Radiological Society of North America (RSNA), in a statement made on the safety of medical imaging during pregnancy, suggested that "MRI and ultrasound (US; sonography) are types of imaging that do not use ionizing radiation and are regarded as safe to the fetus in normal clinical usage, that is, ≤ 3T MRI and without prolonged use of color/power Doppler in the first trimester." As per the US Food and Drug Administration (FDA), MRI has not been studied well enough to be considered nonharmful, although most data suggest this to be accurate.[4] As per the American College of Radiology (ACR) MR guidelines: "Present data have not conclusively documented any deleterious effects of MR imaging exposure on the developing fetus. Therefore, no special consideration is recommended for the first, versus any other, trimester in pregnancy."[5] Much of the risk is theoretic and

based on the exposure of the fetus to the electromagnetic field, potentially creating thermal injury to the fetus.[6,7] There is also concern of auditory complications to the fetus due to the noise from the MR unit. Multiple studies have shown no risk of subsequent hearing loss, however, as with many other MR studies on teratogenicity, they lack long-term follow-up.[8]

Gadolinium-based intravenous contrast agents are used in standard MR imaging in nonpregnant patients. As these agents are water soluble and have the potential to cross the placental barrier, they will enter the amniotic fluid chelated, but through time will dechelate and become toxic resulting in continuous exposure of the fetus while *in utero*. Gadolinium is classified as a category C drug by the FDA and can only be administered if absolutely necessary.[4] The ACR Manual on Contrast Media (2021) states that gadolinium "should be administered only when there is a potential significant benefit to the patient or fetus that outweighs the possible but unknown risk of fetal exposure to free gadolinium ions."[5,9] Much of the data regarding the teratogenic effects of gadolinium are in animal or cell models using higher doses and concentrations and does not necessarily translate to human fetuses. However, Ray and colleagues, in their study conducted in 2016, which aimed to assess the harmful effects of gadolinium during pregnancy, used 12 years of data and over 1,400,000 births and found a substantial increase in the risk of fetal rheumatological, inflammatory, and infiltrative skin conditions with the use of intravenous (IV) gadolinium, but no increased risk of fetal harm with nonenhanced MRI.[8] In addition, recent studies have shown the deposition of gadolinium in the dentate nucleus and globus pallidus of adult nonpregnant patients who have received IV contrast for MR examinations, but the extent and effects of this deposition are of unclear significance to date to our knowledge.

Generally, during pregnancy, noncontrast abdominal and pelvic MR protocols are used for imaging the acute abdomen for nonfetal and nonobstetric causes and rely on fast, multiplanar (typically axial and coronal) heavily T2-weighted sequences performed with and without fat saturation. These are supplemented by gradient-recalled echo (GRE) flow-sensitive sequences along with axial gradient-echo T1 in-phase and out-of-phase sequences. Scanning time is limited as pregnant patients may not tolerate long examinations and often at the authors' institutions, T2 images are obtained in various planes and only a single T1 sequence is obtained primarily to evaluate for hemorrhage. Neither IV nor oral contrast

Table 1
Differential diagnosis for acute abdominal pain in pregnancy (nonobstetric)

Site of Pain	Imaging Modality/Modalities of Choice for Diagnosis or Exclusion
Upper abdomen	

Biliary disease
    Cholelithiasis
    Cholecystitis
	US, noncontrast MR/MRCP as needed

Pancreatitis	US, noncontrast MR as needed
Bowel obstruction	US, noncontrast MR as needed
Hepatic steatosis	US
HELLP syndrome	US, noncontrast MR or CT as needed
Pyelonephritis (flank pain)	US, noncontrast MR as needed
Lower abdomen	
Appendicitis	US, noncontrast MR as needed
Urolithiasis (location of pain varies)	US, noncontrast MR as needed
Cystitis	US
Inflammatory bowel disease	Noncontrast MR
Gynecologic causes (non-obstetrical)	
Ovarian torsion	US, noncontrast MR as needed
Adnexal masses	US, noncontrast MR as needed
Trauma	US (FAST), CT if indicated
Malignancy	US, MR, or CT

Abbreviation: FAST, focused assessment with sonography in trauma.

is given, and a limited number of sequences necessary to establish or exclude a particular diagnosis should be obtained first. Ideally, the interpreting radiologist should review the images before releasing the patient from the MR scanner. The images should be checked for inclusion of the relevant anatomy and for motion artifacts of the mother and the fetus, which could limit diagnostic accuracy.

Use of this type of protocol is sufficient for most of the common acute nonobstetric disorders that can present in pregnancy, particularly appendicitis, urinary tract disorders, and bowel obstruction. Dedicated magnetic resonance cholangiopancreatography (MRCP)/MR urography sequences can also be added as needed. If there is concern for ovarian torsion or other adnexal disorders, noncontrast pelvic MR can be performed without the abdominal component, and similarly abdominal MR alone can be obtained if the consideration is hepatobiliary and pancreatic pathology. For known or suspected inflammatory bowel disease (IBD), either limited sequence noncontrast abdominal and pelvic MR can be performed, or if the patient's condition allows, then MR enterography, with oral but not IV contrast material, can be obtained. In the setting of trauma, very occasionally noncontrast MR is obtained for follow-up, or for initial evaluation in a stable, carefully selected patient following US examination.

Generally, imaging with a 1.5T magnet is preferred as the majority of studies on MR imaging in the pregnant patient have been conducted with this magnetic field strength. 3T magnets are now FDA approved for imaging of pregnant patients, and to our knowledge, no data have suggested potential teratogenic or other negative or adverse effects of the larger field strength magnets. The 3 T magnets, however, are usually avoided due to the theoretic risk of increased thermal energy exposure of the fetus, as well as increased noise produced by these magnets discussed previously (**Table 1**).

Imaging Findings in Disease Processes

Gastrointestinal disease

Appendicitis Appendicitis is the most common nonobstetric cause of acute abdominal pain in the pregnant patient and is the most common nonobstetric indication for surgery in pregnancy. The estimation of the incidence of acute appendicitis in pregnant patients varies widely and has been reported from 1 in 766 pregnancies to 4 in 1000.[10,11] The presenting signs and symptoms are often difficult to discern from the normal abdominal tenderness and nausea of pregnancy as well as many

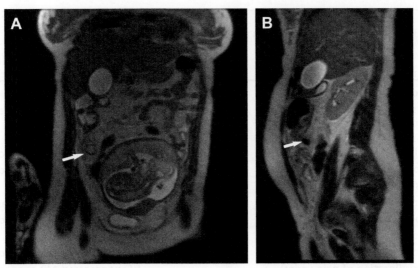

Fig. 1. A 38-year-old woman at 21 weeks gestation presented with recurrent umbilical pain radiating to the right lower quadrant. MR was performed due to concerns of appendicitis. (*A*) Coronal T2 image showed a markedly dilated fluid-filled retrocecal appendix (*arrow*) measuring 2 cm in diameter. (*B*) Sagittal T2 image demonstrated an appendicolith (*arrow*). There were no findings to suggest perforation or abscess on MR. Laparoscopic appendectomy was performed, which revealed perforation with local peritonitis.

other signs and symptoms of pregnancy itself. Identification of the appendix on MR can be difficult in a nonpregnant patient, and it is even more challenging in pregnant patients due to the anatomic changes mentioned previously. Graded-compression US is generally used first, but based on a 5-year, single-institute study analyzing patients in all stages of pregnancy, it has a sensitivity of only 46.1% for the diagnosis of appendicitis in this patient population. Another single-institution study found the sensitivity to be as low as 28.7% when performed in the second and third trimesters of pregnancy. Performing US may also somewhat further delay diagnosis and treatment, which can raise the risk of morbidity and mortality to the fetus.[12,13] A meta-analysis containing data from 2400 patients demonstrated MR to be far superior in the diagnosis of acute appendicitis in pregnant patients, with a sensitivity and specificity of 91.8% and 97.9%, respectively.[14] In the nonpregnant patient population, the nonvisualization of the appendix on MR has been shown to have good negative predictive value in an otherwise good-quality examination. This finding may also be true in pregnancy despite the common cephalad displacement of the appendix, which progresses with advancing pregnancy. A study based on 233 pregnant women over 13 years found no instances of appendicitis when the appendix was not visualized on MR. In addition, the interobserver agreement when assessing for appendicitis in the study was nearly perfect, with a kappa value of 0.917.[15]

In the past, oral contrast was given at some institutions to aid in the diagnosis of acute appendicitis on MR, but it is now most commonly avoided given the documented high sensitivity and specificity of MRI without its administration, as well as the reduction in scanning time with noncontrast-enhanced MR.[14] The normal appendix appears as a tubular blind-ending structure at the base of the cecum and is usually larger than 6 mm in diameter. If larger, then suspicion should be raised for appendicitis (**Fig. 1**A). Shin and colleagues, in a study of 125 patients showed a positive predictive value of 97.6% for identification of a normal appendix when filled with T1 bright content, and therefore, if the appendix is borderline in size (6–7 mm), visualization of bright intraluminal contents of the appendix on T1 may be helpful.[16] Appendiceal wall thickness is also a critical indicator for assessment of appendicitis, and if the wall is thicker than normal (2 mm), then further search for other supportive MR findings of appendicitis is warranted. Once the appendix is correctly identified, the T2 hypointense wall should be well contrasted against the more T2 hyperintense periappendical fat and the intraluminal contents. On T2WI, a bright, fluid-filled, and distended appendix is usually considered abnormal and indicates appendicitis. Periappendical fat inflammation is another strongly supportive finding of appendicitis which is best visualized on T2-weighted fat-suppressed MR images. Appendicoliths can be visualized as low signal structures in the lumen of the appendix on T2-WI (**Fig. 1**B).

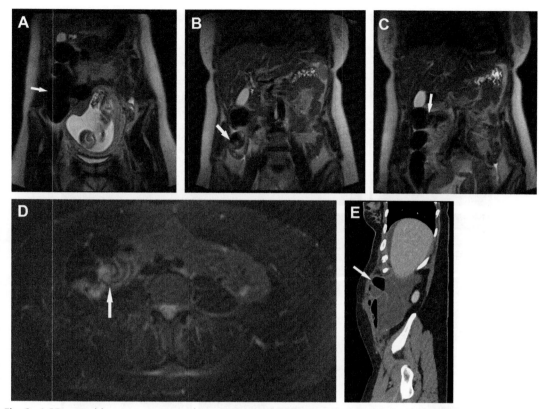

Fig. 2. A 37-year-old woman at 16 weeks gestation with history of ulcerative colitis following total proctocolectomy with reversal of ileostomy and prior small bowel obstruction, presented with abdominal pain and nausea. Coronal HASTE MR image showed dilated small bowel loops measuring up to 4 cm (*arrow*) (*A*) with multiple transition points (*arrows*) (*B, C*). Axial T2 fat-saturated image showed swirling mesenteric vessels (*arrow*) (*D*). These findings suggested a closed-loop small bowel obstruction. The patient was managed conservatively due to immediate improvement in symptoms. (*E*) CT of the abdomen and pelvis with oral and IV contrast performed 6 months post partum demonstrated a subsequent small bowel volvulus (*arrow*), which required surgical intervention.

With acute perforation, a T2 intermediate intensity ill-defined collection can be seen in the expected location of the appendix.

In the nonpregnant patient, leukocytosis is an ancillary finding in the diagnosis of acute appendicitis. However, as mentioned previously, the physiologic leukocytosis found in pregnancy can make this marker less sensitive in the pregnant population. Gentles and colleagues, in a 2020 retrospective study, examined neutrophil count in pregnant patients undergoing MR for suspected acute appendicitis and found that a left shift with neutrophils greater than 70% provided a sensitivity and negative predictive value of 100.0%.[17]

Bowel obstruction and inflammatory bowel disease Small bowel obstruction (SBO) is an uncommon cause of acute abdominal pain in the pregnant patient, but the incidence is somewhat increasing.[18] As in nonpregnant adults, the most common cause of SBO in the pregnant population

is adhesive disease. Additionally, as the incidence of bariatric surgery increases in women of childbearing age, the risk of adhesive disease during pregnancy increases as well.[18] Although US is commonly used for the initial evaluation of suspected bowel obstruction in pregnancy, it has substantial limitations, and therefore, noncontrast MR is the next imaging modality of choice. Although the usual imaging protocol for suspected SBO would include administration of gadolinium, it is not advisable to use in a pregnant patient, as noted above. Accurate interpretations and diagnoses can still be made without IV gadolinium, and MRI will show dilated bowel loops with a transition to bowel decompression, along with any associated complications and underlying etiologies (e.g., strictures, hernia, masses) (**Fig. 2**).

Adhesions can also develop as a complication of IBD. Although the incidence of IBD in pregnancy is similar to that in the nonpregnant population, there may be an increased severity of flare-ups

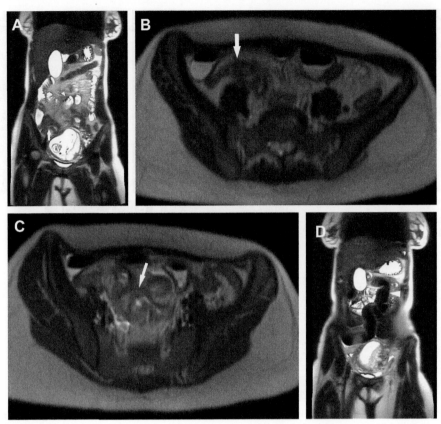

Fig. 3. A 26-year-old woman at 13 weeks gestation with a history of Crohn's disease presented with abdominal pain and emesis. The patient had an MR done elsewhere, which showed fistulizing Crohn's disease with small bowel obstruction that was managed nonoperatively. Coronal (*A*) and axial (*B*) HASTE MR images obtained at the time of admission showed distal ileal thickening (*arrow*), as well as fistualization of multiple bowel loops (*arrow*) (*C*). Proximal dilated small bowel loops, best seen on the coronal images, due to bowel obstruction (*arrowhead*) (*D*) were also noted. The patient was managed conservatively and improved clinically.

during pregnancy for those with preexisting IBD. Additionally, the first severe episode of IBD often occurs during the reproductive years. The MRI protocol for the assessment of the extent of IBD usually includes administration of oral contrast, which allows for better resolution and identification of the bowel wall, but its usage depends on whether the clinical condition of the patient allows for a more prolonged examination. Parameters to consider, specifically for Crohn's disease, include bowel wall edema with a thickness of 3 mm or greater, and stranding of fat planes adjacent to the bowel.[19] Findings may also include high signal intensity of the bowel wall and the fat planes on T2-WI. Complications may include obstruction, stricture, abscess formation, and fistulas (**Fig. 3**). The absence of oral and IV contrast limits MR evaluation of Crohn-related changes as underdistention of the bowel due to the lack of intraluminal contrast may potentially compromise the interpretation of the findings. For example, an inflamed, thickened bowel wall may be mistaken for normal collapsed bowel loops and vice versa; however, studies show that noncontrast MR still allows for meaningful interpretation and diagnosis.[19] Once diagnosed and assessed, appropriate management can be administered.

Hepatobiliary tract emergencies Biliary tract-related diseases causing acute abdominal pain in pregnancy include cholelithiasis and its potential complications, namely, cholecystitis, cholangitis, and pancreatitis. Cholelithiasis has a higher prevalence in pregnant women, thought to be related to biliary stasis and reduced gallbladder contraction.[20] Cholelithiasis alone does not require acute intervention but can eventually lead to a range of complications involving the obstruction of the biliary and pancreatic ductal system. As a result, proper recognition of gallstones and documentation is important. Biliary colic, caused by temporary obstruction of the gallbladder by gallstones,

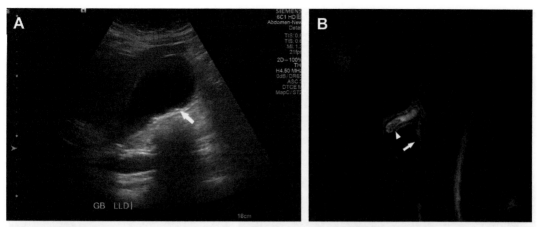

Fig. 4. A 34-year-old woman presented at 3 weeks post partum with right upper quadrant abdominal pain. (*A*) Transabdominal ultrasound showed gallstones (*arrow*) in a distended gallbladder without sonographic evidence of acute cholecystitis. Due to continued pain and elevated liver enzymes, MR/MRCP was performed. (*B*) Coronal thick-slab MRCP showed gallstones (*arrow*) and a large amount of periportal edema (*arrowhead*) diagnostic of cholecystitis. The patient underwent an uncomplicated laparoscopic cholecystectomy.

may arise causing temporary right upper quadrant (RUQ) pain, usually occurring after eating and eventually subsiding when the calculus or calculi pass into the common bile duct (CBD) or return to the gallbladder.

As in nonpregnant patients, US is the initial imaging modality of choice for suspected biliary disease, and usually can accurately reveal biliary dilatation, however, in some patients, findings may be equivocal or nondiagnostic. This is particularly common for choledocholithiasis and pancreatic disease.[21,22] In such instances, MR, and especially MRCP, are commonly used to help clarify any equivocal or inconclusive biliary finding on US (**Fig. 4**). The use of heavily T2-weighted sequences will show bright bile and allow for proper visualization of the biliary and pancreatic ducts, as in nonpregnant patients. In all patients, emergent MRCP may be indicated based on the extent of duct dilation seen on US, or substantial elevation of liver function tests and bilirubin supplementing the US findings.

Gallstones are best recognized on T2-WI as signal voids in the biliary tract. Depending on the stone composition, the MRI appearance is variable. For example, cholesterol stones have low SI on both single-shot fast spin-echo (SSFSE) T2 and 3D fast-spoiled-gradient-echo T1-WI whereas pigment stones usually demonstrate low SI on SSFSE T2 and high SI on 3D fast-spoiled-gradient-echo T1-WI.[23] On MR, biliary obstruction is noted when the intrahepatic biliary ducts measure greater than 3 mm in diameter. However, the absence of dilatation does not exclude obstruction, especially at early stages of the

disease (**Fig. 5**). A CBD diameter of 6 mm or more in a patient without prior cholecystectomy should arouse suspicion for biliary obstruction. Biliary dilation can be easily detected on T2-WI and MRCP as both of these sequences are shown to have very high sensitivity for assessment of biliary dilation and for the demonstration of an obstructive calculus.[24]

A common complication of cholelithiasis is acute cholecystitis, accounting for up to 10% of hospital admissions for acute abdominal pain in any patient population, and is the second most common disease resulting in emergent surgery in the pregnant patient.[3] Approximately 95% of acute cholecystitis results from gallstone impaction in the gallbladder neck, resulting in RUQ pain, fever, nausea, and leukocytosis.[25] The imaging findings of acute cholecystitis are very similar amongst all cross-sectional imaging modalities, and include gallbladder wall thickening, pericholecystic fluid, and gallbladder wall inflammation (see **Fig. 5**).[26,27] Gallbladder wall thickening, greater than 3 mm on T2-weighted images, is not a specific finding as it can also be seen in chronic cholecystitis, malignancy, and various other hepatobiliary pathologies. The use of fat-suppressed T2-WI can help distinguish acute from chronic inflammation, which would suggest acute cholecystitis by the presence of patchy bright foci in the thickened gallbladder wall.[26] The inflammatory process may also spread into the adjacent pericholecystic fat as demonstrated by high pericholecystic signals on fat-suppressed T2-WI. Free pericholecystic fluid, or fluid around the liver creating the C-sign as it

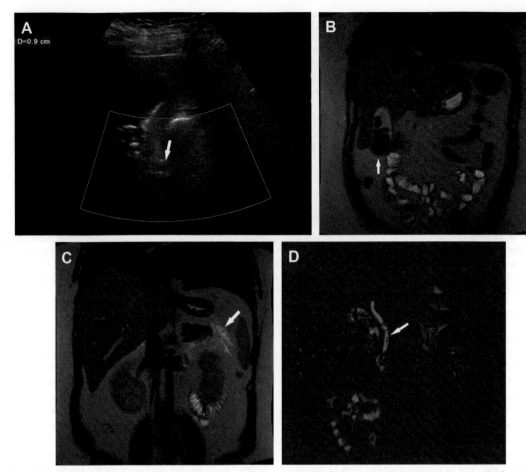

Fig. 5. A 24-year-old woman presented at 11 weeks gestation with post-prandial epigastric pain, leukocytosis, and a serum lipase of 7318 U/L. (*A*) Transabdominal US demonstrated a distended gallbladder with cholelithiasis (not shown) and a dilated common bile duct (CBD) measuring 9 mm (*arrow*). No other imaging findings were present to suggest acute cholecystitis. (*B*) Axial HASTE MR image, as part of an examination performed for further evaluation, demonstrated multiple calculi in the gallbladder (*arrow*) as well as (*C*) mild peripancreatic fluid (*arrow*) and fat stranding, consistent with pancreatitis. There was borderline CBD dilation measuring 7 mm in diameter, best seen on a representative coronal MRCP image (*D*). The patient underwent ERCP with sphincterotomy and common bile duct stent placement and then returned 2 weeks later for cholecystectomy.

traverses between the right side of the liver and abdominal wall or diaphragm, can also aid in establishing the diagnosis.[27] Kiewiet and colleagues in a 2012 meta-analysis that included 5859 patients, showed that the overall sensitivity and specificity of US and MR in the diagnosis of acute cholecystitis were similar, 82% and 81% for US and 86% and 82% for MR, respectively. In their analysis, all studies that compared US and MR directly showed no statistically significant difference in sensitivity or specificity.[27–29]

Cholangitis is another potential complication of cholelithiasis and is also associated with cholecystitis. Though rare in pregnancy, cholangitis arises due to the obstruction of the CBD allowing gastrointestinal bacteria to ascend into the biliary tract. This can have potentially grave consequences,

that is, sepsis leading to death if not treated emergently. Typically, the presentation is described by Charcot's triad of fever, RUQ pain, and jaundice, which may eventually evolve into Reynolds' pentad: Charcot's triad in the setting of shock and delirium. In addition to the clinical presentation and laboratory findings, cholangitis can be diagnosed when the following findings are seen: T2 hypointense intrabiliary material, biliary wall thickening, and hyperintense periportal edema.[30]

Pancreatitis is another potential complication of cholelithiasis, usually primarily diagnosed based on elevated lipase along with epigastric pain. Pancreatitis affects approximately 3 in 10,000 pregnancies, predominately occurring during the third trimester.[31] Once pancreatitis is diagnosed, it carries a fetal mortality rate of 2% to 5%. In

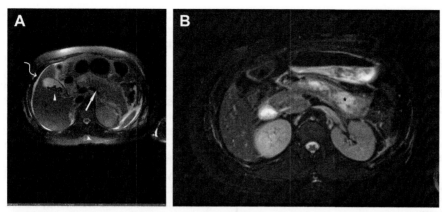

Fig. 6. A 36-year-old woman at 6 weeks gestation presented from an outside hospital for concerns for cholangitis in the setting of gallstone pancreatitis. (*A*) Axial T2 fat-saturated MR image performed on admission revealed diffuse pancreatic edema (*arrow*) with mild ascites (*curved arrow*) consistent with acute pancreatitis. Multiple layered gallstones in the gallbladder (*arrowhead*) were observed. No peripancreatic collection was identified. Six days later a repeat MR was performed due to abnormal liver function tests. (*B*) Axial T2 fat-saturated MR image demonstrated multiple intrapancreatic and peripancreatic collections (*star*) in and adjacent to an edematous pancreas, which was highly consistent with pancreatic and peripancreatic necrosis, ultimately resulting in pregnancy failure.

the nonpregnant population, cross-sectional imaging, particularly CT, is commonly used to confirm the diagnosis and evaluate for any complications. Although anatomic abdominal changes during pregnancy hinder the visualization of the pancreas on US, it is well identified on MRI. On T2-W MRI, pancreatic swelling and peripancreatic edema are seen as high intensity signal along with pancreatic parenchymal enlargement and other signs of biliary obstruction as discussed previously (see **Fig. 5**). In addition, depending on the amount of inflammation, the affected pancreas will have variable loss of its normally high T1 signal intensity, and relatively high SI on T2-weighted MR images, indicates parenchymal edema (**Fig. 6**).[32]

Hemolysis, elevated liver enzymes, low platelete syndrome Hemolysis, elevated liver enzymes, low plateletes (HELLPs) syndrome is a cause of acute abdominal pain specific to pregnancy. This syndrome typically occurs in the third trimester in patients with severe pre-eclampsia or eclampsia and manifests as hemolytic anemia, elevated liver enzymes, and low platelets. Although this condition affects fewer than 1% of pregnancies, it carries serious risk of maternal and perinatal mortality.[33] In the past, HELLP syndrome was managed with prompt delivery; however recently, an individualized approach has been recommended with considerations based on fetal gestational age and maternal-fetal health, without any demonstrable effect on maternal and fetal morbidity and mortality.[34] MR imaging can be used following US to

depict and assess for intra-abdominal complications of the syndrome, particularly intrahepatic and perihepatic hemorrhage and hematomas. Hematoma with acute extravasation will demonstrate high T1 and T2 signal, with eventual loss of T2 signal as the blood products evolve. If a dual-spoiled GRE T1-weighted sequence is included, a blooming artifact is more pronounced on the in-phase images due to progressive dephasing with longer echo times.[33]

Hepatic steatosis Acute fatty liver of pregnancy (AFLP) is an uncommon cause of abdominal pain in pregnancy but was historically potentially fatal and therefore important to identify. Both fetal and maternal mortality rates have greatly improved as the discovery of AFLP as a complication of pregnancy with the current maternal mortality rate at 13%, and the fetal mortality rate at less than 10%.[35] The condition is of unknown etiology to our knowledge, arises late in pregnancy, and is associated with presenting features of hypertension, nausea and vomiting, and abdominal pain. The Swansea criteria is used to establish the diagnosis. If six or more of the criteria listed in **Table 2** are present in the absence of another diagnosis, the diagnosis of AFLP can be made.[36] If MRI is performed, there will be substantial signal loss in the liver on opposed-phase imaging.[18] The current treatment recommendation is prompt delivery of the fetus, and in the majority of patients, normalization of maternal laboratory values usually occurs within a week after delivery.[37]

Table 2 Swansea criteria	
Vomiting	Elevated ammonia
Abdominal pain	Elevated bilirubin
Polydipsia/polyuria	Hypoglycemia
Encephalopathy	Elevated urate
Renal impairment	Leukocytosis
Ascites or liver hyperechogenicity on US	Elevated Transaminases
Microvesicular steatosis on liver biopsy	Coagulopathy

Abbreviation: US, ultrasound.

Genitourinary disease US should be the first imaging modality for evaluation of genitourinary (GU) disease as it has been shown to have a relatively good sensitivity reported between 34% to 95%.[38] The degree of accuracy of US diagnosis depends on the extent of maternal anatomic alterations, demonstrations of the ureteral jets in the bladder, and use of vascular resistive indices.[39] In the pregnant patient, it is important to recognize physiologic occurrence of hydronephrosis and hydroureter due to the compression of the gravid uterus on the ureters, more often affecting the right side and more commonly seen during the late stages of pregnancy. Noncontrast MRI is used when US results are nonspecific or inconclusive, or when sonographic assessment is limited by patient body habitus or bowel gas. MRI is particularly helpful in the evaluation of potential infectious diseases of the GU system.

Urinary tract infections (cystitis and pyelonephritis) Urinary tract infections (UTIs) account for up to 4% of antepartum admission and up to 7% of pregnant women are diagnosed with asymptomatic bacteriuria at some point during their pregnancy.[40] Urinary stasis and vesicoureteral reflux are the predisposing factors for the development of UTI in pregnancy. Vesicoureteral reflux occurs secondary to mass effect from the gravid uterus compressing the urinary tract and as a result of serum progesterone-induced smooth muscle relaxation. Although an easily treated entity, proper identification of a UTI, and more specifically pyelonephritis, is crucial to avoid significant fetal and maternal morbidity. Pregnancy complications associated with inadequately treated UTI include premature labor, anemia, and maternal acute respiratory distress syndrome, which is noted in up to 10% of pregnant patients diagnosed with

pyelonephritis. These complications are thought to be secondary to endotoxin release.[40]

Cystitis, defined as the inflammation of the bladder, presents with dysuria, increased urgency and frequency of urination, and is usually clinically diagnosed with urinary analysis. Generally, imaging does not play a role in the work-up at initial diagnosis but may be useful for persistent or recurrent infections. On MRI, cystitis presents as focal or diffuse irregular mural thickening of the bladder wall with perivesicular fat stranding. These findings may be most apparent on T2-WI if the perivesicular fat is particularly edematous.[41] Ureteritis (inflammation of the ureters), may be seen in association with cystitis, and can be unilateral or bilateral. It is characterized on MR by the presence of diffuse mucosal thickening of the ureters and periureteric fat stranding. Urethritis is relatively rare, and its symptoms may overlap with cystitis. Urethral and periurethral tissue thickening with high SI on T2-WI suggest urethritis on MRI.[41]

Pyelonephritis is the primary cause of septic shock in pregnant patients and as such, is a much more concerning urinary tract disease.[40] Pyelonephritis can either arise from ascending lower urinary tract infection, or may develop as a result of hematogenous spread. Clinical symptoms include those seen with cystitis as well as those involving a systemic inflammatory response including flank pain, nausea, and vomiting. On MRI, the findings of acute pyelonephritis include renal enlargement secondary to edema, perinephric stranding, and free perinephric fluid. Areas of striated cortical signal hyperintensity are also noted on T2-WI (**Fig. 7**).[41–43]

Diffusion-weighted imaging (DWI) has shown to be effective in demonstrating the affected region of the renal parenchyma in patients with pyelonephritis. In a study conducted by Sanga Reddi and colleagues involving 32 subjects, 85% of those with pyelonephritis showed restricted diffusion on DWI.[44] In this study, the apparent diffusion coefficient (ADC) values of the normal renal parenchyma were $1.83 \pm 0.06 \times 10{-3}$ whereas the areas of nephritis had values of $1.20 \pm 0 \, 0.08 \times 10{-3}$. In another study conducted by Goyal and colleagues, accuracy of diagnosis of pyelonephritis with IV contrast-enhanced multidetector CT was compared with IV contrast-enhanced MR with diffusion weighted images obtained pre-contrast administration. Although both modalities showed the ability to correctly reveal pyelonephritis, confidence on MR was significantly higher and reached 100% when DW sequences were obtained, showing statistically significantly restricted diffusion in the nephritic tissue as opposed to the normal renal parenchyma.[45] These results were

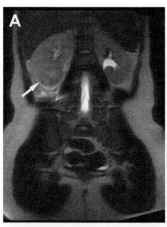
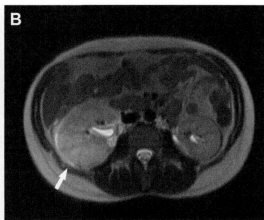

Fig. 7. A 26-year-old woman at 5 weeks gestation by last menstrual period presented with right lower quadrant pain, leukocytosis, and fever. Prior to imaging, the patient was found to be pregnant on routine blood work in the ED, prompting the use of MR instead of CT. Wedge-shaped edema (*arrow*) was demonstrated on HASTE MR in the right kidney on coronal (*A*) and axial (*B*) images, highly consistent with pyelonephritis. The patient was placed on antibiotics with improvement.

also seen in a study conducted by Rathod and colleagues, which compared noncontrast-enhanced CT to DW MRI. In this study, ADC values were used to distinguish between nephritic tissue, normal renal tissue, and abscess. For the diagnosis of nephritis, DW MR had a sensitivity of 95.3%, while non-contrast CT had a sensitivity of 66.7%. Nephritic tissue had statistically significantly lower ADC than normal renal parenchyma,

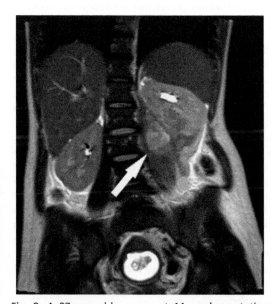

Fig. 8. A 27-year-old woman at 14 weeks gestation presented for follow-up evaluation for a left renal abscess. Coronal T2 MR image demonstrated a 3 cm phlegmonous collection, measured in an oblique transverse direction (*arrow*), with extension into the left psoas muscle.

and abscess had statistically significantly lower ADC then nephritic tissue.[46] With DWI, acute pyelonephritis was seen as patchy hyperintense regions with coinciding regions of low SI on ADC.[46]

Rare complications of pyelonephritis include renal and perinephric abscesses as well as pyonephrosis. Pyonephrosis is defined as a collection of pus and debris in the intrarenal collecting system, which occurs secondary to ureteral obstruction, and is seen in the setting of pyelonephritis due to sloughed papilla. Pyonephrosis is an emergency and typically requires percutaneous urinary drainage. Though US can depict echogenic debris with possible fluid levels in the collecting system, MRI is particularly helpful in the diagnosis of this potentially very serious complication and will demonstrate a thick-walled collecting system with fluid debris levels.[41,42] DWI has shown some promise in helping distinguish pyonephrosis from hydronephrosis, with the former showing lower ADC values, but to the best of our knowledge data is limited to two small studies containing a total combined 7 cases of pyonephrosis.[47,48]

The imaging appearance of renal and perirenal abscesses will depend on their contents. Typically, on MRI, they appear as thick-rimmed complex fluid collections which are hypointense on T1 and hyperintense on T2-WI and are located in the renal cortex or in the perirenal fat with adjacent perinephric stranding (**Fig. 8**). The affected area will tend to have marked restricted signal intensity on ADC images due to the high level of internal debris as compared with a noninfected fluid collection or necrotic mass.[41,44,46] The ADC maps may also be used to help monitor the progression of a renal abscess, as changes on ADC

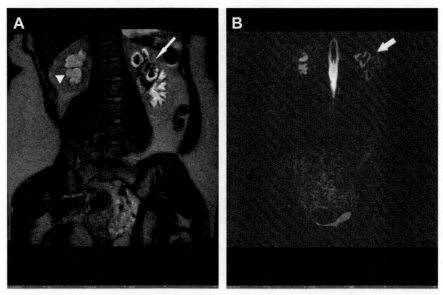

Fig. 9. A 33-year-old woman at 26 weeks gestation presented with abdominal pain. MR was performed due to concerns for appendicitis. (*A*) Coronal T2 MR image demonstrated severe right hydronephrosis (*arrowhead*) secondary to compression from the gravid uterus and mild left hydronephrosis with nephrolithiasis (*arrow*). (*B*) MR urography was then performed for further evaluation and better demonstrated multiple confluent calculi in the left upper pole calyces extending into the proximal pelvis (*arrow*), indicating a staghorn calculus. Also noted again was severe right-sided hydroureteronephrosis without an obstructing calculus.

images can indicate progression or healing.[46,49] In addition, the finding of gas in a collection best demonstrated on susceptibility-weighted images, strongly suggests an abscess, however, the presence of gas in uncommon in non-diabetic patients.

Nephrolithiasis and urolithiasis Urolithiasis, the presence of calculi in the urinary tract, is the leading cause of urologic pain in pregnancy.[50] Many patients with renal urolithiasis are asymptomatic, but those who are symptomatic may present with colicky flank and/or abdominal pain, hematuria, vomiting, and nausea, typically due to the presence of ureteral calculi. Calculi in the urinary tract can cause multiple complications, the more common of which are urinary tract infection and hydroureteronephrosis due to obstruction. In the pregnant patient, especially late in gestation, hydronephrosis and hydroureter of the proximal and middle ureteral segments, particularly of the right kidney, are physiologic, which render analysis for pathologic obstruction difficult.[1] Thus, a nonphysiological cause should be suspected if there is proximal ureteral dilation with tapering in the distal to the middle ureteral segments (**Fig. 9**). The "double kink sign" describes a distal constriction and a collection of a column of urine in the ureter due to pathologic obstruction distal to the physiologic ureteral obstruction of pregnancy.[43,51,52]

MRI is not optimal for the detection of renal calculi with a relatively low sensitivity of 82% and specificity of 98%, when compared with CT which has a sensitivity of 95%.[53] In the pregnant population, MR usually serves as the second-line imaging technique after US; however, the role of US in the evaluation of renal calculi is limited especially if a calculus is located in the mid ureter.[53] Despite its limitations, according to the ACR appropriateness criteria, US remains the first choice modality for evaluation of nephrolithiasis in pregnant patients. In challenging cases, MR urography with an altered protocol can be used in pregnant patients, where T2-static-fluid urography is performed. Typically, this requires multiple acquisitions to obtain adequate images of the entire length of the ureters. Due to their short T2-SI, renal calculi often do not produce high enough signal to be differentiated from adjacent soft tissue and are not detectable on conventional MRI. Larger calculi can be seen as signal voids, however, are not easily distinguishable from ureteral flow void or gas. On MR urography, a complete filling defect with a signal void represents a calculus (see **Fig. 9**).[52]

Gynecologic disease
Ovarian torsion Adnexal torsion complicates approximately 1 in 1800 pregnancies, and most often occurs in the first trimester when the uterus

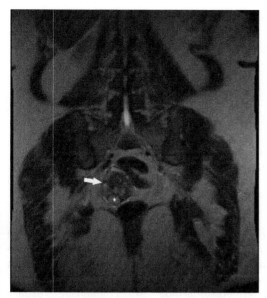

Fig. 10. A 38-year-old woman at 22 weeks gestation presented for further evaluation of a complex right ovarian mass noted on obstetric ultrasound performed 2 weeks earlier (not shown). No normal right ovarian parenchyma was identified at that time. Coronal HASTE MR image demonstrated a 5.5 cm complex right adnexal mass (*arrow*) with macroscopic focal fat measuring 2 cm (*star*), most consistent with a teratoma, and imaging surveillance was recommended. The patient had a cesarean hysterectomy with right salpingo-oophorectomy due to placenta accreta. Pathology of the right ovary demonstrated follicular thyroid neoplasm, most likely to have arisen in struma ovarii.

undergoes the greatest expansion.[54] In most patients, the diagnosis is challenging, and up to 50% of those with suspected adnexal torsion who undergo surgery receive an alternative post-operative diagnosis.[55,56] Accurate diagnosis is important in avoiding any unwarranted surgical procedure during pregnancy while also considering the potential possibility of ovarian necrosis leading to future fertility issues. Among the various forms of adnexal torsion, combined tubo-ovarian torsion, isolated fallopian torsion, and ovarian torsion are the most common. When the ovary twists around its vascular pedicle, venous congestion builds up and edema ensues, eventually leading to arterial supply compromise and infarction.

In all women, most commonly there is a preexisting mass that predisposes the ipsilateral ovary to torsion. Pregnancy-related corpus luteum and ovarian follicles as well as dermoid cysts are common causes of ovarian torsion (**Figs. 10** and **11**); however, torsion can also occur in pregnancy without the presence of an adnexal mass. Although most adnexal masses are asymptomatic, larger masses may produce pain secondary to mass effect, hemorrhage, or rupture, or act as the lead point for ovarian torsion.[57] A corpus luteum is the most common adnexal mass encountered in the first trimester of pregnancy, which in most women will eventually regress, generally by the end of the first trimester. Theca lutein cysts, also known as hyperreactio luteinalis, are formed from hyperplastic theca interna cells, and are thought to arise due to elevated levels of gonadotropins, eventually resolving once the gonadotropin excess is removed. These may occur with multiple gestations, with gestational trophoblastic diseases, or in those undergoing hormonal stimulation for in vitro fertilization and, therefore, are not specific.[58–60] Theca lutein cysts will result in enlarged multicystic ovaries. The cysts tend to be uniform in size, generally affecting both ovaries.

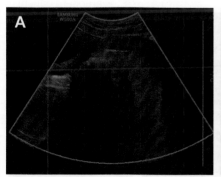
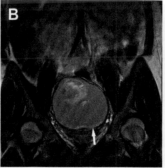
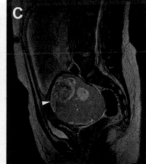

Fig. 11. A 28-year-old woman at 18 weeks gestation presented for further evaluation of a pelvic mass seen on transabdominal US (*A*). Coronal (*B*) and sagittal (*C*) T2 MR images revealed a large circumscribed cystic structure measuring approximately 10 × 8 × 9 cm (CC x AP x TR) (*arrow*) with internal fat–fluid levels (*arrowhead*), indicating a mature cystic teratoma. The decision for surgery was made due to the size of the teratoma causing concerns for uterine dystocia during delivery or eventual rupture secondary to compression from the gravid uterus. Pathology confirmed a benign mature teratoma.

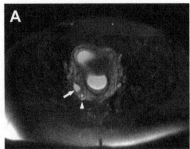
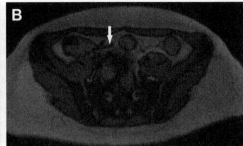

Fig. 12. A 33-year-old woman at 10 weeks gestation presented with right lower quadrant pain. The appendix was not visualized on the initial US. MR was performed for further evaluation. A corpus luteal cyst (*arrow*) was noted on (*A*) axial diffusion MR sequences with peri-cystic fluid (*arrowhead*), indicating rupture. Note the normal appendix on (*B*) axial gradient-echo MR image (*arrow*).

Almost all patients with suspected adnexal masses or abnormalities are initially evaluated with an US examination. A corpus luteum cyst will appear as a unilocular anechoic cyst with a hypervascular rim on color Doppler imaging known as the "ring of fire," which indicates prominent peripheral blood flow.[61] Hemorrhagic corpus luteum can have a fluid debris level or septations, as well as daughter cysts as it ages. Theca lutein cysts are typically large, bilateral collections of thin-walled cysts sometimes referred to as having a "spoke wheel" appearance. On US, they will have normal Doppler flow and lack solid components.[62]

On MR, the corpus luteum is a unilocular cystic structure with crenulated borders, which generally measures up to 3 cm (**Fig. 12**). The fluid compartment will be hypointense on T1-WI and hyperintense on T2-WI.[63] If the cyst becomes hemorrhagic, then high intensity T1-WI with fluid–fluid levels can be expected with corresponding heterogeneous T2 appearance.[59] Hemoperitoneum resulting from cystic rupture may also occasionally be seen but is more often identified in nonpregnant patients. Depending on the age of the bleeding, the appearance may differ on MR. In more acute cases, the T1-WI will show intermediate-to-high signal intensity, usually higher than urine, with an intermediate T2 signal. When this condition is unilateral, it may be mistaken for malignancy. The identification of intermediate T2-signal with high DWI signal residual ovarian parenchyma, along with a consideration of the patient's clinical presentation and laboratory findings, should help differentiate theca lutein cysts from neoplasms.[64]

US is usually the first imaging modality of choice for evaluation of torsion and shows an enlarged, edematous ovary with peripherally displaced follicles, central echogenic parenchyma as a result of edema, and in some cases diminished but high-resistance arterial waveforms on Doppler imaging (**Figs. 13** and **14**). If US interpretations are inconclusive or equivocal, MR is considered.

The most sensitive, but not specific, finding to suggest torsion on MR is ovarian enlargement.

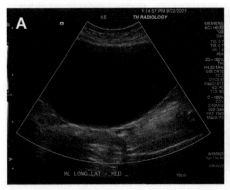
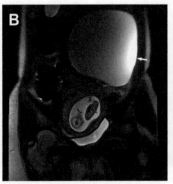
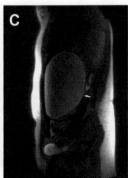

Fig. 13. A 23-year-old woman at 13 weeks gestation presented with left lower quadrant pain. (*A*) Transabdominal US demonstrated a large unilocular midline cyst measuring 14.5 cm in the sagittal plane. Concerns for ovarian torsion were raised due to the inability to definitively identify normal right or left ovarian tissue. Follow-up emergency coronal (*B*) and sagittal (*C*) HASTE MR images demonstrated a large ovarian cyst with smooth, thinned walls (*arrow*), concerning for early torsion. Surgery confirmed a large ovarian cyst, and a torsed but viable ovary.

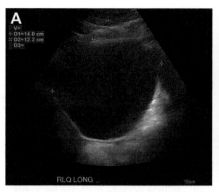
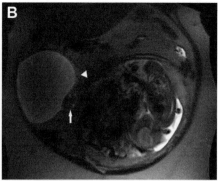

Fig. 14. A 35-year-old woman at 24 weeks with twin gestation presented with stabbing right lower quadrant pain. Transabdominal US demonstrated a large unilocular cyst measuring 14 cm in the sagittal plane with no appreciable color Doppler flow (*A*). No ovarian tissue was identified, raising concern for torsion. Follow-up (*B*) coronal HASTE MR image, as part of an MR examination done emergently, demonstrated the large cyst with an adjacent twisted vascular pedicle (*arrow*) and peri-ovarian fluid (*arrowhead*), which was highly consistent with ovarian torsion.

On T2-WI there is usually high signal intensity in the ovarian stroma due to venous congestion and edema with peripherally displaced follicles. The stromal signal may vary based on the viability of the ovary, as will be described later. Other secondary signs that can aid in establishing the diagnosis include deviation of the uterus toward the affected side, as well as surrounding free pelvic fluid (see **Figs. 13** and **14**). The latter finding can also be seen in those undergoing hormonal stimulation for in vitro fertilization, and therefore, is not specific.[58] Visualization of a heterogeneous, thickened, hyperintense and twisted vascular pedicle on T2-WI can also be seen, that is, the whirlpool sign, which is specific for torsion (see **Fig. 13**).[65,66]

The determination of ovarian viability through imaging is an important step in surgical planning. Normally the lack of IV contrast enhancement in the twisted ovary would substantially aid in diagnosis, but in a pregnant patient, the appearance of the adnexal mass itself can help determine viability. During the early stages of vascular compromise, the cyst/mass will have a thickened smoothed wall, but as arterial supply diminishes and the ovary becomes necrotic, the walls of the cyst/mass become more irregular (see **Fig. 14B**). Ovarian stromal hemorrhage suggests nonviability and is seen as a T1-WI hyperintense signal and intermediate to low T2-WI signal. Restricted diffusion on DWI coinciding with a low ADC suggests necrotic, or hemorrhagic ovarian infarction.[67] The finding of a hypointense perifollicular rim on T2-WI has also been suggested as an indicator for severe ischemic injury and loss of ovarian viability.[65,66,68]

Trauma The current standard of care for evaluation of traumatic injury in a pregnant patient

includes US examination (the focused assessment with sonography in trauma [FAST] examination) followed by CT if clinically indicated. CT may be underutilized or not used quickly enough due to concerns for the effects of radiation on the fetus. The radiation dose of a CT of the abdomen and pelvis is approximately 25 mGy depending both on body habitus and the specific imaging techniques utilized for a particular patient.[69] The ACR designates a maximum of 50 mGy exposure to a fetus, a threshold under which no risk to fetal development or viability has been reported at any stage of pregnancy.[70] In the setting of trauma, the health of the mother is the primary consideration and there should be no hesitation in using CT imaging if clinically appropriate. The role of MRI in the initial evaluation of abdominal or pelvic trauma is currently very limited. The length of examination is the main limiting factor since delaying diagnosis in trauma patients increases the risk of morbidity and mortality. At the authors' institutions, MRI has very occasionally been performed in this setting when the mother refuses CT examination. In such situations, MRI can be considered if the mother and the fetus are believed to be clinically stable and are monitored sufficiently while MR is being performed. MRI can also be considered in follow-up imaging after initial evaluation of trauma to limit cumulative radiation exposure although to the best of our knowledge there is currently no clear understanding of the potential cumulative risk to the fetus.

SUMMARY

Imaging evaluation of pregnant patients with acute abdominal pain can be challenging and establishing an accurate clinical diagnosis may be difficult for a variety of reasons, particularly late in pregnancy. Noncontrast MR remains a safe and accurate diagnostic imaging examination, often following an initial inconclusive US examination, and can be used in most settings to avoid ionizing radiation exposure. Efficient and accurate diagnosis of acute disease processes is necessary to limit risk of adverse events for both the mother and the fetus. All radiologists should be familiar with the current guidelines for performing and accurately interpreting MR imaging of the pregnant patient.

CLINICS CARE POINTS

- MR imaging using a less than 3T magnet is considered safe in pregnancy.
- Gadolinium is avoided for potential risk of future rheumatologic conditions in the fetus.
- MR has a reported overall sensitivity of 91.8% and a specificity of 97.9% in the diagnosis of acute appendicitis in the pregnant patient.
- As the incidence of bariatric surgery among women of child-bearing age increases, so does the risk of adhesional disease, which can put such individuals at risk for small bowel obstruction.
- Noncontrast magnetic resonance cholangiopancreatography can be performed following US, if needed, for hepatobiliary emergencies.
- Evidence of biliary obstruction is indicated by dilated biliary ducts on both US and MRI.
- MR evidence of acute cholecystitis includes a distended, thickened gallbladder wall and the presence of patchy bright signals in the wall, best seen on fat-suppressed T2-WI.
  - The inflammatory process may also spread into the adjacent pericholecystic fat, as demonstrated by high pericholecystic signals on the same images.
- On MR imaging, the findings of acute pyelonephritis include renal enlargement secondary to edema, perinephric stranding, and free perinephric fluid.
  - Low apparent diffusion coefficient (ADC) values can help identify nephritic tissue and abscess.
  - ADC values have been used to monitor renal abscess progression.
- MR is less sensitive for the identification of renal and ureteral calculi than CT.

  - MR urography, that is, T2-static-fluid urography, avoids the use of IV contrast while allowing for good visualization of the ureters.
- Calculi will be seen as signal voids.
- Normal physiologic hydroureter is suggested by right-sided midureteral tapering with distal collapse.
- The most sensitive finding to suggest ovarian torsion on MR is ovarian enlargement.
  - T2-WI will demonstrate a high–signal-intensity ovary with peripherally oriented follicles secondary to stromal venous congestion and edema.
  - Low ADC values suggest necrotic ovarian tissue.
- Ovarian torsion can occur in pregnancy with or without a specific adnexal mass as a lead point.
- The most common ovarian "mass" in pregnancy is a corpus luteum.
- US followed by CT is the standard of care for pregnant patients with traumatic injuries; the role for MRI remains limited in the trauma setting.

DISCLOSURE

Dr M. Moshiri: Editor RSNA Case Collection; The remaining authors have nothing to disclose.

REFERENCES

1. Bhatia P, Chhabra S. Physiological and anatomical changes of pregnancy: implications for anaesthesia. Indian J Anaesth 2018;62(9):651–7.
2. Soma-Pillay P, Catherine NP, Tolppanen H, et al. Physiological changes in pregnancy. Cardiovasc J Afr 2016;27(2):89–94.
3. Juhasz-Böss I, Solomayer E, Strik M, et al. Abdominal surgery in pregnancy—an interdisciplinary challenge. Dtsch Ärztebl Int 2014;111(27–28):465–72.
4. Grainger D, Safety Guidelines for Magnetic Resonance Imaging Equipment in Clinical Use." MHRA Regulating Medicines and Medical Devices, 2021, February, 86.
5. Kanal E, Barkovich AJ, Bell C, et al. ACR guidance document for safe MR practices. Am J Roentgenol 2007;188(6):1447–74.
6. Marycz K, Kornicka K, Röcken M. Static magnetic field (SMF) as a regulator of stem cell fate – new perspectives in regenerative medicine arising from an underestimated tool. Stem Cell Rev Rep 2018; 14(6):785–92.

7. Milunsky A, Ulcickas M, Rothman KJ, et al. Maternal heat exposure and neural tube defects. JAMA 1992; 268(7):882–5.

8. Ray JG, Vermeulen MJ, Bharatha A, et al. Association between mri exposure during pregnancy and fetal and childhood outcomes. JAMA 2016;316(9):952–61.

9. American College of Radiology, Committee on Drugs and Contrast Media. ACR manual on contrast media. 2015. Available at. http://www.acr.org/~/link. aspx?_id=29C40D1FE0EC4E5EAB6861BD213 793E5&_z=z. Accessed January 30, 2022.

10. Andersen B, Nielsen TF. Appendicitis in pregnancy: diagnosis, management and complications. Acta Obstet Gynecol Scand 1999;78(9):758–62.

11. Zingone F, Sultan AA, Humes DJ, et al. Risk of acute appendicitis in and around pregnancy: a population-based cohort study from england. Ann Surg 2015;261(2):332–7.

12. Lehnert BE, Gross JA, Linnau KF, et al. Utility of ultrasound for evaluating the appendix during the second and third trimester of pregnancy. Emerg Radiol 2012;19(4):293–9.

13. Shetty MK, Garrett NM, Carpenter WS, et al. Abdominal computed tomography during pregnancy for suspected appendicitis: a 5-year experience at a maternity hospital. Semin Ultrasound CT MR 2010; 31(1):8–13.

14. Kave M, Parooie F, Salarzaei M. Pregnancy and appendicitis: a systematic review and meta-analysis on the clinical use of MRI in diagnosis of appendicitis in pregnant women. World J Emerg Surg 2019;14:37.

15. Tsai R, Raptis C, Fowler KJ, et al. MRI of suspected appendicitis during pregnancy: interradiologist agreement, indeterminate interpretation and the meaning of non-visualization of the appendix. Br J Radiol 2017;90(1079):20170383.

16. Shin I, An C, Lim JS, et al. T1 bright appendix sign to exclude acute appendicitis in pregnant women. Eur Radiol 2017;27(8):3310–6.

17. Gentles JQ, Meglei G, Chen L, et al. Is neutrophilia the key to diagnosing appendicitis in pregnancy? Am J Surg 2020;219(5):855–9.

18. Moreno CC, Mittal PK, Miller FH. Nonfetal imaging during pregnancy: acute abdomen/pelvis. Radiol Clin North Am 2020;58(2):363–80.

19. Stern MD, Kopylov U, Ben-Horin S, et al. Magnetic resonance enterography in pregnant women with Crohn's disease: case series and literature review. BMC Gastroenterol 2014;14(1):146.

20. de Bari O, Wang TY, Liu M, et al. Cholesterol cholelithiasis in pregnant women: pathogenesis, prevention and treatment. Ann Hepatol 2014;13(6):728–45.

21. Zahur Z, Jeilani A, Fatima T, et al. Transabdominal ultrasound: a potentially accurate and useful tool for detection of choledocholithiasis. J Ayub Med Coll Abbottabad JAMC 2019;31(4):572–5.

22. Burrowes DP, Choi HH, Rodgers SK, et al. Utility of ultrasound in acute pancreatitis. Abdom Radiol 2020;45(5):1253–64.

23. Tsai HM, Lin XZ, Chen CY, et al. MRI of gallstones with different compositions. AJR Am J Roentgenol 2004;182(6):1513–9.

24. Nandalur KR, Hussain HK, Weadock WJ, et al. Possible biliary disease: diagnostic performance of high-spatial-resolution isotropic 3D T2-weighted MRCP. Radiology 2008;249(3):883–90.

25. Kimura Y, Takada T, Kawarada Y, et al. Definitions, pathophysiology, and epidemiology of acute cholangitis and cholecystitis: Tokyo guidelines. J Hepatobiliary Pancreat Surg 2007;14(1):15–26.

26. Watanabe Y, Nagayama M, Okumura A, et al. MR imaging of acute biliary disorders. Radiographics 2007;27(2):477–95.

27. Håkansson K, Leander P, Ekberg O, et al. MR imaging in clinically suspected acute cholecystitis: a comparison with ultrasonography. Acta Radiol 2000;41(4):322–8.

28. Kiewiet JJS, Leeuwenburgh MMN, Bipat S, et al. A Systematic review and meta-analysis of diagnostic performance of imaging in acute cholecystitis. Radiology 2012;264(3):708–20.

29. Oh KY, Gilfeather M, Kennedy A, et al. Limited abdominal MRI in the evaluation of acute right upper quadrant pain. Abdom Imaging 2003;28(5):643–51.

30. Park MS, Yu JS, Kim YH, et al. Acute cholecystitis: comparison of MR cholangiography and US. Radiology 1998;209(3):781–5.

31. Eddy JJ, Gideonsen MD, Song JY, et al. Pancreatitis in pregnancy: a 10 year retrospective of 15 Midwest hospitals. Obstet Gynecol 2008;112(5):1075–81.

32. Miller FH, Keppke AL, Dalal K, et al. MRI of pancreatitis and its complications: part 1, acute pancreatitis. Am J Roentgenol 2004;183(6):1637–44.

33. Plowman RS, Javidan-Nejad C, Raptis CA, et al. Imaging of pregnancy-related vascular complications. Radiographics 2017;37(4):1270–89.

34. Sibai BM. Diagnosis, controversies, and management of the syndrome of hemolysis, elevated liver enzymes, and low platelet count. Obstet Gynecol 2004;103(5):981–91.

35. Nelson DB, Yost NP, Cunningham FG. Acute fatty liver of pregnancy: clinical outcomes and expected duration of recovery. Am J Obstet Gynecol 2013;209(5):456.

36. Ch'ng CL, Morgan M, Hainsworth I, et al. Prospective study of liver dysfunction in pregnancy in Southwest Wales. Gut 2002;51(6):876–80.

37. Brady CW. Liver disease in pregnancy: what's new. Hepatol Commun 2020;4(2):145–56.

38. Katz DS, Klein MAI, Ganson G, et al. Imaging of abdominal pain in pregnancy. Radiol Clin North Am 2012;50(1):149–71.

39. Baheti AD, Nicola R, Bennett GL, et al. Magnetic resonance imaging of abdominal and pelvic pain

in the pregnant patient. Magn Reson Imaging Clin N Am 2016;24(2):403–17.

40. Habak PJ, Griggs J. Urinary tract infection in pregnancy. In: StatPearls. StatPearls Publishing; 2021. Available at. http://www.ncbi.nlm.nih.gov/books/NBK537047/. Accessed December 5, 2021.

41. El-Ghar MA, Farg H, Sharaf DE, et al. CT and MRI in urinary tract infections: a spectrum of different imaging findings. Medicina (Mex). 2021;57(1):32.

42. Craig WD, Wagner BJ, Travis MD. Pyelonephritis: radiologic-pathologic review. Radiographics 2008; 28(1):255–76.

43. Leyendecker JR, Gorengaut V, Brown JJ. MR imaging of maternal diseases of the abdomen and pelvis during pregnancy and the immediate postpartum period. Radiographics 2004;24(5):1301–16.

44. Sanga Reddi B, Bodagala V, Lakshmi A, et al. Diffusion weighted MR imaging in the diagnosis of acute pyelonephritis and its complications: a prospective observational study. J Dr NTR Univ Health Sci 2019;8(3):170.

45. Goyal A, Sharma R, Bhalla AS, et al. Diffusion-weighted MRI in inflammatory renal lesions: all that glitters is not RCC. Eur Radiol 2013;23(1):272–9.

46. Rathod SB, Kumbhar SS, Nanivadekar A, et al. Role of diffusion-weighted MRI in acute pyelonephritis: a prospective study. Acta Radiol 2015;56(2):244–9.

47. Cova M, Squillaci E, Stacul F, et al. Diffusion-weighted MRI in the evaluation of renal lesions: preliminary results. Br J Radiol 2004;77(922):851–7.

48. Chan JH, Tsui EY, Luk SH, et al. MR diffusion-weighted imaging of kidney: differentiation between hydronephrosis and pyonephrosis. Clin Imaging 2001;25(2):110–3.

49. Faletti R, Cassinis MC, Fonio P, et al. Diffusion–weighted imaging and apparent diffusion coefficient values versus contrast–enhanced MR imaging in the identification and characterisation of acute pyelonephritis. Eur Radiol 2013;23(12):3501–8.

50. Pedro RN, Das K, Buchholz N. Urolithiasis in pregnancy. Int J Surg 2016;36:688–92.

51. Spencer JA, Chahal R, Kelly A, et al. Evaluation of painful hydronephrosis in pregnancy:: magnetic resonance urographic patterns in physiological dilatation versus calculous obstruction. J Urol 2004; 171(1):256–60.

52. Grenier N, Pariente JL, Trillaud H, et al. Dilatation of the collecting system during pregnancy: physiologic vs obstructive dilatation. Eur Radiol 2000;10(2):271–9.

53. Brisbane W, Bailey MR, Sorensen MD. An overview of kidney stone imaging techniques. Nat Rev Urol 2016;13(11):654–62.

54. Spalluto L, Woodfield C, DeBenedectis C, et al. MR imaging evaluation of abdominal pain during pregnancy: appendicitis and other nonobstetric causes. Radiographics 2012;32:317–34.

55. Cohen SB, Weisz B, Seidman DS, et al. Accuracy of the preoperative diagnosis in 100 emergency laparoscopies performed due to acute abdomen in nonpregnant women. J Am Assoc Gynecol Laparosc 2001;8(1):92–4.

56. Melcer Y, Maymon R, Pekar-Zlotin M, et al. Clinical and sonographic predictors of adnexal torsion in pediatric and adolescent patients. J Pediatr Surg 2018; 53(7):1396–8.

57. Hakoun AM, AbouAl-Shaar I, Zaza KJ, et al. Adnexal masses in pregnancy: an updated review. Avicenna J Med 2017;7(4):153–7.

58. Asch E, Wei J, Mortele KJ, et al. Magnetic resonance imaging performance for diagnosis of ovarian torsion in pregnant women with stimulated ovaries. Fertil Res Pract 2017;3:13.

59. Telischak NA, Yeh BM, Joe BN, et al. MRI of adnexal masses in pregnancy. Am J Roentgenol 2008; 191(2):364–70.

60. Zhang H. Bilateral theca-lutein cysts in one pregnant woman at MRI. Int J Clin Med Images 2014;1(1). Available at. https://www.imagejournals.org/articles/bilateral-thecalutein-cysts-in-one-pregnant-woman-at-mri-mimicking-the-cystadenoma-21.html. Accessed December 2, 2021.

61. Bonde AA, Korngold EK, Foster BR, et al. Radiological appearances of corpus luteum cysts and their imaging mimics. Abdom Radiol N Y 2016;41(11): 2270–82.

62. Edell H, Shearkhani O, Rahmani MR, et al. Incidentally found hyperreactio luteinalis in pregnancy. Radiol Case Rep 2018;13(6):1220–3.

63. Foti PV, Attinà G, Spadola S, et al. MR imaging of ovarian masses: classification and differential diagnosis. Insights Imaging 2015;7(1):21–41.

64. Takeuchi M, Matsuzaki K, Nishitani H. Manifestations of the female reproductive organs on mr images: changes induced by various physiologic states. Radiographics 2010;30(4):e39.

65. Iraha Y, Okada M, Iraha R, et al. CT and MR imaging of gynecologic emergencies. Radiographics 2017; 37(5):1569–86.

66. Dawood MT, Naik M, Bharwani N, et al. Adnexal torsion: review of radiologic appearances. Radiographics 2021;41(2):609–24.

67. Kato H, Kanematsu M, Uchiyama M, et al. Diffusion-weighted imaging of ovarian torsion: usefulness of apparent diffusion coefficient (ADC) values for the detection of hemorrhagic infarction. Magn Reson Med Sci 2014;13(1):39–44.

68. Gomes MM, Cavalcanti LS, Reis RL, et al. Twist and shout: magnetic resonance imaging findings in ovarian torsion. Radiol Bras 2019;52(6):397–402.

69. Raptis CA, Mellnick VM, Raptis DA, et al. Imaging of trauma in the pregnant patient. Radiographics 2014; 34(3):748–63.

70. Thy-Scint.pdf. Available at. https://www.acr.org/-/media/ACR/Files/Practice-Parameters/Thy-Scint.pdf. Accessed January 17, 2022.

Pediatric Emergency MRI

Maria Gabriela Figueiro Longo, MD[a],*, Camilo Jaimes, MD[b],
Fedel Machado, MD[b], Jorge Delgado, MD[c], Michael S. Gee, MD, PhD[a]

KEYWORDS

- Emergency radiology • Pediatric radiology • Emergency MRI • Stroke • Appendicitis

KEY POINTS

- The need to minimize the exposure of children to ionizing radiation has led to increased utilization of MRI as an alternative modality to computed tomography for evaluation of pediatric patients in the emergency room setting.
- The evolution of the MR technology has improved access to MRI in the emergency room due to reduced acquisition time, decreased motion sensitivity, and improved spatial resolution.
- The development of short pediatric MR protocols that could encompass the most common diagnoses seen in the emergency room would improve access to MR and patient care overall.

INTRODUCTION

There is an overall increase in the use of imaging in the pediatric emergency room (ER) setting, primarily ultrasound (US) and MRI, which is accompanied by a reduction in computed tomography (CT) examinations performed.[1] One of the main reasons for the increase in the use of US and MRI is the increasing awareness among patients, families, and health care providers of the risks of ionizing radiation.[1–3] Previous large epidemiologic studies have shown an association between ionizing radiation exposure and potential future risk of cancer, particularly in children who have a higher proportion of dividing cells and a longer latency period postexposure.[4–6] Current ionizing radiation doses associated with pediatric CT are substantially reduced due to advances in CT technology,[7] and ongoing efforts such as the Imaging Gently and Image Wisely campaigns have focused attention on minimizing risks of ionizing radiation when ordering imaging studies in children.[8,9] MRI has emerged as an alternate nonionizing radiation cross-sectional imaging modality to CT in children as it provides higher contrast evaluation of the visceral organs.[10] Advances in MRI technology have led to shortened scan time, decreased

motion sensitivity, and improved spatial resolution.[1,11] With increased access to MRI in the ER setting, the goal of this article is to review major applications of MR in pediatric ER patients, including MR imaging findings of the most common pathologies, and to discuss optimized pediatric MR protocols and future trends in emergency pediatric imaging.

CHOOSING BETWEEN COMPUTED TOMOGRAPHY AND MR IN THE EMERGENCY ROOM SETTING

Some of the main advantages of the use of MR over CT, aside from the lack of ionizing radiation, include superior contrast resolution; potential avoidance of the need for intravenous cannulation and intravenous contrast (important for patients with poor renal function, history of allergy, or difficult vascular access); and potentially avoiding the need for multiple imaging tests.[3,11] The use of intravenous gadolinium-based contrast agents is rarely necessary for most emergency MR indications.[11,12]

Disadvantages of MRI compared with CT include higher financial cost and more limited scanner availability, particularly off-hours.

[a] Division of Pediatric Radiology, Massachusetts General Hospital, Harvard Medical School, 55 Fruit Street, Boston, MA 02114, USA; [b] Department of Radiology, Boston Children's Hospital, Harvard Medical School, 300 Longwood Avenue, Boston, MA 02115, USA; [c] Division of MSK Radiology, Massachusetts General Hospital, Harvard Medical School, 55 Fruit Street, Boston, MA 02114, USA
* Corresponding author.
E-mail address: mfigueirolongo@mgh.harvard.edu

Magn Reson Imaging Clin N Am 30 (2022) 533–552
https://doi.org/10.1016/j.mric.2022.05.004
1064-9689/22/© 2022 Elsevier Inc. All rights reserved.

Abbreviations	
CAIPI	controlled aliasing in parallel imaging
FLAIR	Fluid-attenuated inversion recovery
DWI	diffusion-weighted imaging
SWI	Susceptibility weighted imaging
SPACE	sampling perfection with application-optimized contrasts using different flip angle evolution
IAC	internal acoustic canal
MOG-AD	Myelin oligodendrocyte glycoprotein antibody-associated disease
NMO-SD	Neuromyelitis optica spectrum disorder
hCG	human chorionic gonadotropin
STIR	short tau inversion recovery
GRE	gradient echo sequences
ERCP	Endoscopic retrograde cholangiopancreatography
MIP	maximum intensity projection
FSE	fast spin-echo
ADC	apparent diffusion coefficient maps
DTI	Diffusion tensor imaging
TOF	time of flight
ASL	arterial spin labeling
CBF	Cerebral blood flow

Moreover, MRI scan times are substantially longer (20–30 min or more) compared with CT (1–2 s), which can be prohibitive for infants and young children below 6 year old who cannot lie still in the scanner without sedation or for hemodynamically unstable patients.[13] Finally, patients with certain metallic implants and other devices cannot undergo MRI.[3,11]

PROTOCOL OPTIMIZATION AND NEW TECHNIQUES

New image acquisition and reconstruction techniques have led to decreased MR scan times and increased use of MR in the ER, especially in the pediatric population.[14] Techniques such as parallel imaging acceleration are already widely used in the clinical setting, which relies on acquiring and encoding spatial information from multiple receiver coil elements simultaneously, leading to a reduction in acquisition time.[15] More recently, the combination of parallel imaging with controlled aliasing in all three spatial directions (Wave-CAIPI) has led to up to fivefold acceleration in the acquisition time of three-dimensional volumetric images.[16–19] Acquiring imaging faster is helpful to decrease the motion artifacts and improve pediatric patient compliance with MRI. Additional techniques such as radial non-Cartesian k-space sampling can be applied to the thoracic and abdomen to decrease respiratory motion artifact by dispersion along multiple noncoherent phase encoding directions. Radial techniques also improve image contrast through oversampling of the center of k-space.[13] Additional strategies have been tested to correct motion prospectively using a marker-less tracking system, which can continuously update the imaging field-of-view based on the patient's motion.[20] Finally, deep learning-based reconstruction algorithms have recently been approved for clinical use to improve signal-to-noise ratio and image sharpness, enabling shorter scan times, thinner slice acquisition, and improved volumetric resolution.[21,22]

NEURO APPLICATIONS
Arterial Ischemic Stroke

Pediatric arterial ischemic stroke (pAIS) is defined as a focal injury to the brain parenchyma resulting from disruption of normal arterial supply occurring in a child between the ages of 29 days and 18 years.[23] The estimated incidence of pAIS ranges between 4.6 and 6.4 per 100,000 children.[24] The etiology, course, and prognosis of pAIS differ dramatically from those of adults. In children, the most common risk factors for arterial infarcts are intra- and extracranial arteriopathies and congenital heart disease. This highlights the fact that imaging plays a crucial role in diagnosing and establishing the cause of the infarct.

The high sensitivity and specificity of DWI to diagnose ischemia makes MRI the preferred modality in the evaluation of children with focal neurologic symptoms.[25] Given the potential for low patient compliance, it is convenient to acquire the DWI as the first sequence in the protocol. T2-

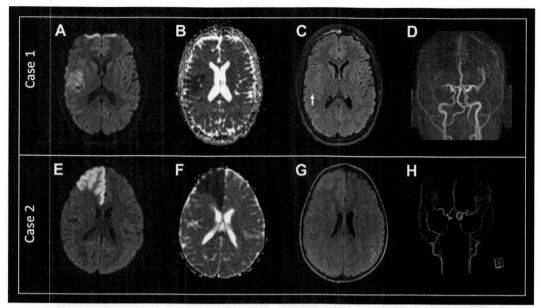

Fig. 1. *Pediatric arterial ischemic stroke. Case 1:* a 12-year-old boy with acute stroke secondary to a paradoxic embolism through a patent foramen ovale associated with immobility (muscular dystrophy). Axial diffusion (*A*) and ADC (*B*) show decreased diffusivity in the right MCA territory. Axial FLAIR (*C*) shows no hyperintense signal, confirming a hyperacute timeframe; the signal in distal vessels represents slow flow (*arrow*). Three-dimensional MIP from a TOF MRA (*D*) shows a cutoff in a proximal right M2. *Case 2:* acute infarct in a 3-year-old boy with bilateral steno-occlusive changes of the ICA. Axial diffusion (*E*) and ADC (*F*) show acute ischemia in the ACA and MCA territories. Axial T2W FLAIR (*G*) shows a hyperintense signal in the infarct core, suggestive of at least 6 h of evolution. Three-dimensional MIP from a time-of-flight MRA (*H*) shows a loss of signal in the ICA termini bilaterally.

weighted (T2W) and T2W FLAIR allow further evaluation of the brain parenchyma, which can help estimate the acuity of the infarct; even though the progression of findings may vary slightly between children and adults, it is generally accepted that appreciable T2 prolongation develops within the brain parenchyma after at least 6 hours of ischemia (**Fig. 1**).[26] SWI or T2* sequences can help identify blood products and potentially clot within a vessel. Owing to the frequent association of pAIS with arteriopathies, all patients should undergo MR angiography (MRA), preferably with non-contrast sequences such as the time-of-flight technique (see **Fig. 1**D, H).

A common arteriopathy of childhood is moyamoya disease. Morphologically, this presents as varying degrees of narrowing (steno-occlusive changes) of the internal carotid artery (ICA) termini with the proliferation of lenticulo-striate collaterals. The involvement in moyamoya is frequently bilateral, although asymmetry is common; posterior circulation involvement is rare but occurs in severe cases and virtually always in association with anterior circulation disease. In this population, infarcts cluster in the cerebral watershed territories.[27] A different type of arteriopathy, known as transient cerebral arteriopathy of

childhood, is a focal (unilateral) narrowing of the ICA terminus with extension into the adjacent A1 or M1 segments. The cause is rarely identified and it has been postulated that it could be the result of a postinfectious arteritis.[28] A similar pattern of focal and unilateral narrowing of the ICA can also be seen with intracranial dissections, although a history of trauma can frequently be elucidated. Other systemic arteriopathies, such as fibromuscular dysplasia, or immune-mediated arteritis (vasculitis) can also cause infarcts. Post-contrast imaging of the vessel wall and the brain parenchyma can help in the evaluation of cases where there is a high suspicious of an active vasculitis.[29]

An important difference between adult and pediatric patients is the relatively high prevalence of stroke-like conditions (stroke mimics) in patients who present with acute onset focal neurologic deficits. In this setting, MRI is even more valuable as it provides a one-stop shop to evaluate for acute ischemia or establish an alternative diagnosis. Conditions leading to focal neurologic deficits in children that can mimic pAIS include complex migraines, seizures, intracranial hemorrhages, demyelinating lesions, and tumors (**Fig. 2**).

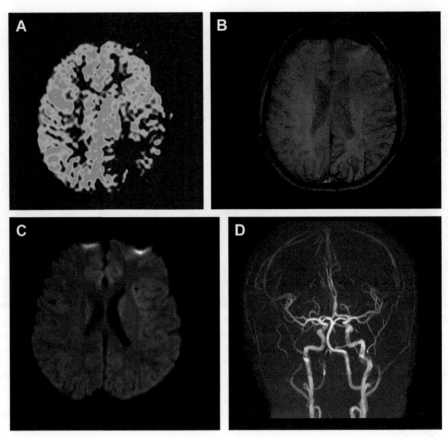

Fig. 2. *Stroke mimic.* Hemiplegic migraine in a 13-year-old girl presenting with slurred speech and weakness in the right side of the body. Axial ASL (*A*) shows decreased CBF in the left posterior quadrant of the brain. Axial SWI (*B*) shows the prominence of the venous structures in the same distribution, representing increased deoxyhemoglobin from increased oxygen extraction. Axial DTI (*C*) and 3D MIP from a TOF MRI (*D*) are normal.

Infection

Infections of the central nervous system (CNS) frequently exist as a continuum that involves the meninges and the parenchyma. A multitude of microorganisms, including viruses, bacteria, and parasites can affect the CNS, often resulting in non-focal neurologic deficits such as altered mental status, encephalopathy, seizures, and headaches. The high soft-tissue contrast of MRI is particularly helpful in identifying subtle areas of edema in the parenchyma, subtle enhancement, or changes in diffusivity. Similarly, incomplete suppression of fluid signal on T2W FLAIR or leptomeningeal enhancement on post-contrast T1-weighted (T1W) images or post-contrast T2W FLAIR are sensitive markers of the meningeal involvement (**Fig. 3**).

Viral meningitis is the most common CNS infection and the causative organisms are frequently enteroviruses.[30] The findings on MRI may be subtle or absent, and cerebrospinal fluid (CSF) analysis may be the only evidence of the disease.

Purulent collections are not a feature of viral infections and strongly suggest the presence of either a primary bacterial infection or a superinfection. Herpes encephalitis is common among adolescents and young adults and presents with characteristic restricted diffusion in the mesial temporal lobes and other limbic structures; occasionally, petechial hemorrhage coexists. The MRI appearance of viral encephalitis is nonspecific and pleomorphic. Varying degrees of asymmetric parenchymal inflammation, without or with enhancement, can be present; involvement of the deep gray nuclei is frequent. Many arboviruses (eastern equine encephalitis, western equine encephalitis, *Venezuelan*, among others) and *flaviviruses* (*Powassan*) affect children (**Fig. 4**). In general, the prognosis of encephalitis tends to be worse than that of isolated meningitis as the areas of parenchymal involvement can evolve to gliosis and encephalomalacia.

The incidence of bacterial meningitis has largely decreased with the widespread utilization of meningococcal and pneumococcal vaccines.

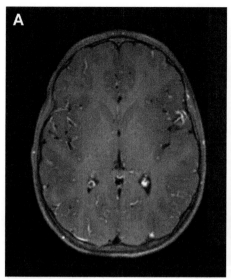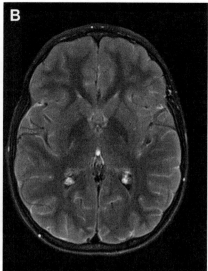

Fig. 3. *Meningitis.* Meningitis in a 7-year-old girl with headache and fever. Axial T1W SPACE (*A*) and 2D FLAIR (*B*) after contrast show diffuse leptomeningeal enhancement. Note that FLAIR is exquisitely sensitive to the T1 shortening effects of gadolinium-based contrast agents and can aid in the detection of subtle leptomeningeal pathology.

Bacterial meningoencephalitis presents with severe areas of leptomeningeal and parenchymal inflammation and frequently shows purulent contents. A common complication of bacterial meningitis is labyrinthitis; enhancement of the cochlea, vestibule, or semicircular canals portends a poor auditory prognosis as these areas typically progress to labyrinthitis ossificans. Vascular complications can also occur, leading to localized arterial ischemia and less frequently venous ischemia.[31]

Inflammatory Diseases

Acute disseminated encephalomyelitis (ADEM) is a monophasic inflammatory disorder that commonly affects children and can involve the brain and spinal cord. The incidence is estimated to be 0.4 per 100,000 person-years. ADEM can occur at any age, with a peak incidence between 5 and 8 years of age. In most cases, the event is precipitated by a recent viral infection, bacterial infection, or immunization.[32] Typical imaging features include T2W FLAIR hyperintense, multifocal, rounded, relatively large, and ill-defined lesions, which affect the cerebral white matter in an asymmetric manner (**Fig. 5**). Involvement of adjacent gray matter structures is common, and enhancement is variable.[33]

Acute Cranial Neuropathies

Deficits of cranial nerve require investigation with contrast-enhanced MRI. Imaging should include high-resolution cisternographic imaging (T2W SPACE or constructive interference steady state) covering the cranial nerve of concern and high-resolution T1W post-contrast imaging. Leptomeningeal enhancement along the nerves can be a sign of inflammation or infection. Differential considerations include Lyme meningitis and sarcoid.[34] Occasionally, a lesion in a nerve, such as a schwannoma, can be identified. Abnormal enhancement localized to the fundus of the IAC and the labyrinthine segment of the facial nerve can be seen in Bell's palsy.[35] It is important to ensure that the protocol provides whole-brain coverage in at least some of the sequences, preferably the fluid-sensitive sequences. Many brain tumors (eg, diffuse intrinsic pontine glioma) can present with acute-onset cranial neuropathies and therefore, the whole-brain parenchyma needs to be screened.[36]

Optic neuritis is a unique form of cranial neuropathy that carries a specific differential diagnosis. Frequently, optic neuritis can be seen as the first manifestation of an inflammatory brain disorder (clinically isolated syndrome) or a manifestation of established multiple sclerosis, MOG-AD, or NMO-SD. Imaging should include high-resolution fat-suppressed (FS) fluid-sensitive sequences and post-contrast imaging through the orbits (**Fig. 6**). A first presentation of optic neuritis should always prompt the imaging of the whole brain to look for possible clues of an underlying immune-mediated disorder.

Seizures

Seizures are a common indication of emergent neuroimaging. The incidence of nonfebrile

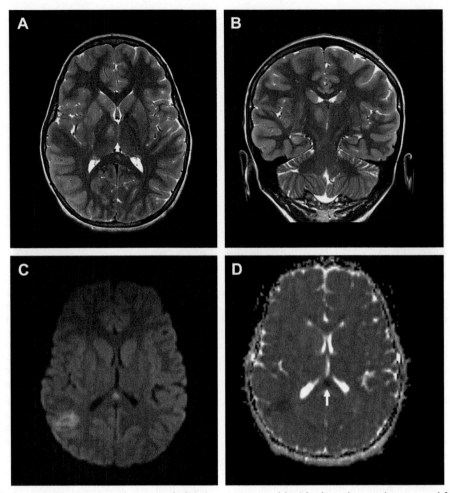

Fig. 4. *Viral meningitis. Powazza* virus encephalitis in an 11-year-old with altered mental status and fever. Axial (*A*) and coronal T2W (*B*) images show edema in the right greater than the left basal ganglia and in the right temporal and parietal cortex, which also seems swollen. Axial diffusion (*C*) and ADC (*D*) show restricted diffusion in the right parietal cortex and right insula consistent with cytotoxic edema; restricted diffusion in the splenium of the corpus callosum (*arrow*) is consistent with a focus of excitotoxic injury. No abnormal enhancement was seen.

unprovoked seizures in children ranges from 30 per 100,000 person-years in the late teenage years to 204 per 100,000 person-years during infancy.[37] Febrile seizures are even more common, as they have been reported to occur in up to 2% of all children.[38] The pretest probability of positive findings on imaging varies depending on whether the seizure was a nonfebrile unprovoked seizure, a febrile seizure, and as a function of clinical presentation. The American College of Radiology (ACR) recommends the use of MRI in cases of post-traumatic seizures, focal seizures (either ictal or postictal semiology), prolonged status epilepticus or intractable seizures, and in children who failed to return to baseline after the event.[39] Children with febrile seizures that fully resolve, generally do not require any imaging. There is currently no consensus on whether a first-time generalized

seizure with complete recovery requires emergent imaging; some providers defer an MRI until obtaining results from an electroencephalogram or may favor a head CT as a screening modality (**Fig. 7**).

Shunt Failure

The causes of obstructive hydrocephalus in children are varied and include posthemorrhagic hydrocephalus, postinfectious hydrocephalus, congenital malformations, and tumors. The most common strategies to treat pediatric hydrocephalus are the use of a ventriculoperitoneal (VP) shunt or with an endoscopic third ventriculostomy (ETV). VP shunts are effective in providing a low resistance route for CSF drainage; however, children with shunts endure a lifelong risk of shunt failure due to disconnection, obstruction, or malfunction

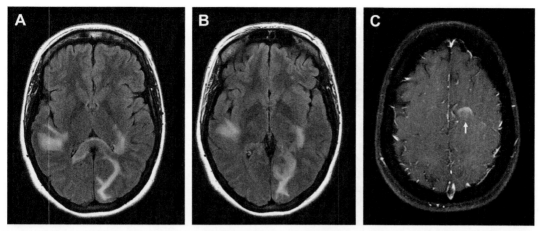

Fig. 5. *ADEM* in an 8-year-old patient 1 week after an upper respiratory infection. Axial FLAIR images (*A, B*) show asymmetric and multifocal white matter lesions with some involvement of adjacent gray matter structures. Post-contrast T1W image (*C*) with fat suppression shows patchy enhancement in the left frontal lobe (*arrow*).

of the tubing, reservoir, and valve. The advent of ultrafast MRI sequences, including single-shot T2W (ssT2W), has led to an increase in the utilization of MRI to monitor ventricular size and diagnose shunt failure. Even in uncooperative children, ssT2W frequently suffices and a CT can be avoided, thus sparing the child unnecessary radiation exposure (**Fig. 8**). Endoscopic third ETV has emerged as a preferred alternative to shunt catheters, whenever the obstruction can be bypassed by this approach. Heavily T2W sequences (eg,: high-resolution T2W SPACE) accentuate the dephasing associated with CSF flow and enable confirmation of patency of the ETV.

Nontraumatic Spinal Emergencies

MRI vastly outperforms CT in the diagnosis of spinal pathology and consequently is the first-line imaging modality whenever an acute myelopathy is suspected. Although the physical examination of the patient often localizes the sources of the neurologic complaints to the spinal cord and may even provide a level for the symptoms, imaging is frequently required to establish an etiologic diagnosis. Tumors, inflammatory myelopathies (transverse myelitis), and cord hemorrhage can all result in acute neurologic deficits that are indistinguishable. A distinct pediatric entity, known as acute flaccid myelitis (AFM), can have a dramatic

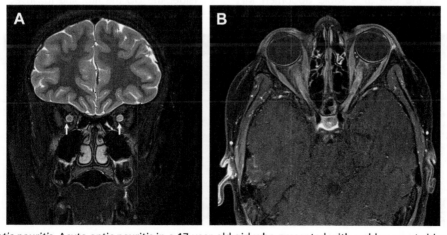

Fig. 6. *Optic neuritis.* Acute optic neuritis in a 17-year-old girl who presented with sudden onset vision changes. Coronal fat-suppressed (FS) T2W image (*A*) shows a hyperintense signal in the optic nerves bilaterally (*arrows*). Axial post-contrast FS T1W (*B*) shows long-segment enhancement in the anterior aspect of the optic nerves (intraorbital and canalicular). The pattern is suggestive of MOG-AD which was later confirmed. No brain abnormalities were present at the time of diagnosis.

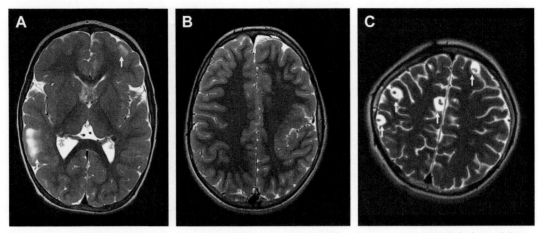

Fig. 7. *Seizure.* Epileptogenic lesions in three different patients with seizures. Axial T2W (*A*) shows bilateral cortical tubers (*arrows*) and subependymal nodules in a patient with Tuberous sclerosis. Axial-W T2 (*B*) shows an extensive cortical malformation in the left perisylvian region. Axial T2W (*C*) shows multiple cystic lesions with a calcified scolex, consistent with neurocysticercosis (*arrows*).

presentation. Outbreaks of AFM occurred in 2014 and 2018, in association with an outbreak of upper respiratory infections secondary to enterovirus.[40] Affected children developed a rapidly progressive flaccid paralysis consistent with lower motor-neuron involvement. MRI findings include longitudinally extensive T2 prolongation centered in the central gray matter and anterior horns and enhancement of the ventral nerve roots. Enhancement of cranial nerves and T2 prolongation in the brainstem are common associated findings (**Fig. 9**).[41]

BODY APPLICATIONS

Small single-center studies have shown the cost-effectivity of the use of a rapid abdomen MR

protocols in the evaluation of abdominal pain in children in an ER setting.[11,12,42] Although these are small noncontrolled studies, the possibility of using a "universal" abdomen MR protocol to cover the most common pathologies in the emergency setting may have the potential to supplant the use of the CT at the emergency in the pediatric population.[11,12]

Appendicitis

The initial evaluation in cases of suspected appendicitis is based on the clinical risk assessment (low, intermediate, or high) using one of the available clinical scales, which helps risk-stratify patients who will need investigation by imaging.[43–45] The ACR appropriateness criteria consider the US the first line for investigation of

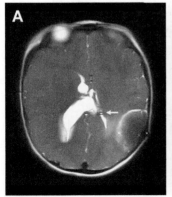
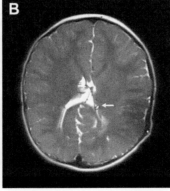
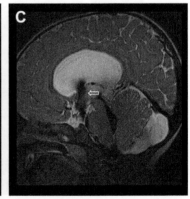

Fig. 8. *Shunt evaluation.* Shunt failure in a 3-year-old boy with Chiari II and prior ventriculitis. Axial single-shot T2W FSE (*A*) shows distension of the right lateral ventricle and right periatrial transependymal edema, which are new relative to the prior ventricular check MRI (*B*). A left parietal ventricular catheter is noted (*arrows*). Sagittal T2W SPACE (*C*) in a different patient shows a dephasing jet through the floor of the third ventricle, showing patency of the endoscopic third ventriculostomy (open *arrow*).

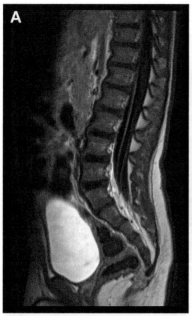
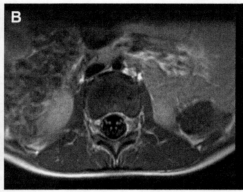

Fig. 9. Acute flaccid myelitis in a 3-year-old boy with sudden-onset lower extremity weakness in the setting of a recent gastrointestinal infection who tested positive for *Enterovirus-D68*. Sagittal (*A*) and axial T1W (*B*) images after contrast show enhancement of the anterior nerve roots.

patients with an intermediate or high risk of appendicitis. Contrast-enhanced CT or rapid abdominal MR are both considered appropriate in cases the US is equivocal or nondiagnostic.[46] At the authors' institutions, unenhanced abdomen MR is recommended as second-line imaging follow-up for equivocal US. Some studies have suggested that the accuracy of abdominal CT compared with MR for the diagnosis of appendicitis is similar in the pediatric population.[47–51] Likely the improved spatial resolution and contrast enhancement of CT balance the superior tissue contrast of MRI. Moreover, the implementation and development of faster MR sequences have great potential to increase the spatial resolution of MR improving, even more, the method's sensitivity.[48,52]

The MRI findings suggestive of acute appendicitis include the following:

- Thickening of the appendix (>6 mm in outer diameter);
- Fluid-filled appendix;
- Appendiceal wall thickening;
- Presence of appendicolith;
- Periappendiceal edema or fluid (T2W hyperintensity, better seen in the FS sequences) (**Fig. 10**).[3,12,53]

MR is also used to rule out complications, including perforation or abscess. The signs that suggest perforation include appendiceal wall discontinuity (direct sign), presence of free air, decompressed appendix, and presence of an abscess.[12,50] Standard appendiceal MR protocols are short (<5 min) and consist of axial and coronal ssT2W images with and without FS, without oral or intravenous contrast.[54] This protocol is designed for children 5 years and older who are able to tolerate MR without the need for sedation. Optional sequences include diffusion-weighted imaging, radial T2W fast spin echo, and T1W FS post-contrast imaging. The use of diffusion-weighted imaging may slightly increase the sensitivity of MR for the diagnosis of appendicitis, although no large study has been performed. In cases positive for appendicitis, it is common to see increased diffusivity in the appendix.[12,55] Post-contrast sequences are also optional, as the overall additional scanning time does not seem to result in significantly improved sensitivity.[47,49,51,55,56] Radial T2W can improve tissue contrast for detecting appendiceal and periappendiceal inflammation.

Inflammatory Bowel Disease

Magnetic resonance enterography (MRE) is not routinely performed in the ER setting for multiple reasons, including long acquisition time, requirement for oral contrast preparation, and limited window of time for image acquisition once the patient is ready. Standard abdominal MR or CT without oral contrast typically provides enough information to

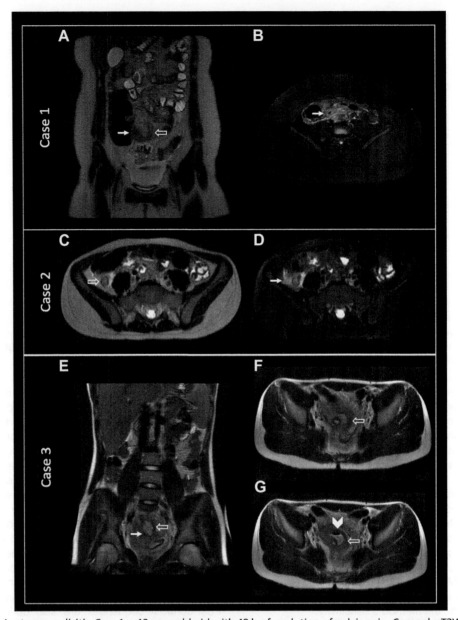

Fig. 10. *Acute appendicitis. Case 1:* a 12-year-old girl with 48 h of evolution of pelvic pain. Coronal ssT2W (*A*) and axial ssT2W FS (*B*) images show a fluid-filled appendix with diffuse wall thickening (*open arrow*). An appendico-lith is noted at the base of the appendix (*arrow*), and periappendiceal T2W hyperintense signal suggestive of in-flammatory changes, better seen in the FS sequence (*B*). *Case 2:* an 11-year-old boy with right lower quadrant pain and fever. Axial ssT2W (*C*) and axial ssT2W FS (*D*) images showing the importance of fat suppression to show periappendiceal inflammatory changes that are almost imperceptive in the non-FS sequence (*C*) and exuberant in the FS sequence (*arrow*). *Case 3:* a 15-year-old boy with lower abdominal pain over the past 7 days, slightly better in the last few hours. Coronal (*E*) and axial (*F, G*) ssT2W images show complicated appendicitis. There is an area of discontinuity in the appendiceal wall at the tip (*arrow*)—direct sign of rupture—associated with an adjacent collection (*open arrow*), with air–fluid level (*head arrow*).

evaluate inflammatory bowel disease (IBD) activity and penetrating disease complications requiring intervention. Pelvic MRI can also be performed for focused detection of fistulizing perianal Crohn's disease in patients with perianal symptoms.

Because IBD patients (and Crohn's disease patients in particular) may be at higher risk of needed serial CT scans over time for symptomatic evaluation, abdominal MRI can be considered in the ER setting for patients at high risk for penetrating

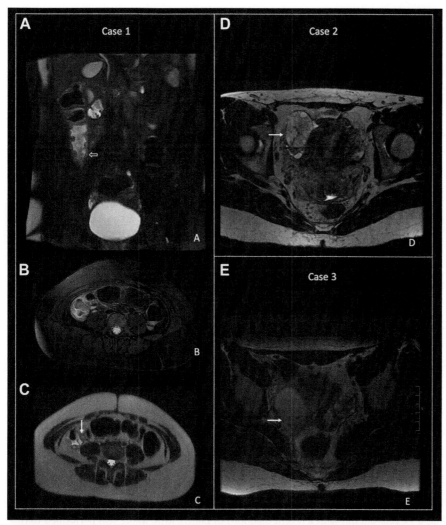

Fig. 11. *Differential diagnosis of acute appendicitis.* The appendix was visualized in all cases and was normal-appearing (not included in the figure). *Case 1:* a 14-year-old girl with right lower quadrant pain and diarrhea. Coronal T2W FS (*A*), axial T2W FS (*B*), and axial T2W (*C*) images show submucosal edema in the ascending colon (*open arrow*), with pericolonic T2W hyperintense signal representing inflammatory changes (*A, B*), with circumferential wall thickening of the terminal ileum (*arrow*), suggestive of enterocolitis. In association with the clinical history and distribution of the lesions, the possibility of inflammatory bowel disease was raised and subsequently confirmed. *Case 2:* an 18-year-old girl with acute right lower quadrant pain. Axial T2W image (*D*) shows an asymmetrically enlarged right ovary (left ovary was not included in the image), with peripheral follicles, and central T2W hypointensity, likely secondary to interstitial hemorrhage. *Case 3:* a 16-year-old girl with subacute pelvic pain. Axial T2W image (*E*) shows a cystic right adnexal lesion, with T2W shading (*arrow*) suggesting layering blood products, which may present hemorrhagic ovarian cyst versus endometrioma.

disease complications.[57] IBD is also one of the main differentials of appendicitis (**Fig. 11**).[50,56]

MR features of active IBD include bowel wall thickening >3 mm, bowel wall edema (increased T2W signal intensity compared with muscle) or hyperenhancement on enteric phase (55–70 s) post-contrast images, vasa recta engorgement, perienteric edema/inflammation, and bowel wall diffusion restriction.[3,12,58] Inflammatory enterocolitis can be difficult to distinguish from infectious

enterocolitis without clinical correlation, especially in the first episode, and may be considered mainly based on the distribution (eg, isolated terminal ileitis) or appearance (prominent perienteric inflammation), although no finding is specific.

Pelvic Pain

The first-line imaging modality for diagnosis of pelvic pain in pediatric female patients in the ER is

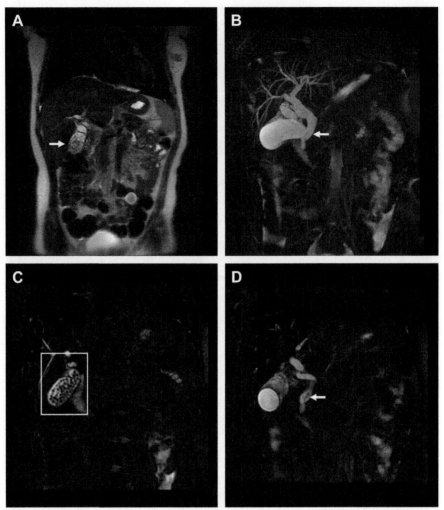

Fig. 12. *MRCP,* a 14-year-old girl with a recent diagnosis of pancreatitis. MRCP was performed to rule out biliary obstruction. Coronal T2W (*A*) and coronal (*C*) MRCP show filing defects in the gallbladder consistent with chole-lithiasis (*arrow* in *A* and square in *C*). Three-dimensional MIP MRCP reconstruction (*B*) shows dilation of the common bile duct (*arrow*). Coronal MRCP (*D*) shows filling defects within the common bile duct. The diagnosis of biliary pancreatitis was made and the biliary tree was treated with ERCP and stone removal.

pelvic US,[59] although female pelvic pathology is often incidentally identified on patients that undergo appendicitis MR due to right lower quadrant pain.[12,50,56]

Adnexal lesions causing hemorrhage

Adnexal lesions associated with hemorrhage in post-menarchal girls include hemorrhagic ovarian cysts, ectopic pregnancy, and endometrioma. Hemorrhagic cysts may cause pain during the luteal menstrual phase and, in some cases, can rupture, leading to hemoperitoneum. On MR hemorrhagic cysts are typically T1W hyperintense and show variable T2W signal, often with retractile clot noted in its wall (see **Fig. 11**). Endometriomas can

have an overlapping appearance with hemorrhagic cysts, although more often are more T1W hyperintense and T2W hypointense than hemorrhagic cysts. If the cyst is ruptured with hemoperitoneum, the main differential is ectopic pregnancy, which is excluded based on the β-hCG status in most cases.[12]

Ovarian torsion

Although the diagnosis of ovarian torsion is primarily clinically associated with US findings, the symptoms could be nonspecific in the pediatric population and incidentally found in the MR performed for other reasons. The MR findings of ovarian torsion consist in the following:

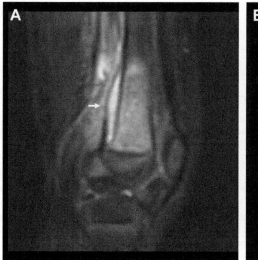
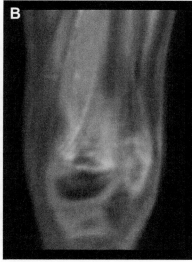

Fig. 13. *Osteomyelitis,* a 5-year-old boy investigating hematogenous osteomyelitis involving the distal femur. Sagittal STIR (*A*) and T1W FS post-contrast (*B*) images show bone marrow edema and enhancement of the distal femoral metaphysis. Subperiosteal abscess is noted in the dorsal aspect of the femur (*arrow*). There is no trans-physeal extension, which occurs almost exclusively below the age of 18 months, when there is communication between epiphyseal and metaphyseal vessels. After this age, the physis act as a barrier that limits infection spread, as noted in this case.

- Asymmetrically enlarged ovary, with peripherally distributed follicles;
- Twisted vascular pedicle (whirlpool sign and pathognomonic);
- Ovarian hemorrhage, which is initially seen as a T2W hypointense rim surrounding the perifollicular region or in the interstitium (see **Fig. 11**).[3,12,53,60]

The presence of an adnexal mass (eg, teratoma) as a leading point for torsion is not essential for the diagnosis but should be excluded. Other causes as ovarian hypermobility can lead to torsion in the absence of underlying adnexal lesions.[60,61]

Pancreaticobiliary Pathology: Magnetic Resonance Cholangiopancreatography

Another clinical indication for abdominal MR in the ED is for investigation of patients with suspected cholestasis.[62] We use an abbreviated noncontrast magnetic resonance cholangiopancreatography (MRCP) protocol, reserving post-contrast sequence for cases with suspicion of cholangitis, which may show enhancement of the wall of the biliary tree.[62] The MRCP is a heavily T2W (TE range 500–1000 msec) fluid-sensitive volumetric sequence, which is helpful to visualize the biliary tree for detection of obstructing stones (**Fig. 12**) or strictures.[12,63] For detection of biliary obstruction, MRCP is more sensitive than the CT or US[64] and has similar accuracy to endoscopic

retrograde cholangiopancreatography.[63,65] Therefore, MRCP may be considered as the first line of investigation in patients with cholestasis and concern for biliary stone or other obstructing process.[62]

MUSCULOSKELETAL APPLICATIONS

In the ED, the most common musculoskeletal pathology requiring MRI evaluation in children is osteomyelitis with or without associated septic arthritis. Although traumatic musculoskeletal injuries are well-evaluated by MRI in the pediatric population, MRI is not generally performed at the ED as it does not alter acute diagnosis or management, and therefore will not be included in this article.

Osteomyelitis and septic arthritis occur most commonly in patients younger than 5 years and can have a nonspecific clinical presentation, being common symptoms including fever, irritability, and refusal to bear weight on the involved extremity. Both entities share similar causative organisms: *Staphylococcus aureus* is the most common agent, and *Kingella kingae* has increasing recognition of a common pathogen below 4 years of age.[66–68] The most frequent cause of osteomyelitis in children is hematogenous seeding of bacteria into the bone during episodes of transient bacteremia.[69] Direct inoculation of bacteria from open fractures or surgical interventions is less common.[68,70]

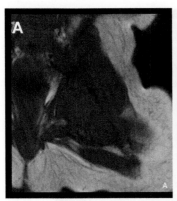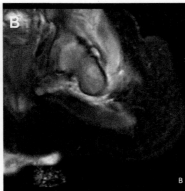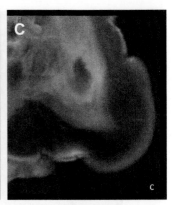

Fig. 14. *Osteomyelitis.* MR imaging in a 46-day-old boy with osteomyelitis and soft tissue abscess. Coronal T1W (*A*) image shows low signal intensity within the whole bone marrow included in the field of view due to hemato-poietic bone marrow. Coronal STIR (*B*) image shows only faintly increased T2W signal intensity in relation to the adjacent hyperintense bone marrow. There is extensive soft tissue edema and a fluid collection. Coronal post-contrast T1W FS (*C*) image adds to the confidence of osteomyelitis diagnosis by showing a large soft tissue abscess.

Hematogenous Osteomyelitis

In the pediatric skeleton, the most common locations for hematogenous spread are the highly vascularized metaphysis. The metaphysis contains terminal vessels at the metaphyseal–physeal interface, where bacteria get stranded.[71] Most cases of hematogenous osteomyelitis occur in the metaphysis of long bones as femur, tibia, and humerus, in this order.[68,69] Other areas involved in osseous growth known as metaphyseal equivalents such as the osseocartilaginous interphase at the epiphyseal ossification centers, triradiate cartilage, sacroiliac joints, ischiopubic synchondrosis, and periphery of round bones in the hands and feet show the similar vascular structure and, therefore, are susceptible to hematogenous seeding.[72] These metaphyseal equivalents are especially important to evaluate in the pelvis, where a common pattern of disease is having extensive soft tissue edema with minimal osseous findings.[71]

From the initial source of infection in the metaphysis, the infection can spread into the adjacent osseous diaphysis or epiphysis, to the subperiosteal space, and within the joint or into the adjacent soft tissues. Infection from the metaphysis into the epiphysis occurs almost exclusively below the age of 18 months, when there is communication between epiphyseal and metaphyseal vessels. The presence of these vessels is also believed to be the reason for the higher incidence of septic arthritis in this age group. After this age, the physis act as a barrier that limits infection spread (**Fig. 13**).[73]

In the pediatric population, evaluation with MRI should include a combination of T1W and FS fluid-sensitive sequences (eg, T2W FS or STIR) in short-axis and long-axis planes. The use of gadolinium contrast is not needed for osteomyelitis diagnosis but can be helpful in infants and children younger than 18 months for the detection of epiphyseal cartilage infection.[74,75] Of note, epiphyseal secondary ossification centers can normally show diminished enhancement and comparison with the asymptomatic contralateral limb may help in questionable cases.[76] The detection of osteomyelitis in neonates and young infants is challenging due to extremely low T1W signal intensity and relatively high signal intensity of fluid-sensitive sequences from hematopoietic bone marrow. The use of contrast-enhanced imaging and close attention to periosteal and soft tissue findings aid in the detection of disease in this age group (**Fig. 14**).[71] In older children with more ossified epiphyses and increased fatty bone marrow, the use of contrast does not seem to improve the accuracy for the diagnosis of osteomyelitis[75,77]; however, it can be helpful to rule out associated periosteal abscess needing surgical drainage. Some authors advocate for the use of an extended field of view in patients below the age of 5 years to detect the source of infection, possible multifocal infection, or other causes that could explain the patient's symptoms.[71,75,78]

Septic Arthritis

Septic arthritis is considered an orthopedic urgency with delay in diagnosis and treatment resulting in irreversible joint damage.[66,79] Septic arthritis most frequently occurs in large joints of the lower extremities with up to 80% of cases involving the hip or knee.[79] Most cases occur from direct hematogenous spread. However, secondary septic arthritis infection spread from adjacent

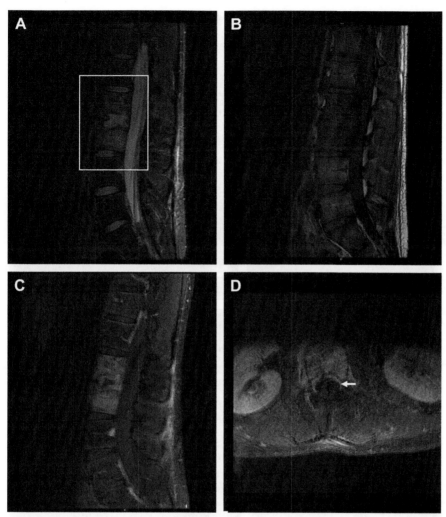

Fig. 15. *Discitis and osteomyelitis,* an 18-year-old boy with a history of 2 months of lower back pain. Sagittal STIR (*A*) and T1W (*B*) images show marrow edema in the L2 and L3 vertebral bodies, with erosion of the L2–L3 end-plates (square). Note that there is no significant loss of disk height due to the presence of fluid within the disk. Sagittal I1W fat-suppressed (FS) post-contrast image (*C*) shows enhancement of the areas of marrow edema and surrounding the intervertebral disk. Axial T1W FS post-contrast image (*D*) shows an extension of the inflammatory findings, with the enhancement of the psoas muscles and ventral epidural space (*arrow*).[87]

osteomyelitis into the joint is not uncommon, reaching frequencies as high as 60% to 80% in infants with hip or shoulder septic arthritis.[80] The knee is unlikely to have this phenomenon as the metaphysis is extraarticular.[79] From the imaging perspective, the most important finding is joint effusion. The lack of joint effusion on MRI or US examination can generally exclude septic arthritis.[81] Additional imaging criteria have proven unreliable to exclude infection in the setting of joint effusion. Given the lack of additional specific imaging findings, emergent arthrocentesis is warranted. Owing to the common coexistence of septic arthritis and osteomyelitis, some authors advocate for the use of MRI in most cases.[82]

Spine

Discitis with or without osteomyelitis

Discitis is the infection of the intervertebral disk. Different from adults, pediatric patients can have primarily infection of the disk with extension to the adjacent endplates due to the presence of vascular channels in the disks that disappear later in life.[83,84]

Based on ACR appropriateness criteria, spine MR with contrast is the first line in the investigation of discitis.[85] Classic MR findings include the following:

- Loss of the normal T2W hyperintense signal of the disk;[84]

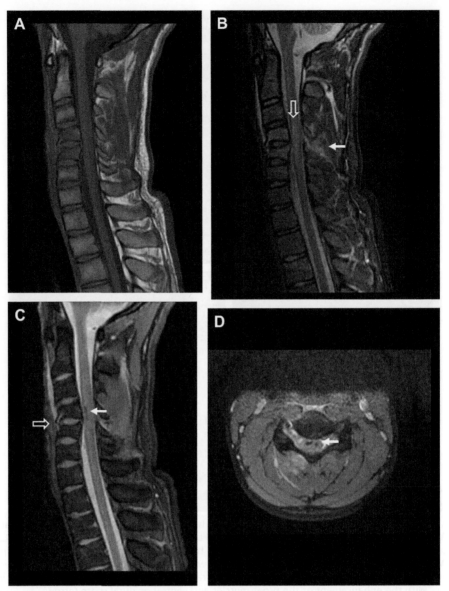

Fig. 16. *Spinal trauma,* a 16-year-old boy with weakness of the upper extremities post-motor vehicle accident. Sagittal T1W (*A*), sagittal STIR (*B*), sagittal T2W GRE (*C*), and axial T2W GRE (*D*) images show hyperflexion three-column injury at the C4–C5 level, with compression fractures of the anterior aspect of the C4 and C5 vertebral bodies, leading to retropulsion toward to the spinal canal and cord compression at that level, with signs of hemorrhagic cord contusion (open *arrow* in *B*, and *arrow* in *C* and *D*). There is associated injury in the anterior longitudinal ligament (*open arrow* in *C*) and in the interspinous ligaments (*arrow* in *B*) as well as a small prevertebral hematoma.

- Decreased intervertebral disk height, although some cases can have normal or increased height due to the presence of abscess within the disk;[84,86]
- Hyperenhancement of the disk and adjacent vertebral body (not always present);
- T1W hypointensity/T2W hyperintensity in the adjacent vertebrae (marrow edema) if there is associated osteomyelitis.[84]

MR is also used to rule out complications, including extension to the paraspinal muscles, disk extrusion, epidural abscess, and cord compression (**Fig. 15**).[84,86] Indeed, Shifrin and colleagues[87] found that paraspinal edema and psoas edema are highly sensitive and specific, respectively, for the MRI detection of spinal epidural abscess. They concluded that "familiarity with the findings for spinal epidural abscess at unenhanced

MRI could help expedite further definitive evaluation when the contrast agent is not administered."[87]

Ligament and cord injury

Spine MR is not the first line of investigation in patients with suspicion of spine trauma[88] but may be considered as a follow-up study in patients with suspected cord compression/contusion or ligamentous injury.[89] Children are more prone to injuries of the cervical spine compared with adults because of the disproportional larger head for body size, laxity of the ligaments, and weaker paravertebral musculature.[90] The main MR findings are as follows:

- Anterior and posterior longitudinal ligaments injury;
- Intervertebral disk rupture;
- Muscular and interspinal ligament tears;
- Shearing of the subepiphyseal growth zone of the vertebral endplates (**Fig. 16**).[91]

Spine MR also allows the evaluation of cord integrity, which has a good correlation with the neurologic prognosis. Major cord hemorrhages have profoundly poor outcomes, minor hemorrhages are associated with partial recovery of function, and isolated cord contusions tend to recover completely.[91]

SUMMARY

Technological advances to reduce acquisition time, decrease motion sensitivity, and improve image contrast and spatial resolution have led to an increase in the use of MR in pediatric patients in the ER setting. MR applications in the pediatric population continue to increase, including neuro, body, and musculoskeletal indications. The increase of MR use in the pediatric population in the emergency setting helps to decrease radiation exposure while improving diagnostic accuracy for acute pathology.

CLINICS CARE POINTS

- The involvement in moyamoya is frequently bilateral, although asymmetry is common; posterior circulation involvement is rare but occurs in severe cases and virtually always in association with anterior circulation disease. In this population, infarcts cluster in the cerebral watershed territories.

- Acute disseminated encephalomyelitis typical imaging features include T2-weighted (T2W) FLAIR hyperintense, multifocal, rounded, relatively large, and ill-defined lesions, which affect the cerebral white matter in an asymmetric manner. Involvement of adjacent gray matter structures is common, and enhancement is variable.

- Optic neuritis is a unique form of cranial neuropathy that carries a specific differential diagnosis. Frequently, optic neuritis can be seen as the first manifestation of an inflammatory brain disorder (clinically isolated syndrome) or a manifestation of established multiple sclerosis, MOG-AD, or NMO-SD.

- MR is the imaging modality of choice in pediatric patients with clinical suspicion of acute appendicitis with equivocal ultrasound. Appendicitis MR protocols rely on motion-insensitive single-shot T2W sequences and can be performed without oral or intravenous contrast.

- Extension of osteomyelitis across physis occurs almost exclusively below the age of 18 months, when there is communication between epiphyseal and metaphyseal vessels. After this age, the physis act as a barrier that limits the spread of infection.

- Different from adults, pediatric patients with discitis can have primarily infection of the disk with extension to the adjacent endplates because of the presence of vascular channels in the disks that disappear later in life.

REFERENCES

1. Marin JR, Rodean J, Hall M, et al. Trends in use of advanced imaging in pediatric emergency departments, 2009-2018. JAMA Pediatr 2020;174(9): 2009–18.
2. Kulaylat AN, Moore MM, Engbrecht BW, et al. An implemented MRI program to eliminate radiation from the evaluation of pediatric appendicitis. J Pediatr Surg 2015;50(8):1359–63.
3. Ditkofsky NG, Singh A, Avery L, et al. The role of emergency MRI in the setting of acute abdominal pain. Emerg Radiol 2014;21(6):615–24.
4. Mathews JD, Forsythe AV, Brady Z, et al. Cancer risk in 680 000 people exposed to computed tomography scans in childhood or adolescence: Data linkage study of 11 million Australians. BMJ 2013; 346(7910):1–18.
5. Pearce MS, Salotti JA, Little MP, et al. Radiation exposure from CT scans in childhood and subsequent risk of leukaemia and brain tumours: A retrospective cohort study. Lancet 2012;380(9840): 499–505.
6. Hong JY, Han K, Jung JH, et al. Association of Exposure to Diagnostic Low-Dose Ionizing Radiation with

Risk of Cancer among Youths in South Korea. JAMA Netw Open 2019;2(9):1–11.

7. Gottumukkala R, Gee M, Hampilos P, et al. Current and Emerging Roles of Whole-Body MRI in Evaluation of Pediatric Cancer Patients. Radiographics 2019;39(2):516–34.

8. American Academy of Pediatrics. Choosing Wisely. Available at: https://www.choosingwisely.org/societies/american-academy-of-pediatrics/. Accessed October 10, 2022.

9. American College of Radiology, Choosing Wisely. Available at: https://www.choosingwisely.org/societies/american-college-of-radiology/. Accessed October 6, 2022.

10. Jaimes C, Yang E, Connaughton P, et al. Diagnostic equivalency of fast T2 and FLAIR sequences for pediatric brain MRI: a pilot study. Pediatr Radiol 2020; 50(4):550–9.

11. Desoky S, Udayasankar UK. Unenhanced MRI for abdominal pain in the pediatric emergency department: Point - Safe and comprehensive assessment while reducing delay in care. Am J Roentgenol 2021;216(4):874–5.

12. Warner J, Desoky S, Tiwari HA, et al. Unenhanced MRI of the Abdomen and Pelvis in the Comprehensive Evaluation of Acute Atraumatic Abdominal Pain in Children. Am J Roentgenol 2020;215(5): 1218–28.

13. Harrington SG, Jaimes C, Weagle KM, et al. Strategies to perform magnetic resonance imaging in infants and young children without sedation. Pediatr Radiol 2021. https://doi.org/10.1007/s00247-021-05062-3.

14. Kozak BM, Jaimes C, Kirsch J, et al. Mri techniques to decrease imaging times in children. Radiographics 2020;40(2):485–502.

15. Griswold MA, Jakob PM, Heidemann RM, et al. Generalized Autocalibrating Partially Parallel Acquisitions (GRAPPA). Magn Reson Med 2002;47(6): 1202–10.

16. Conklin J, Longo MGF, Cauley SF, et al. Validation of highly accelerated WAVE-CAIPI SWI compared with conventional SWI and T2*-weighted gradient recalled-echo for routine clinical brain MRI at 3T. AJNR Am J Neuroradiol 2019;40(12):2073–80.

17. Polak D, Cauley S, Huang SY, et al. Highly-accelerated volumetric brain examination using optimized wave-CAIPI encoding. J Magn Reson Imaging 2019;50(3):961–74.

18. Tabari A, Conklin J, Figueiro Longo MG, et al. Comparison of ultrafast wave-controlled aliasing in parallel imaging (CAIPI) magnetization-prepared rapid acquisition gradient echo (MP-RAGE) and standard MP-RAGE in non-sedated children: initial clinical experience. Pediatr Radiol 2021;51(11):2009–17.

19. Conklin J, Tabari A, Figueiro Longo MG, et al. Evaluation of Highly Accelerated Wave-CAIPI Susceptibility-Weighted Imaging (SWI) in the Non-Sedated

Pediatric Setting: Initial experience. In: Conference: Society of Pediatric Radiology. ; 2019.

20. Slipsager J, Glimberg S, Højgaard L, et al. Comparison of prospective and retrospective motion correction in 3D-encoded neuroanatomical MRI. Magn Reson Med 2021. https://doi.org/10.1002/mrm.28991.

21. McMillan AB, Estowski L, Cashen TA, et al. Accelerated whole-body imaging with uniform fat-suppression and deep-learning reconstruction. In: Conference: ISMRM & SMRT Annual Meeting Exhibition. Utah, May 15-20, 2021.

22. Bash S, Thomas M, Fund M, et al. Deep-Learning Reconstruction Improves Quality of Clinical Brain and Spine MR Imaging. In: Radiological Society of North America 2019 Scientific Assembly and Annual Meeting. Chicago (IL), December 1-6, 2019.

23. Khala A, Michael I, Fullerton H, et al. Pediatric Stroke Imaging. Pediatr Neurol 2019;176(3):139–48.

24. Agrawal N, Johnston SC, Wu YW, et al. Imaging data reveal a higher pediatric stroke incidence than prior us estimates. Stroke 2009;40(11): 3415–21.

25. Sorensen AG, Wu O, Copen WA, et al. Human acute cerebral ischemia: Detection of changes in water diffusion anisotropy by using MR imaging. Radiology 1999;212(3):785–92.

26. Allen LM, Hasso AN, Handwerker J, et al. Sequence-specific MR imaging findings that are useful in dating ischemic stroke. Radiographics 2012;32(5):1285–97.

27. Li J, Jin M, Sun X, et al. Imaging of Moyamoya Disease and Moyamoya Syndrome: Current Status. J Comput Assist Tomogr 2019;43(2):257–63.

28. Fullerton HJ, Stence N, Hills NK, et al. Focal cerebral arteriopathy of childhood: Novel severity score and natural history. Stroke 2018;49(11):2590–6.

29. Song JW, Lehman L, Rivkin M, et al. Serial vessel wall MR imaging of pediatric tuberculous vasculitis. Neurol Clin Pract 2019;9(6):459–61.

30. Meningitis and Encephalitis Fact Sheet | National Institute of Neurological Disorders and Stroke. Available at: https://www.ninds.nih.gov/Disorders/Patient-Caregiver-Education/Fact-Sheets/Meningitis-and-Encephalitis-Fact-Sheet https://www.ninds.nih.gov/Disorders/Patient-Caregiver-Education/Fact-Sheets/Meningitis-and-Encephalitis-Fact-Sheet. Accessed December 12, 2021.

31. Prabhu SP, Young-Poussaint T. Pediatric central nervous system emergencies. Neuroimaging Clin N Am 2010;20(4):663–83.

32. Chvojka M, Gut J, Jiránek M. Acute disseminated encephalomyelitis. Pediatr Pro Praxi 2020;21(5): 369–73.

33. Krupp LB, Tardieu M, Amato MP, et al. International Pediatric Multiple Sclerosis Study Group criteria for pediatric multiple sclerosis and immune-mediated

central nervous system demyelinating disorders: revisions to the 2007 definitions. Mult Scler J 2013; 19(10):1261–7.

34. Agarwal R, Sze G. Neuro-lyme disease: MR imaging findings. Radiology 2009;253(1):167–73.

35. Kim IS, Shin SH, Kim J, et al. Correlation between MRI and operative findings in Bell's palsy and Ramsay Hunt syndrome. Yonsei Med J 2007;48(6): 963–8.

36. Srikanthan D, Taccone MS, Van Ommeren R, et al. Diffuse intrinsic pontine glioma: current insights and future directions. Chin Neurosurg J 2021;7(1):1–11.

37. Åndell E, Tomson T, Carlsson S, et al. The incidence of unprovoked seizures and occurrence of neurodevelopmental comorbidities in children at the time of their first epileptic seizure and during the subsequent six months. Epilepsy Res 2015;113:140–50.

38. Duffner PK, Berman PH, Baumann RJ, et al. Clinical practice guideline - Neurodiagnostic evaluation of the child with a simple febrile seizure. Pediatrics 2011;127(2):389–94.

39. Trofimova A, Milla SS, Ryan ME, et al. ACR Appropriateness Criteria® Seizures-Child. J Am Coll Radiol 2021;18(5):S199–211.

40. Fatemi Y, Chakraborty R. Acute Flaccid Myelitis: A Clinical Overview for 2019. Mayo Clin Proc 2019; 94(5):875–81.

41. Maloney JA, Mirsky DM, Messacar K, et al. MRI findings in children with acute flaccid paralysis and cranial nerve dysfunction occurring during the 2014 enterovirus D68 outbreak. AJNR Am J Neuroradiol 2015;36(2):245–50.

42. Hagedorn KN, Hayatghaibi SE, Levine MH, et al. Cost Comparison of Ultrasound Versus MRI to Diagnose Adolescent Female Patients Presenting with Acute Abdominal/Pelvic Pain Using Time-Driven Activity-Based Costing. Acad Radiol 2019;26(12): 1618–24.

43. Saucier A, Huang EY, Emeremni CA, et al. Prospective evaluation of a clinical pathway for suspected appendicitis. Pediatrics 2014;133(1):e88–95.

44. Goldman RD, Carter S, Stephens D, et al. Prospective Validation of the Pediatric Appendicitis Score. J Pediatr 2008;153(2):278–82.

45. Santillanes G, Simms S, Gausche-Hill M, et al. Prospective evaluation of a clinical practice guideline for diagnosis of appendicitis in children. Acad Emerg Med 2012;19(8):886–93.

46. Koberlein GC, Trout AT, Rigsby CK, et al. ACR Appropriateness Criteria® Suspected Appendicitis-Child. J Am Coll Radiol 2019;16(5):S252–63.

47. Kinner S, Pickhardt PJ, Riedesel EL, et al. Diagnostic accuracy of MRI versus CT for the evaluation of acute appendicitis in children and young adults. Am J Roentgenol 2017;209(4):911–9.

48. Johnson AK, Filippi CG, Andrews T, et al. Ultrafast 3-T MRI in the evaluation of children with acute lower abdominal pain for the detection of appendicitis. Am J Roentgenol 2012;198(6):1424–30.

49. Duke E, Kalb B, Arif-Tiwari H, et al. A systematic review and meta-Analysis of diagnostic performance of MRI for evaluation of acute appendicitis. Am J Roentgenol 2016;206(3):508–17.

50. Dillman JR, Gadepalli S, Sroufe NS, et al. Equivocal pediatric appendicitis: Unenhanced MR imaging protocol for nonsedated children-a clinical effectiveness study. Radiology 2016;279(1):216–25.

51. Repplinger MD, Pickhardt PJ, Robbins JB, et al. Prospective comparison of the diagnostic accuracy of MR imaging versus CT for acute appendicitis. Radiology 2018;288(2):467–75.

52. James K, Duffy P, Kavanagh RG, et al. Fast acquisition abdominal MRI study for the investigation of suspected acute appendicitis in paediatric patients. Insights Imaging 2020;11(1):1–11.

53. Naffaa L, Barakat A, Baassiri A, et al. Imaging acute non-traumatic abdominal pathologies in pediatric patients: A pictorial review. J Radiol Case Rep 2019;13(7):29–43.

54. Moore MM, Kulaylat AN, Hollenbeak CS, et al. Magnetic resonance imaging in pediatric appendicitis: a systematic review. Pediatr Radiol 2016;46(6): 928–39.

55. Bayraktutan Ü, Oral A, Kantarci M, et al. Diagnostic performance of diffusion-weighted MR imaging in detecting acute appendicitis in children: Comparison with conventional MRI and surgical findings. J Magn Reson Imaging 2014;39(6):1518–24.

56. Koning JL, Naheedy JH, Kruk PG. Diagnostic performance of contrast-enhanced MR for acute appendicitis and alternative causes of abdominal pain in children. Pediatr Radiol 2014;8:948–55.

57. Duigenan S, Gee MS. Imaging of pediatric patients with inflammatory bowel disease. Am J Roentgenol 2012;199(1):907–15.

58. Mojtahed A, Gee MS. Magnetic resonance enterography evaluation of Crohn disease activity and mucosal healing in young patients. Pediatr Radiol 2018;48(9):1273–9.

59. Bhosale PR, Javitt MC, Atri M, et al. ACR Appropriateness Criteria® Acute Pelvic Pain in the Reproductive Age Group. Ultrasound Q 2016;32(2):108–15.

60. Ngo AV, Otjen JP, Parisi MT, et al. Pediatric ovarian torsion: a pictorial review. Pediatr Radiol 2015; 45(12):1845–55.

61. Oltmann SC, Fischer A, Barber R, et al. Cannot exclude torsion-a 15-year review. J Pediatr Surg 2009;44(6):1212–7.

62. Hindman N, Arif-Tiwari H, Kamel I, et al. ACR Appropriateness Criteria® Radiologic Jaundice. J Am Coll Radiol 2019;16(5S):S126–40.

63. Choi JY, Jeong ML, Jae YL, et al. Navigator-triggered isotropic three-dimensional magnetic resonance cholangiopancreatography in the diagnosis

of malignant biliary obstructions: Comparison with direct cholangiography. J Magn Reson Imaging 2008;27(1):94–101.

64. Maurea S, Caleo O, Mollica C, et al. Valutazione diagnostica comparativa tra colangio-pancreatografia RM, ecografia e TC in pazienti con patologia del sistema bilio-pancreatico. Radiol Med 2009;114(3): 390–402.

65. Kolodziejczyk E, Jurkiewicz E, Pertkiewicz J, et al. MRCP Versus ERCP in the Evaluation of Chronic Pancreatitis in Children: Which is the Better Choice? Pancreas 2016;45(8):1115–9.

66. Erkilinc M, Gilmore A, Weber M, et al. Current Concepts in Pediatric Septic Arthritis. J Am Acad Orthop Surg 2021;29(5):196–206.

67. Dodwell ER. Osteomyelitis and septic arthritis in children: Current concepts. Curr Opin Pediatr 2013; 25(1):58–63.

68. Pääkkönen M, Peltola H. Bone and Joint Infections. Pediatr Clin North Am 2013;60(2):425–36.

69. Dartnell J, Ramachandran M, Katchburian M. Haematogenous acute and subacute paediatric osteomyelitis. J Bone Joint Surg Br 2012;94 B(5):584–95.

70. Hu AC, Ng WKY. Orbital Osteomyelitis in the Pediatric Patient. J Craniofac Surg 2021;32(1):206–9.

71. Jaramillo D, Dormans JP, Delgado J, et al. Hematogenous osteomyelitis in infants and Children: Imaging of a Changing Disease. Radiology 2017;283(3): 629–43.

72. Nixon GW. Hematogenous osteomyelitis of metaphyseal-equivalent locations. Am J Roentgenol 1978;130(1):123–9.

73. Offiah A. Acute osteomyelitis, septic arthritis and discitis: differences between neonates and older children. Eur J Radiol 2006;60(2):221–32.

74. Browne LP, Guillerman RP, Orth RC, et al. Community-acquired staphylococcal musculoskeletal infection in infants and young children: Necessity of contrast-enhanced MRI for the diagnosis of growth cartilage involvement. Am J Roentgenol 2012; 198(1):194–9.

75. Pugmire BS. Role of MRI in the diagnosis and treatment of osteomyelitis in pediatric patients. World J Radiol 2014;6(8):530–7.

76. Johnson DP, Hernanz-Schulman M, Martus JE, et al. Significance of epiphyseal cartilage enhancement defects in pediatric osteomyelitis identified by MRI with surgical correlation. Pediatr Radiol 2011;41(3): 355–61.

77. Averill LW, Hernandez A, Gonzalez L, et al. Diagnosis of osteomyelitis in children: Utility of fat-suppressed contrast-enhanced MRI. Am J Roentgenol 2009;192(5):1232–8.

78. Lindsay AJ, Delgado J, Jaramillo D, et al. Extended field of view magnetic resonance imaging for suspected osteomyelitis in very young children: is it useful? Pediatr Radiol 2019;49(3):379–86.

79. Brown DW, Sheffer BW. Pediatric Septic Arthritis: An Update. Orthop Clin North Am 2019;50(4):461–70.

80. Montgomery CO, Siegel E, Blasier RD, et al. Concurrent septic arthritis and osteomyelitis in children. J Pediatr Orthop 2013;33(4):464–7.

81. Eich GF, Superti-Furga A, Umbricht FS, et al. The painful hip: Evaluation of criteria for clinical decision-making. Eur J Pediatr 1999;158(11):923–8.

82. Monsalve J, Kan JH, Schallert EK, et al. Septic arthritis in children: Frequency of coexisting unsuspected osteomyelitis and implications on imaging work-up and management. Am J Roentgenol 2015; 204(6):1289–95.

83. Dunbar JAT, Sandoe JAT, Rao AS, et al. The MRI appearances of early vertebral osteomyelitis and discitis. Clin Radiol 2010;65(12):974–81.

84. Rodriguez DP, Poussaint TY. Imaging of back pain in children. AJNR Am J Neuroradiol 2010;31(5): 787–802.

85. Booth TN, Iyer RS, Falcone RA, et al. ACR Appropriateness Criteria® Back Pain—Child. J Am Coll Radiol 2017;14(5):S13–24.

86. Ledermann HP, Schweitzer ME, Morrison WB, et al. MR imaging findings in spinal infections: Rules or myths? Radiology 2003;228(2):506–14.

87. Shifrin A, Lu Q, Lev MH, et al. Paraspinal edema is the most sensitive feature of lumbar spinal epidural abscess on unenhanced MRI. Am J Roentgenol 2017;209(1):176–81.

88. Kadom N, Palasis S, Pruthi S, et al. ACR Appropriateness Criteria® Suspected Spine Trauma-Child. J Am Coll Radiol 2019;16(5):S286–99.

89. Beckmann NM, West OC, Nunez D, et al. ACR Appropriateness Criteria ® Suspected Spine Trauma. J Am Coll Radiol 2019;16(5):S264–85.

90. Chang PT, Yang E, Swenson DW, et al. Pediatric Emergency Magnetic Resonance Imaging: Current Indications, Techniques, and Clinical Applications. Magn Reson Imaging Clin N Am 2016;24(2):449–80.

91. Pang D. Spinal cord injury without radiographic abnormality in children, 2 decades later. Neurosurgery 2004;55(6):1325–42.

ED MRI: Safety, Consent, and Regulatory Considerations

Ruhani Doda Khera, MD, MBA[a],*, Joshua A. Hirsch, MD[b], Karen Buch, MD[c],
Sanjay Saini, MD, MBA[d]

KEYWORDS

- MR safety • Emergency MRI • MRI screening • MR accidents • MR consent • MRI safety zones

KEY POINTS

- MRI safety hazards are composed of projectiles from ferrous metals, burns and tissue heating, nerve stimulation, acoustic noise, and MR contrast reactions.
- Careful site layout—Four-zone design of MRI sites helps in creating a more secure access to Zone IV (machine room) that has the strongest magnetic field.
- MR personnel training—Level I and Level II personnel should meet annual training requirements to help ensure a safe MR environment. Non-MR personnel are always supervised by MR personnel, who maintain a close watch, especially on persons and objects entering Zones III and IV.
- MR compatibility device labeling marks all equipment in close vicinity of the MRI as MRI safe, MRI conditional, and MRI unsafe.
- MR screening helps elicit the previous history of trauma with ferromagnetic objects, implants and devices, jewelry, contrast allergy, and kidney disease.

Abbreviations	
ED	Emergency Department
MR	IMagnetic Resonance Imaging
RF	Radiofrequency
ACR	American College of Radiology
ISMRM	International Society of Magnetic Resonance in Medicine
ABMRS	American Board of Magnetic Resonance Safety
SAR	Specific Absorption Rate
ICD	Implantable Cardioverter Defibrillator
TJC	The Joint Commission
NSF	Nephrogenic systemic fibrosis
ICU	Intensive Care Unit
CT	Computed Tomography
BLS	Basic Life Support
CPR	Cardiopulmonary Resuscitation

[a] Department of Radiology, Massachusetts General Hospital and Harvard Medical School, Austen2 (222), 55 Fruit Street, Boston, MA 02114, USA; [b] Department of Radiology, Massachusetts General Hospital and Harvard Medical School, Gray 2, Neuro-Interventional Radiology, 55, Fruit Street, Boston, MA 02114, USA; [c] Department of Radiology, Massachusetts General Hospital and Harvard Medical School, Gray 2 (241K), 55, Fruit Street, Boston, MA 02114, USA; [d] Department of Radiology, Massachusetts General Hospital and Harvard Medical School, Austen 2 (222), 55, Fruit Street, Boston, MA 02114, USA
* Corresponding author. Department of Radiology, Massachusetts General Hospital and Harvard Medical School, Austen2 (222), Massachusetts General Hospital, 55 Fruit Street, Boston, MA 02114, USA
E-mail address: rdodakhera@mgh.harvard.edu
Twitter: @RuhaniDodaKhera (R.D.K.)

Magn Reson Imaging Clin N Am 30 (2022) 553–563
https://doi.org/10.1016/j.mric.2022.04.011
1064-9689/22/© 2022 Elsevier Inc. All rights reserved.

mri.theclinics.com

INTRODUCTION

Over the last two decades, there has been a substantial increase in the use of advanced diagnostic imaging services in emergency departments (EDs).[1] Multiple studies have established an appropriate role for emergency MRI in conditions, such as stroke, transient ischemic attack, pulmonary embolism, spinal cord compression, appendicitis, cardiovascular emergencies, and trauma patients.[2–9] According to The Joint Commission Comprehensive Stroke Center Certification, MRI should be available at all times, 24/7 for emergency evaluation of stroke in ED patients.[10] Although an ED MRI affects operations downstream with an increased ED length of stay, the extra amount of time can be justified by reduced hospital admission rates, for example, by ruling out stroke patients.[10] Various safety hazards are posed to patients and staff members by MRI. These comprise magnetic forces on metals, burns and tissue heating, nerve stimulation, bioeffects, acoustic noise, and contrast reactions.[11] The constant static magnetic field has the potential for accidents if metals, adornments, implants, and other inadvertent sources are present within or near the field.[11] This may be, especially, problematic in an emergency setting. MR personnel should be aware of the principles of magnetism and electromagnetic fields to maintain a safe environment, and effective screening measures must be in place to provide a safe examination experience.[12]

DISCUSSION

Twenty years ago, an MRI accident in Valhalla, NY, took the life of a 6-year-old boy, named Michael Columbini. An oxygen tank was pulled into the MRI bore, crushing the boy's skull.[13] Although MRI is a generally safe and noninvasive examination, the strong magnetic and radio frequency (RF) electromagnetic fields are necessary for imaging pose inherent risks. Projectiles from ferrous metal and induced currents leading to potential burns can cause serious consequences and even death.[14–18] It is therefore essential to address underlying safety issues and concerns. Numerous published resources are available to assist radiology departments in establishing an effective safety program, such as the American College of Radiology (ACR),[19] the International Society of Magnetic Resonance in Medicine,[20] and the American Board of Magnetic Resonance Safety (ABMRS).[21]

MRI ZONES

The static magnetic field declines at a rate of approximately $1/distance^3$.[17] All MRI suites are divided into four zones to ensure safety (**Fig. 1**). Zones are labeled from I to IV; Zone I is the furthest from the scanner, and Zone IV is the scanner itself.[22] Zones III and IV are restricted to MRI staff only. All MR sites must make sure that the physical layout integrates means to prevent the general public and auxiliary hospital staff from accidentally moving into a prohibited area.[12]

1. *Zone I*: This area can be freely accessed by the general public. Zone I allows patients, health care workers, and all other employees of the MR site to access the MR environment.
2. *Zone II:* This area is the interface between a freely accessible Zone I and tightly secure Zones III and IV. In this area, patients are always under supervision. MRI preparation including medical history, screening questions, and gowning is done in this area.
3. *Zone III*: In this area, free access by unscreened non-MR personnel or ferromagnetic objects can result in serious injury or death. Zone III is entirely under the supervision of Level II MR personnel, and only screened persons are permitted in this area.
4. *Zone IV*: This area is the machine room itself and has the strongest magnetic field. It is marked with a red light and a "The Magnet is Always On" signage.

The ACR requires all MR sites to use either badge swipe access or keypads at the entry to Zones III and IV.[23] It is important that entries to Zones III and IV are closed at all times, and the failure to do so can lead to serious accidents.[14,17,19,20] Any individual entering Zones III and IV should be changed into MRI Pocketless Scrubs. This includes technologists, floor nurses, and physicians. A full change of attire (that includes undergarments) is required for patients. This also applies to any accompanying guardians. Improperly changing a patient can cause burns and heating.

MRI PERSONNEL

There are two types of MRI personnel:

Level I Personnel: Employees who have received formal education in general MR safety concepts and screening procedures and are aware of how to function safely in the MR site are designated as Level I personnel, for example, MRI site office staff, patient aides.[23]

Level II Personnel: Employees who have advanced knowledge of MRI and the safety risks involved (such as the potential for RF-related burns or thermal loading and neuromuscular excitation resulting from rapidly changing gradients)

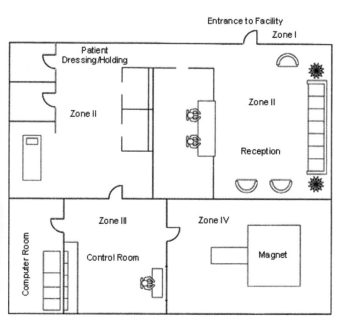

Fig. 1. MRI site layout showing the four zones recommended by ACR. (*From* ACR safety zones https://www.acr.org/Clinical-Resources/Radiology-Safety/MR-Safety; with permission.)

are referred to as Level II personnel. These employees are responsible for making sure that the MRI site is safe at all times, for example, MRI technologists, MRI nurses, and radiologists.

Non-MRI Personnel: All other facility staff who have not undergone MRI safety training within the last 12 months, including patients and visitors, are designated as Non-MRI personnel. They are not allowed unsupervised access to the MRI room.[23]

MRI COMPATIBILITY LABELING

To prevent accidents, institutions have a policy of labeling all equipment that is likely to come in the vicinity of an MRI as MR safe, conditional, or unsafe (**Fig. 2**).[24] With the increasing use of 3.0 T and higher strength magnets, it is imperative that one never assumes MR compatibility or safety information for an object unless there is clear, written documentation.[25]

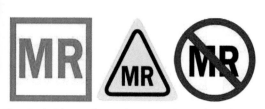

Fig. 2. Guidance for Industry and Food and Drug Administration Staff, U.S Food and Drug Administration. Document issued on May 20, 2021. https://www.fda.gov/media/74201/download

1. MR Safe: These items are composed of electrically nonconductive, nonmetallic, and nonmagnetic materials and pose no safety issues in the MR environment. Such items can be brought into the scanner room if marked properly with an "MRI Safe" label.
2. MR Conditional: These items pose no threats when scanned under specific conditions mentioned in the labeling or product manuals. Some of these items can be taken inside Zone IV, whereas some cannot. Some items can only be taken into a 1.5 T room. It is advised to always check and match the MRI safety labeling with the MRI system for static field strength, maximum spatial field gradient, dB/dt limitations (usually only applicable to active implants), specific absorption rate limits, anatomic location of isocenter, scan duration, and any other conditions needed for safe use of the device (eg, restrictions on the types of coils that may be used or device settings).[21]
3. MR Unsafe: These items are ferromagnetic in nature and should not enter the screened patient holding area or MRI room.[26]

PATIENT SCREENING IN EMERGENCY

In an emergent setting, all patients and accompanying non-MR personnel may be screened only once provided it is done by a Level II MR personnel.[21] Level II personnel ask questions regarding metal implants, ferromagnetic foreign body penetration, orbital trauma, intracranial

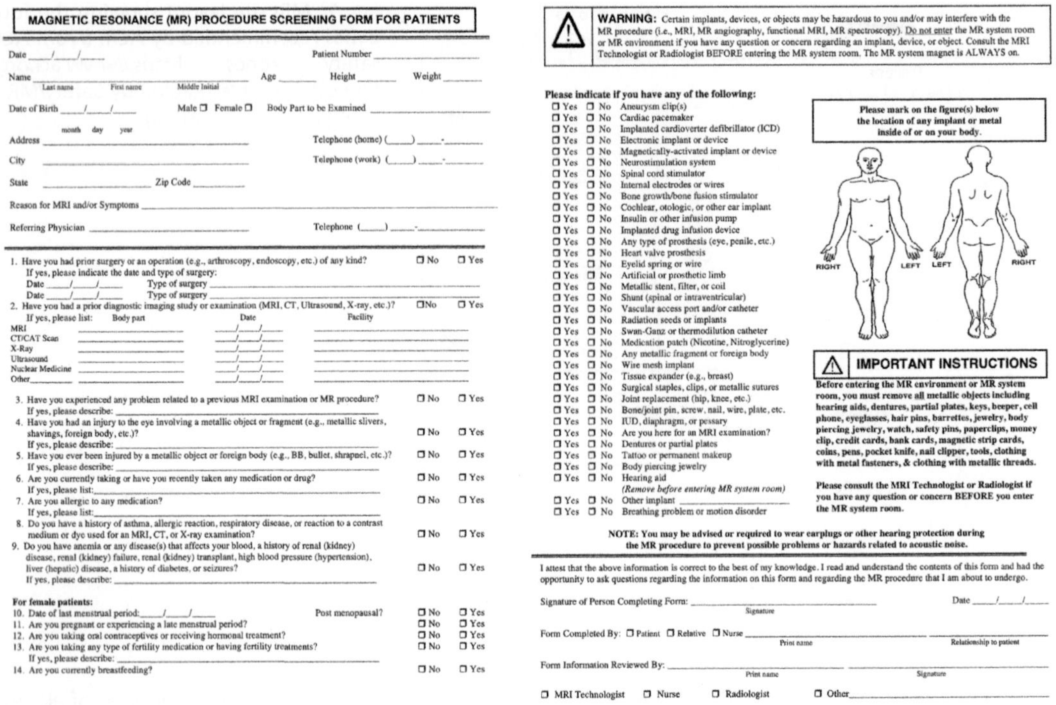

MAGNETIC RESONANCE (MR) PROCEDURE SCREENING FORM FOR PATIENTS

Date ___/___/___ Patient Number ________

Name ________ (Last name, First name, Middle Initial) Age ____ Height ____ Weight ____

Date of Birth ___/___/___ (month day year) Male ☐ Female ☐ Body Part to be Examined ________

Address ________ Telephone (home) (___) ___-____

City ________ Telephone (work) (___) ___-____

State ________ Zip Code ________

Reason for MRI and/or Symptoms ________

Referring Physician ________ Telephone (___) ___-____

1. Have you had prior surgery or an operation (e.g., arthroscopy, endoscopy, etc.) of any kind? ☐ No ☐ Yes
   If yes, please indicate the date and type of surgery:
   Date ___/___/___ Type of surgery ________
   Date ___/___/___ Type of surgery ________
2. Have you had a prior diagnostic imaging study or examination (MRI, CT, Ultrasound, X-ray, etc.)? ☐No ☐ Yes
   If yes, please list: Body part / Date / Facility
   MRI
   CT/CAT Scan
   X-Ray
   Ultrasound
   Nuclear Medicine
   Other____
3. Have you experienced any problem related to a previous MRI examination or MR procedure? ☐ No ☐ Yes
   If yes, please describe: ________
4. Have you had an injury to the eye involving a metallic object or fragment (e.g., metallic slivers, shavings, foreign body, etc.)? ☐ No ☐ Yes
   If yes, please describe: ________
5. Have you ever been injured by a metallic object or foreign body (e.g., BB, bullet, shrapnel, etc.)? ☐ No ☐ Yes
   If yes, please describe: ________
6. Are you currently taking or have you recently taken any medication or drug? ☐ No ☐ Yes
   If yes, please list: ________
7. Are you allergic to any medication? ☐ No ☐ Yes
   If yes, please list: ________
8. Do you have a history of asthma, allergic reaction, respiratory disease, or reaction to a contrast medium or dye used for an MRI, CT, or X-ray examination? ☐ No ☐ Yes
9. Do you have anemia or any disease(s) that affects your blood, a history of renal (kidney) disease, renal (kidney) failure, renal (kidney) transplant, high blood pressure (hypertension), liver (hepatic) disease, a history of diabetes, or seizures? ☐ No ☐ Yes
   If yes, please describe: ________

For female patients:

10. Date of last menstrual period: ___/___/___ Post menopausal? ☐ No ☐ Yes
11. Are you pregnant or experiencing a late menstrual period? ☐ No ☐ Yes
12. Are you taking oral contraceptives or receiving hormonal treatment? ☐ No ☐ Yes
13. Are you taking any type of fertility medication or having fertility treatments? ☐ No ☐ Yes
    If yes, please describe: ________
14. Are you currently breastfeeding? ☐ No ☐ Yes

WARNING: Certain implants, devices, or objects may be hazardous to you and/or may interfere with the MR procedure (i.e., MRI, MR angiography, functional MRI, MR spectroscopy). Do not enter the MR system room or MR environment if you have any question or concern regarding an implant, device, or object. Consult the MRI Technologist or Radiologist BEFORE entering the MR system room. The MR system magnet is ALWAYS on.

Please indicate if you have any of the following:

☐ Yes ☐ No Aneurysm clip(s)
☐ Yes ☐ No Cardiac pacemaker
☐ Yes ☐ No Implanted cardioverter defibrillator (ICD)
☐ Yes ☐ No Electronic implant or device
☐ Yes ☐ No Magnetically-activated implant or device
☐ Yes ☐ No Neurostimulation system
☐ Yes ☐ No Spinal cord stimulator
☐ Yes ☐ No Internal electrodes or wires
☐ Yes ☐ No Bone growth/bone fusion stimulator
☐ Yes ☐ No Cochlear, otologic, or other ear implant
☐ Yes ☐ No Insulin or other infusion pump
☐ Yes ☐ No Implanted drug infusion device
☐ Yes ☐ No Any type of prosthesis (eye, penile, etc.)
☐ Yes ☐ No Heart valve prosthesis
☐ Yes ☐ No Eyelid spring or wire
☐ Yes ☐ No Artificial or prosthetic limb
☐ Yes ☐ No Metallic stent, filter, or coil
☐ Yes ☐ No Shunt (spinal or intraventricular)
☐ Yes ☐ No Vascular access port and/or catheter
☐ Yes ☐ No Radiation seeds or implants
☐ Yes ☐ No Swan-Ganz or thermodilution catheter
☐ Yes ☐ No Medication patch (Nicotine, Nitroglycerine)
☐ Yes ☐ No Any metallic fragment or foreign body
☐ Yes ☐ No Wire mesh implant
☐ Yes ☐ No Tissue expander (e.g., breast)
☐ Yes ☐ No Surgical staples, clips, or metallic sutures
☐ Yes ☐ No Joint replacement (hip, knee, etc.)
☐ Yes ☐ No Bone/joint pin, screw, nail, wire, plate, etc.
☐ Yes ☐ No IUD, diaphragm, or pessary
☐ Yes ☐ No Are you here for an MRI examination?
☐ Yes ☐ No Dentures or partial plates
☐ Yes ☐ No Tattoo or permanent makeup
☐ Yes ☐ No Body piercing jewelry
☐ Yes ☐ No Hearing aid *(Remove before entering MR system room)*
☐ Yes ☐ No Other implant ________
☐ Yes ☐ No Breathing problem or motion disorder

Please mark on the figure(s) below the location of any implant or metal inside of or on your body.

RIGHT LEFT LEFT RIGHT

IMPORTANT INSTRUCTIONS

Before entering the MR environment or MR system room, you must remove all metallic objects including hearing aids, dentures, partial plates, keys, beeper, cell phone, eyeglasses, hair pins, barrettes, jewelry, body piercing jewelry, watch, safety pins, paperclips, money clip, credit cards, bank cards, magnetic strip cards, coins, pens, pocket knife, nail clipper, tools, clothing with metal fasteners, & clothing with metallic threads.

Please consult the MRI Technologist or Radiologist if you have any question or concern BEFORE you enter the MR system room.

NOTE: You may be advised or required to wear earplugs or other hearing protection during the MR procedure to prevent possible problems or hazards related to acoustic noise.

I attest that the above information is correct to the best of my knowledge. I read and understand the contents of this form and had the opportunity to ask questions regarding the information on this form and regarding the MR procedure that I am about to undergo.

Signature of Person Completing Form: ________ (Signature) Date ___/___/___

Form Completed By: ☐ Patient ☐ Relative ☐ Nurse ________ (Print name) ________ (Relationship to patient)

Form Information Reviewed By: ________ (Print name) ________ (Signature)

☐ MRI Technologist ☐ Nurse ☐ Radiologist ☐ Other________

Fig. 3. MR screening form. (*From* mrisafety.com, courtesy of Dr. Frank Shellock; with permission.)

aneurysm clips, pacemakers/implantable cardioverter defibrillator, kidney disease, contrast allergy, and pregnancy/breastfeeding before any patient is brought into the machine room. Patient screening information must be recorded in radiology assessment before bringing the subject into the scanner room. **Fig. 3** shows a list of MR safety screening questions. If a patient or accompanying non-MR personnel have a metal implant, the make and model number have to be reviewed

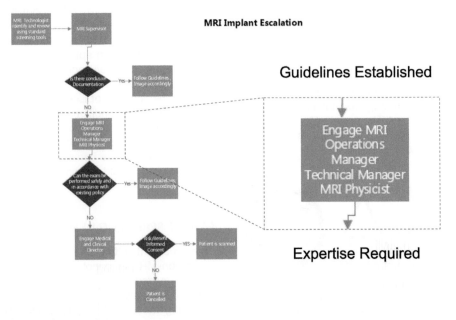

Fig. 4. Implant escalation policy.

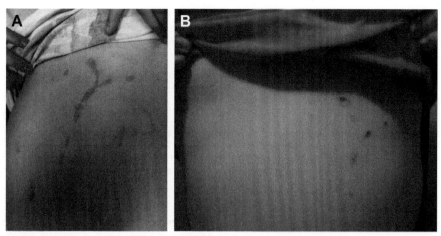

Fig. 5. RF burns on patient's anterior abdominal wall at (*A*) 2 hours and (*B*) 2 weeks after MRI. (*Courtesy of* Jeremy Herrington, MHA, RT(R) (MR), Boston, MA.)

in the MRI safety hand book by Level II Personnel. If there is no documentation for the patient, a radiologist makes the determination as to whether the patient can be scanned or not based on a risk versus benefit assessment with the referring ED physician. Based on the necessity of the examination, a whole-body scout CT or plain film x-rays may be obtained to determine the presence or lack of implanted devices. Commonly encountered implants in the ED setting include cardiac pacemakers and defibrillators, cardiac stents, and retained ballistic fragments.[27–29] Information on implants or consents must be documented in radiology assessment before a patient is brought into MRI. There are no exceptions. **Fig. 4** elaborates on various steps in an implant escalation policy.

After a thorough screening, the patient is escorted to the dressing area and changes completely into hospital attire (eg, gowns/robes/pants/footwear). This step is extremely important to avoid RF burns (**Fig. 5**) because of heating in case metal or metallic fibers are present in personal clothing. Serious incidents have been reported with athletic clothes, underwear, and other antimicrobial metallic solution-infused clothing.[30] It is also advised to remove medication patches, electrocardiogram patches, pulse oximeter sensors, and jewelry before the examination to reduce the risk of burns. Careful consideration must also be given to transport equipment and medical assistance devices, particularly in the ED. Ferrous metal detectors are used at some MRI sites as an added layer of protection, for example, at the changing room/scanner entrance.[31] From a workflow perspective, the

two-table model is critical in the ED because there may not be enough time, and technologists could be potentially scanning a patient while setting up another.

Final Stop or Time-Out Process

A recent recommendation in the ACR guidance document on MR safety states the use of a final stop or a time-out process.[30] This practice guideline ensures that MR personnel conduct a final concluding review with patients, employees, and equipment to make sure all metallic objects have been removed or evaluated and all safety measures are in place.[32,33]

SPECIAL PATIENT POPULATIONS
Claustrophobia

Claustrophobia may increase the level of distress and anxiety, especially in an emergency. In such cases, an appropriately screened family member or guardian may be allowed to remain with the patient during scanning. The ACR Manual suggests techniques such as offering a warm blanket, maintaining verbal and physical contact with the patient during the scan, using appropriate headphones and music, positioning the patient feet first instead of head first, offering bright lights in the room, and using relaxation techniques, such as controlled breathing, a shorter MRI protocol, and lastly antianxiety medication.[21] Patient anxiolysis, analgesia, sedation, and anesthesia should be carried out according to the ACR,[34] the American Society of Anesthesiologists,[35–37] and The Joint Commission (TJC) standards.[38]

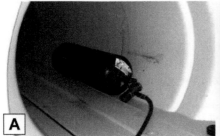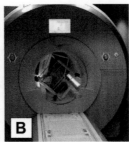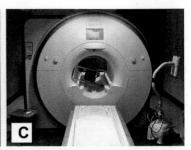

Fig. 6. (*A*) MR Accident. An MR unsafe oxygen cylinder seen within the bore of an MR scanner. (*B*) Non-MR compatible laundry cart and (*C*) stepping stool within the bore of an MRI scanner. (*Courtesy of* Jeremy Herrington, MHA, RT(R) (MR), Boston, MA.)

Pregnant Patients

In case the patient is pregnant, avoiding gadolinium-based MR contrast agents is prudent.[39] However, the risk–benefit ratio is weighed by a radiologist based on an individual case-by-case basis while considering the institutional contrast policy.[21]

Pediatric/Minor Patients

Pediatric age group patients may not give reliable history. To increase the possibility of avoiding all potential dangers, Level II personnel are tasked with questioning teenagers and older children twice: once in the absence of parents/guardians and once in their presence. It is prudent to change them into gowns before entering Zone IV and ensure that no metallic toys or objects enter the scanner room. Extra care should be taken to avoid taking their personal pillows, stuffed animals, or comfort items into Zone II. Neonates and younger children require temperature monitoring for hypo and hyperthermia, and MR compatible temperature monitors are available.[21]

Nonambulatory Patients

High-risk and nonambulatory patients present more challenges for MRI scanning. These patients should be moved with all care only in an MR Conditional wheelchair or stretcher.[21] Metallic objects, such as needles or small oxygen tanks, may be accidentally transported into the machine room (**Fig. 6**). When possible, transfer of these patients to the MR table should be done in Zone III (eg, via a detachable MR table).

Unconscious, Unresponsive, or Altered Level of Consciousness Patients

These groups of patients pose a grave challenge to ED MRI imaging, particularly related to managing acute or subacute stroke imaging and cord compression studies. The 2020 ACR Manual of

MR safety mentions that for patients who are unconscious, unresponsive, or with an altered level of consciousness, their family members/guardians must complete a written MR safety screening questionnaire before patients' entry into Zone III.[21] In case there is no reliable history and the MRI is critically urgent, it is advised that a plain film radiograph be obtained (unless a recent radiograph/CT/MR of the same area is available) to exclude potentially harmful metallic foreign bodies, implants, or devices.

CONTRAST SAFETY

Nephrogenic systemic fibrosis (NSF) is a feared and rare complication associated with gadolinium-based MRI contrast agents in patients which is almost exclusively seen in patients with renal impairment. NSF typically develops weeks-to-months following gadolinium administration and most commonly involves the dermis (extremities, trunk, and face). Additional organs may be involved, eventually leading to death.[40] Histopathologically, NSF resembles eosinophilic fasciitis/scleromyxedema. On clinical examination, the skin appears hyperpigmented and indurated with subcutaneous edema. Patients may report pain, pruritis, tightness, and a burning sensation.

Gadolinium-based contrast material with lower levels of stability is associated with higher risks of NSF. There are three groups of gadolinium-based contrast agents, classified by the ACR based on the associated risk of developing NSF: Group I—highest risk, Group II—very low risk, and Group III—likely very low risk.[38] The ACR Committee on Drugs and Contrast Media considers the risk of NSF among patients administered standard doses of group II contrast media sufficiently low or nonexistent such that kidney function screening is now optional before use. Furthermore, group II contrast media may be administered to high-risk patients with renal screening or contacting the referring provider.

Indeed, some institutions are currently using the newer macro-cyclic agents such as Dotarem and Gadavist without strict adherence to an estimated glomerular filtration rate of 30 mL/min/1.73 m^2. A complete chart enumerating the different gadolinium-based intravascular contrast agents is provided in Appendix A, page 125 of the 2021 ACR Manual on Contrast Media.[41]

The ACR guidance document on contrast safety recommends that all patients with a history of asthma, allergic respiratory disorders, and previous iodinated or gadolinium-based contrast reactions should be closely followed as they are at an increased risk of an adverse reaction.[25]

MRI CONSENT

For patients undergoing a clinical MRI scan, informed consent is obtained from patients with implantable medical devices, metallic accessories which cannot be removed, as well as body-piercing jewelry (necklaces, earrings, transdermal-piercings, and so forth), which are unable to be removed. Note that gold and platinum wedding bands that are unable to be removed before the MRI scan do not necessitate informed consent. The informed consent procedure is initiated after patients note metallic devices/accessories/jewelry which is unable to be removed, the MRI technologist has used a handheld metal detector to test for ferromagnetic properties, and all additional precautions have been taken to reduce the risk of burns and overheating of tissue in these patients. The patient then signs an acknowledgment form indicating he/she understands the risk of tissue burns, vibration, and pulling of the metallic device/accessory/jewelry. If the patient is not alert and oriented and is unable to communicate with the MR technologist, a risk versus benefit conversation should be undertaken between the radiologist and the responsible clinical service. This conversation between the radiologist and clinical team should be documented in the patient's electronic medical record. A sample of this consent form is shown in **Fig. 7**.

MEDICAL RESUSCITATION

Codes are never run inside the MRI room. Never bring a crash cart into the machine room! In case of a medical emergency such as cardiac or respiratory arrest within Zone IV that requires urgent resuscitation or medical intervention, properly trained and certified MR personnel should begin cardiopulmonary resuscitation or basic life support as soon as possible although the patient is being urgently removed from Zone IV to a predetermined, magnetically safe location. The priority should be stabilizing the patient with basic life support with cardiac compressions and manual ventilation while evacuating the patient as quickly as possible from the MR room, which might limit safe resuscitative efforts. It is not advised to quench the magnet for such a medical emergency as the process can easily take longer than a minute while introducing new threats, as it is necessary to evacuate Zone IV, when possible, for an intentional quench.[21,22]

EMERGENCY RESPONSE

In case of an emergent call, a specific MR personnel is designated to ensure the safety of firefighters, code or rapid-response teams, and other emergent services. ACR recommends that all fire alarms, cardiac arrests, or other emergent service response calls initiating from the MR site must be forwarded concurrently to a specifically designated MR personnel at the facility. This individual should be present on-site before the arrival of the emergent responders to make sure that they do not have unrestricted access to Zones III and IV.[21,22]

REGULATORY CONSIDERATIONS

TJC[42] and the ACR[19] regularly publish updated standards of care for MR safety. TJC requires maintenance and documentation of annual MR safety training for technologists, management and documentation of patient safety issues such as NSF, implants, claustrophobia, and so forth with corrective action for each instance, and documentation of all ferromagnetic and thermal injuries.[11] The ACR MRI accreditation program evaluates staff qualifications, safety policies, quality control, and image quality.[43] For the ACR, although the MR physician is required to focus efforts on policies and procedures addressing clinical safety issues such as contrast use and sedation, the MR scientist evaluates the MR safety program (including access restriction, signage, screening procedures, and cryogen safety) and inspects the system's physical and mechanical integrity.[11] State regulations related to MR safety may vary on a regional basis in the United States, and it is important for institutions to maintain comprehensive and cogent policies and procedures.

MR SAFETY ROLES

To maintain a safe MR environment, an MR medical director, a safety officer, and a safety expert must be designated by the current clinical

MRI Screening- Jewelry Acknowledgement Form

Patient:

I am unable to remove my jewelry prior to my MRI study. The MRI technologist has informed me of the possibility of pulling, twisting, or heating of my jewelry during the MRI study and the risk that this may result in injury, particularly to the structures near the jewelry. The jewelry may also alter the magnetic field in the MRI and reduce the quality of the images.

I understand the above risks. The MRI technologist has reviewed with me how to use the emergency squeeze ball. If I experience pulling, heating, or other sensation at the body part where the item of jewelry is located, I will immediately squeeze the emergency squeeze ball.

Patient:

_____   _____   _____   _____ AM/PM
　　Signature　　　　　　　　　Print Name　　　　　　　Date　　　　Time

Technologist:
Circle one

☐　The patient's jewelry was not removed despite best attempts or because patient refused.

☐　Possibility of heating or motion of jewelry was discussed with the patient prior to the MRI.

☐　MRI technologist reviewed use of emergency squeeze ball prior to entering MRI.

☐　MRI technologist instructed the patient to squeeze the emergency squeeze ball in the event of pulling, heating, or any other sensation, particularly at the site of the item of jewelry.

☐　Patient was counseled to contact their physician, the MRI department, or seek emergency medical treatment in the event that an injury appears after the MRI exam.

Technologist:

_____   _____   _____   _____ AM/PM
　　Signature　　　　　　　　　Print Name　　　　　　　Date　　　　Time

Fig. 7. Informed consent—jewelry acknowledgment form.

standard of practice.[11] Recently, the ABMRS [20] created a safety certification process for each of these positions. The medical director (MR physician) ensures all safety guidelines are defined, enforced, and adhered to. The safety officer (MRI operating technologist) is responsible for safe MR operation while also monitoring the surrounding environment. The safety expert (scientist or engineer) helps in mitigating any risks and concerns. A safety officer must always be present on the site.[21,22]

MR SAFETY POLICIES AND PROCEDURES

All emergency MR sites must maintain device-specific safety policies irrespective of magnet field strength. These policies must be regularly reviewed alongside any changes to device and/or site safety parameters, such as upgrades to hardware/software that may affect gradient capabilities or RF duty cycles. At the time of review, national and international standards should be considered before any local guidelines and policies are established.[21]

SUMMARY

MRI is a noninvasive diagnostic tool with underlying safety concerns because of its strong magnetic and RF electromagnetic fields. It plays a significant role in ED patients with stroke, transient ischemic attack, cardiovascular emergencies, trauma, and so forth. The four-zone layout of an MR site enhances the secure access to the main scanner room. MR personnel should undergo annual safety training to help ensure a safe environment for patients and site staff. Level II MR personnel have more advanced training than Level I MR personnel. Screening is the main process that ensures safety for multiple teams working in the ED. The screening questionnaire requires information on implants, devices, ferromagnetic objects, and previous trauma by a metallic foreign body, body piercing, contrast allergy, pregnancy, kidney disease, and previous surgery. Some patient populations require special considerations before and during an MRI scan. Codes are never run in the machine room, and all efforts are made to move the patient into a safe area outside of Zone IV while simultaneously trying to resuscitate the patient. An active safety team with effective policies and procedures is imperative for the smooth functioning of the ED MRI.

CLINICS CARE POINTS

- MRI is a generally safe, noninvasive investigation that has its own risk profile unique from many other diagnostic studies.
- Appropriate screening, careful site layout, personnel training, control of access to Zones III and IV, and device labeling can alleviate most MRI accidents.
- Informed consent can be used to share risk profiles with patients.
- Codes are never run in the scanner room. In case of a medical emergency within Zone IV, trained and certified MR personnel initiate BLS (Basic Life Support) or CPR (Cardiopulmonary Resuscitation) simultaneously although the patient is urgently removed from Zone IV to a predetermined, magnetically safe location.
- The Joint Commission and the American College of Radiology publish the updated standards of care for MR safety on a regular basis and are excellent resources for maintaining a safe MR environment.

DISCLOSURE

Dr J. A. Hirsch is a consultant for Medtronic and Persica and has received grant funding from Neiman Health Policy Institute (both non-related). The remaining authors have nothing to disclose.

REFERENCES

1. Redd V, Levin S, Toerper M, et al. Effects of fully accessible magnetic resonance imaging in the emergency department. Acad Emerg Med 2015; 22:741–9.
2. Gerischer LM, Fiebach JB, Scheitz JF, et al. Magnetic resonance imaging–based versus computed tomography–based thrombolysis in acute ischemic stroke: comparison of safety and efficacy within a cohort study. Cerebrovasc Dis 2013;35(3):250–6.
3. Forster A, Gass A, Kern R, et al. Brain imaging in patients with transient ischemic attack: a comparison of computed tomography and magnetic resonance imaging. Eur Neurol 2012;67(3):136–41.
4. Revel MP, Sanchez O, Couchon S, et al. Diagnostic accuracy of magnetic resonance imaging for an acute pulmonary embolism: results of the "IRM-EP" study. J Thromb Haemost 2012;10(5):743–50.
5. Larsson EM, I Ioltas S, Crongvist S, et al. Comparison of myelography, CT myelography and magnetic resonance imaging in cervical spondylosis and disk herniation. Pre- and postoperative findings. Acta Radiol 1989;30(3):233–9.
6. Cobben L, Groot I, Kingma L, et al. A simple MRI protocol in patients with clinically suspected appendicitis: results in 138 patients and effect on outcome of appendectomy. Eur Radiol 2009;19(5):1175–83.
7. Lipinski MJ, McVey CM, Berger JS, et al. Prognostic value of stress cardiac magnetic resonance imaging in patients with known or suspected coronary artery disease: a systematic review and meta-analysis. J Am Coll Cardiol 2013;62(9):826–38.
8. Leurent G, Langella B, Fougerou C, et al. Diagnostic contributions of cardiac magnetic resonance imaging in patients presenting with elevated troponin, acute chest pain syndrome and unobstructed coronary arteries. Arch Cardiovasc Dis 2011;104(3): 161–70.

9. Akhtar JI, Spear RM, Senac MO, et al. Detection of traumatic brain injury with magnetic resonance imaging and S-100B protein in children, despite normal computed tomography of the brain. Pediatr Crit Care Med 2003;4(3):322–6.

10. The Joint Commission. Advanced Certification Comprehensive Stroke Centers. Available at: https://www.jointcommission.org/accreditation-and-certification/certification/certifications-by-setting/hospital-certifications/stroke-certification/advanced-stroke/comprehensive-stroke-center/. Accessed November 19, 2021.

11. Cross NM, Hoff MN, Kanal KM. Avoiding MRI-Related Accidents: A Practical Approach to Implementing MR Safety. J Am Coll Radiol 2018;15(12):1738–44.

12. Kimbrell V. Elements of Effective Patient Screening to Improve Safety in MRI. Magn Reson Imaging Clin N Am 2020;28(4):489–96.

13. Kraly C. AHRA 2011: Industry Slow to Columbini MRI Lessons?. In: Diagnostic imaging. 2011. Available at: https://www.diagnosticimaging.com/view/ahra-2011-industry-slow-colombini-mri-lessons 2011. Accessed November 26, 2021.

14. Peck P. Fatal MRI accident is first of its kind. In: WebMD. 2001. Available at: https://www.webmd.com/a-to-z-guides/news/20010801/fatal-mri-accident-is-first-of-its-kind#1. Accessed Novemeber 26, 2021.

15. Henderson JM, Tkach J, Phillips M, et al. Permanent neurological deficit related to magnetic resonance imaging in a patient with implanted deep brain stimulation electrodes for parkinson's disease: casereport. Neurosurgery 2005;57(5):E1063.

16. Greenberg TD, Hoff MN, Gilk TB, et al, ACR Committee on MR Safety. ACR guidance document on MR safe practices: updates and critical information. J Magn Reson Imaging 2020;51(2):331–8.

17. Biederman RW, Doyle M, Yamrozik J. Cardiovascular MRI tutorial: lectures and learning. Philadelphia: Lippincott Williams & Wilkins; 2007.

18. Calamante F, Ittermann B, Kanal E, et al. Recommended responsibilities for management of MR safety. J Magn Reson Imaging 2016;44:1067–9.

19. ACR. MR Safety. American College of Radiology. Available at: https://www.acr.org/Clinical-Resources/Radiology-Safety/MR-Safety. Accessed Novemner 26, 2021.

20. MR safety guidance, documents and links. ISMRM; 2019. Available at: https://www.ismrm.org/mr-safety-links/mr-safety-resources-page/. Accessed November 25, 2021.

21. American Board of Magnetic Resonance Safety. Home page. Available at: https://www.abmrs.org. Accessed November 25, 2021.

22. American College of Radiology. ACR manual on MR safety. 2020. Available at: https://www.acr.org/-/media/ACR/Files/Radiology-Safety/MR-Safety/Manual-on-MR-Safety.pdf. Accessed November 18, 2021.

23. Kanal E, Borgstede JP, Barkovich JA, et al. American College of Radiology White Paper on MR Safety: 2004 Update and Revisions. Am J Roentgenol 2004;182(5):1111–4.

24. ASTM International. ASTM F2503-20 standard practice for marking medical devices and other items for safety in the magnetic resonance environment. ASTM International; 2020. Available at: https://www.astm.org/f2503-20.html. Accessed November 25, 2021.

25. Kanal E, Barkovich JA, Bell C, et al, Expert Panel on MR Safety. ACR guidance document on MR safe practices: 2013. J Magn Reson Imaging 2013;37(3):501–30.

26. Jabehdar Maralani P, Schieda N, Hecht EM, et al. MRI safety and devices: An update and expert consensus. J Magn Reson Imaging 2020;51:657–74.

27. Nazarian S, Hansford R, Rahsepar AA, et al. Safety of Magnetic Resonance Imaging in Patients with Cardiac Devices. N Engl J Med 2017;377(26):2555–64.

28. Schenk CD, Gebker R, Berger A, et al. Review of safety reports of cardiac MR-imaging in patients with recently implanted coronary artery stents at various field strengths. Expert Rev Med Devices 2021;18(1):83–90.

29. Ditkofsky N, Colak E, Kirpalani A, et al. MR imaging in the presence of ballistic debris of unknown composition: a review of the literature and practical approach. Emerg Radiol 2020;27(5):527–32.

30. Pietryga JA, Fonder MA, Rogg JM, et al. Invisible metallic microfiber in clothing presents unrecognized MRI risk for cutaneous burn. Am J Neuroradiol 2013;34(5):E47–50.

31. Frederickson TW, Lambrecht JE. Using the 2018 guidelines from the joint commission to kickstart your hospital's program to reduce opioid-induced ventilatory impairment. In: Anesthesia patient safety foundation. 2018. Available at: https://www.apsf.org/article/using-the-2018-guidelines-from-the-joint-commission-to-kickstart-your-hospitals-program-to-reduce-opioid-induced-ventilatory-impairment/. Accessed November 25, 2021.

32. Sawyer-Glover AM, Shellock FG. Pre-MRI procedure screening: recommendations and safety considerations for biomedical implants and devices. J Magn Reson Imaging 2000;12(1):92–106.

33. Shellock FG, Alberto S. MRI Safety Update 2008: Part 2, Screening Patients for MRI. Am J Roentgenol 2008;191(4):1140–9.

34. American College of Radiology; Society of Interventional Radiology. ACR-SIR practice parameter for adult sedation/analgesia. Revised. 2015. Available at: https://www.acr.org/-/media/ACR/Files/Practice-Parameters/Sed-Analgesia.pdf?la=en. Accessed November 25, 2021.

35. Committee on Standards and Practice Parameters, American Society of Anesthesiologists, Standards for basic anesthetic monitoring, 2015, American Society of Anesthesiologists, (approved by the ASA House of Delegates on October 21, 1986, last amended on October 20, 2010, and last affirmed on October 28, 2015). Available at: https://www.asahq.org/standards-and-guidelines/standards-for-basic-anesthetic-monitoring.

36. Committee on Standards and Practice Parameters, American Society of Anesthesiologists, Standards for postanesthesia care, 2009, American Society of Anesthesiologists, (approved by the ASA House of Delegates on October 27, 2004 and last amended on October 21, 2009). Available at: https://www.asahq.org/standards-and-guidelines/standards-for-postanesthesia-care.

37. Committee on Standards and Practice Parameters, American Society of Anesthesiologists, Statement on non-operating room anesthetizing locations, 2018, American Society of Anesthesiologists, (approved by the ASA House of Delegates on October 19, 1994, last amended on October 16, 2013, and reaffirmed on October 17, 2018). Available at: https://www.asahq.org/standards-and-guidelines/statement-on-nonoperating-room-anesthetizing-locations.

38. The Joint Commission, Report no. TX 2-2: standards and intents of sedations and anesthesia care. Comprehensive Accreditation Manual for Hospitals, 2002, Joint Commission on Accreditation of Healthcare Organizations. Available at: https://www.jointcommission.org/standards/standard-faqs/ambulatory/provision-of-care-treatment-and-services-pc-000001645/3.

39. Kallmes DF, Watson RE Jr. Gadolinium administration in undetected pregnancy: cause for alarm? Radiology 2019;293(1):201–2.

40. Grobner T. Gadolinium–a specific trigger for the development of nephrogenic fibrosing dermopathy and nephrogenic systemic fibrosis? Nephrol Dial Transpl 2006;21(4):1104–8.

41. American College of Radiology. Manual on contrast media. 2021. Available at: https://www.acr.org/-/media/ACR/Files/Clinical-Resources/Contrast_Media.pdf. Accessed November 25, 2021.

42. The Joint Commission. Compliance checklist: Joint commission's imaging standards. 2020. Available at: https://www.jointcommission.org/-/media/tjc/documents/accred-and-cert/ahc/imaging-checklist.pdf. Accessed November 25, 2021.

43. American College of Radiology. MRI accreditation. Available at: https://www.acraccreditation.org/Modalities/MRI. Accessed November 25,2021.

Emerging Techniques and Future Directions
Fast and Portable Magnetic Resonance Imaging

Min Lang, MD[a], Otto Rapalino, MD[a], Susie Huang, MD, PhD[a,b],
Michael H. Lev, MD[a], John Conklin, MD, MS[a,*], Lawrence L. Wald, PhD[a,b]

KEYWORDS

- Emergency department • Magnetic resonance imaging • Fast MRI • Portable MRI • Brain imaging

KEY POINTS

- Fast MRI methods decrease scan times by reducing the amount of time required to acquire the k-space data, acquiring less k-space data (under sampling), or a combination of the two.
- Fast brain MRI protocols are particularly useful in motion-prone patients such as pediatric patients or adults with altered mental status.
- Point-of-care and portable MRI methods offer the possibility to reduce costs, relax siting constraints, and extend the diagnostic power of MRI to the bedside for patient diagnosis and monitoring in acute care settings.

INTRODUCTION

This article focuses on emerging technologies that have the potential to improve the speed, efficiency, and availability of MRI in emergency settings, specifically, fast MRI and portable MRI. Although these technologies have been topics of research interest for some time, the past several years have seen increasing efforts toward clinical evaluation and adoption of fast MRI and portable MRI in the emergency department and other acute care settings. These techniques are increasingly adopted in clinical research studies, and we anticipate will play an increasing role in emergency radiology over the coming decade.

An increasing number of hospitals are moving toward 24/7 availability of on-site MRI, which is currently required by The Joint Commission for Comprehensive Stroke Center certification.[1] While stroke may be the most compelling indication needing improved MRI speed and availability for neuroimaging in the emergency setting (see R.

Gilberto González's article, "Diffusion MRI of Large Vessel Occlusion Ischemic Stroke for Treatment Selection," in this issue), improved MRI could also add value in the diagnosis, prognosis, and management of a wide variety of acute intracranial pathology (see Damien Galanaud and Rajiv Gupta's article, "MR Imaging for Acute Central Nervous System Pathologies and Presentations in Emergency Department," in this issue). Furthermore, its lack of ionizing radiation makes MRI a safer choice for pediatric and pregnant patients (see Abigail Stanley and colleagues' article, "Magnetic Resonance Imaging of Acute Abdominal Pain in the Pregnant Patient"; and Maria Gabriela Figueiro Longo and colleagues' article, "Pediatric Emergency Magnetic Resonance Imaging," in this issue).

The use of MRI in the emergency department has traditionally been limited by availability, long scan times, and sensitivity to motion.[2] Lack of timely scanner availability or delays induced by

[a] Department of Radiology, Massachusetts General Hospital, 55 Fruit Street, Boston, MA 02114, USA;
[b] Athinoula A. Martinos Center for Biomedical Imaging, 149 13th Street, Charleston, MA 02129, USA
* Corresponding author. Blake SB0029A, 55 Fruit Street, Boston, MA 02114.
E-mail address: john.conklin@mgh.harvard.edu

Magn Reson Imaging Clin N Am 30 (2022) 565–582
https://doi.org/10.1016/j.mric.2022.05.005

the difficulty transporting a patient to the MRI suite can prolong inpatient hospital stays and negatively impact hospital revenue and patient/provider satisfaction.[3,4] Long MRI scan times require longer booking slots, limiting patient throughput and potentially delaying diagnosis and management. Long scan times are also associated with higher sensitivity to motion, a particular challenge in the emergency department.

For all these reasons, techniques to improve the efficiency of clinical brain MR examinations have gained increasing attention. Past efforts to develop ultrafast brain MRI examinations suffered from artifacts and poor image quality, limiting robust clinical use across multiple contrasts. Recent advances in MR technology have led to the development of accelerated acquisition techniques that have the comparable diagnostic quality to conventional sequences.[5–9] Decreased acquisition time has the further benefit of reducing image degradation due to patient motion and has shown value for optimizing workflow and throughput.[10]

Complimentary to the benefits of increasing the speed of the conventional examination, portable MRI used at the point-of-care is emerging as a revolutionary technology with the potential to bring rich diagnostic information directly to the patient's bedside. This paradigm shift requires dramatic changes in the hardware design, clinical workflow, and potential applications of MRI in the emergency setting.

This article will review ultrafast MR technologies and portable MRI systems (including the first FDA approved and commercially available portable MRI scanner), and the major clinical use cases in the emergency department setting.

ULTRAFAST MR TECHNOLOGY

From some historical perspective, fast imaging has not always been motivated by the desire to rapidly evaluate critically ill patients in the emergency setting. Echoplanar imaging (EPI) was first described by Sir Peter Mansfield in 1977, far before the technology became commercially available and successful. Ian Pykett and Richard Rzedzian, both of whom trained under Mansfield, founded Advanced NMR in the 1980s, a company to develop EPI technology for cardiac imaging. Advanced NMR installed its first EPI dedicated gradient system at the Massachusetts General Hospital in 1990.[11] Early applications of EPI focused on cardiac motion in an attempt to freeze the motion of the beating human heart. However, the technology truly exploded with the advent of dynamic time-series imaging of brain hemodynamics by Bruce Rosen and Arno Villringer at the MGH-NMR Center, and became a ubiquitous research tool after the discovery of the blood oxygen level dependent (BOLD) effect and the application of EPI to enable functional MRI of human brain activations.[12–14] The development functional MRI, diffusion MRI and dynamic susceptibility contrast (DSC) perfusion MRI spurred the wide clinical and commercial adoption of EPI brain imaging. However, it has only been in the past few years that the hardware, pulse sequence development, and acquisition strategies have emerged to allow ultrafast multi-contrast brain imaging entirely based on EPI.[15,16]

However, EPI is just one of the many fast imaging strategies that have been used to facilitate fast brain imaging.[5–9,17–19] These techniques typically fall into 3 broad categories: (1) faster image data acquisition, (2) acquisition of less imaging data (ie, under-sampling), or (3) a combination of both (**Fig. 1**). The fundamental principles for achieving short scan time have been known for some time, but successful implementation requires gradient improvements, adequate coil sensitivity, sequence development, and reconstruction algorithms. Advances in these diverse technologies for faster clinical scanning have propelled them to the forefront of clinical imaging in recent years. An overview of the major approaches for fast MRI follows later in discussion.

Ultrafast Spoiled Gradient Echo

Gradient echo (GRE) imaging readouts use 2 gradients that are opposite in direction in rapid succession. The first dephasing gradient accelerates the dephasing and squelching of the free induction decay (ie, artificially shortens T2*).[20,21] The second rephasing gradient, which is opposite in polarity but same in strength, reverses the phase scramble to generate a GRE. In the course of the unscrambling, a single line of k-space data is collected. To acquire k-space lines as fast as possible, ultrafast GRE uses a very small flip angle, as low as 5° to 10°, very short repetition time (TR), and short echo time (TE). In comparison, conventional spin-echo sequences use flip angles close to 90° and 180° for the excitation and refocusing pulses, respectively, very short repetition time (TR) and short echo time (TE). Unfortunately, short TR and small flip angles can result in decreased tissue contrast. To preserve T1 contrast, a magnetization preparation pulse, commonly a 180° inversion pulse, is often applied at the beginning of acquisition, that is, Magnetization Prepared RApid Gradient Echo (MP-RAGE) as initially described by Mugler in 1990.[22]

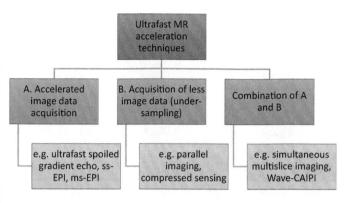

Fig. 1. Ultrafast MR acceleration techniques. CAIPI, controlled aliasing in parallel imaging; ms-EPI, multishot echoplanar imaging; ss-EP, single-shot echoplanar imaging.

Optimized k-space filling can be performed following variable trajectories (linear, centric, square-spiral or elliptical spiral). As ultrafast GRE depends on the T2* decay, it is susceptible to field inhomogeneity.

Echo-Planar Imaging

EPI has developed dramatically since it was first described by Mansfield in 1977 and is now used clinically to achieve rapid acquisition of images in 20 to 100 msec per slice.[23] Unlike conventional spin-echo sequences whereby one line of k-space is acquired with each TR, EPI acquires multiple lines of k-space after a single RF pulse. To achieve this, the frequency-encoding gradient oscillates from a positive to a negative amplitude, continuously producing the dephasing and rephasing phenomena described under the GRE image. Thus, rather than a single GRE forming (as in GRE), a continuous GRE train is formed, each providing a line of k-space data. The echo train length, also known as the EPI factor, is the number of k-space lines encoded in a single shot and is an important determinate of acquisition speed. Other prepared contrasts such as a spin-echo (to achieve T1- or T2-weighted imaging), inversion recovery, and diffusion sensitizing gradients can also be applied immediately prior to the EPI readout.

There are 2 main types of EPI—single-shot and multi-shot. In single-shot EPI (ss-EPI), all the needed k-space lines for a 2D image are acquired after a single RF excitation, and the k-space lines are filled by an echo train with multiple gradient reversals. A constant phase-encoding gradient was used in the original EPI technique resulting in zigzag filling of k-space. This has been nearly completely replaced by the newer "Blipped" technique, whereby each echo is phase-encoded by its own "blip" which advances the k_y line location at the end of each readout, resulting in rectilinear sampling of k-space.[24,25]

In multi-shot EPI (ms-EPI), the k-space data are acquired in multiple segments ("shots"), with each shot acquiring a fraction of the total k-space.[25] The shots are repeated until the full set of k-space data is collected. As fewer k-space lines are collected per shot, there is less time to build up phase errors.[26] This results in reduced image distortion from regions of the head whereby the tissue adversely affects the field homogeneity and causes a susceptibility artifact. Because of the image distortion and as higher resolution scans require more k-space coverage, ms-EPI has been the preferred way to acquire high-resolution EPI scans (at a cost of increased scan time and increased sensitivity to motion). **Figs. 2** demonstrate example images of msEPI sequences compared with conventional reference sequences.

Parallel Imaging

One way to speed up the acquisition is to acquire, for example, only every other or every third k-space line (k-space undersampling). Undersampling k-space reduces the image FOV in the undersampled direction. This causes aliasing artifact unless directly addressed in the image reconstruction through a parallel imaging reconstruction such as SENSitivity Encoding (SENSE) or GeneRalized Autocalibrating Partial Parallel Acquisition (GRAPPA) which utilize multiple receiver coils with known placements and sensitivities to determine where the MR signal arises and "undo" the aliasing. The positional information provided by the multichannel phased-array coils supplements the incomplete k-space data and prevents aliasing.[27,28] The parallel imaging acceleration factor, R, is the ratio of k-space data required for a full y sampled image to that acquired in the undersampled image. It is also the factor by which the image acquisition is sped up compared with the conventional approach. An acceleration factor of 1.5 to 4 is commonly used.[19]

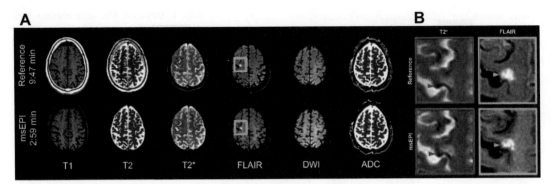

Fig. 2. *(A)* ms-EPI MR sequences (T1-weighted, T2/T2*-weighted, FLAIR, DWI/ADC) compared to a conventional reference clinical protocol based on turbo-spine echo (TSE) brain MR sequences in a patient with old cortical infarct in the right precentral gyrus with associated hemosiderin staining. *(B)* The red magnification box demonstrates similar conspicuity of hemosiderin staining in the right precentral gyrus (red arrowheads). The blue magnification box demonstrates a similar appearance of FLAIR hyperintensity in the right precentral gyrus, suggestive of the old cortical infarct (blue arrowheads). No DWI hyperintensity was seen on the MSEPI or conventional images.

There are 2 general reconstruction classes of parallel imaging reconstructions. The first being image domain reconstruction (reconstruct then correct), which unfold images using a coil-sensitivity map from the aliased image.[19] The second method is k-space domain reconstruction (correct then reconstruct), whereby the under-sampled k-space information is auto-calibrated before Fourier transformation. In both cases, the image suffers an SNR reduction due to 2 factors; (1) the reduced data from having acquired fewer k-space lines, and (2) a noise amplification in the image reconstruction due to imperfect spatial information supplied by the array coil geometry. The first scales simply as the square root of the acceleration factor R, and the second factor is termed the "geometry factor" or g-factor and is typically between 1 and 3, although it can become very large if too much acceleration is attempted.

Simultaneous Multislice Imaging

While conventional parallel imaging speeds up the acquisition by omitting in-plane phase encoding steps, some acquisitions can also be sped up by encoding multiple slices simultaneously. The principle underlying simultaneous multislice (SMS), also known as a multiband imaging, is the simultaneous excitation and readout of multiple slice planes to reduce TR and acquisition time and/or extend slice coverage in a given TR.[29] SMS is most widely used for EPI sequences as simultaneous slice acquisition directly translates to shorter TR in most cases, although SMS versions of turbo spin-echo and GRE sequences have also recently been introduced and are commercially available.

The acceleration achieved with SMS is similar to standard parallel imaging, but there are a few subtle differences arising from operating on the slice selection process rather than the phase encoding. For example, the RF power demand and thus SAR concern is higher in SMS as it uses a high peak-power composite RF pulse for multi-slice excitation.[29] But SMS incurs less SNR penalty than conventional parallel imaging methods as k-space is not under-sampled (so there is no $\sqrt{R}$ SNR penalty). If the g-factor of the acquisition is near unity, there is little to no penalty in SNR; a substantial advantage of SMS over conventional parallel imaging. This is because SMS acceleration does not reduce the echo train length, number of phase-encoding steps, or number of k-space samples. SMS can introduce artifacts, such as the spread of signal across simultaneously acquired slices, termed inter-slice leakage, which can amplify the effects of motion.[30,31] While methods to reduce inter-slice leakage such as slice-GRAPPA have been developed, inter-slice leakage artifacts can still occur and affect diagnostic quality.[32] **Fig. 3** demonstrates an example of SMS accelerated DWI and ADC image pairs.

Wave-Controlled Aliasing in Parallel Imaging

Volumetric imaging has become increasingly important in neuroimaging for surgical planning and assessment of various pathologies such as brain tumors.[33] Acquisition times, however, are often long and greatly increase the total examination time. Parallel imaging is often applied to reduce the acquisition time of volumetric sequences. In conventional 3D parallel imaging, the image data can be under-sampled in the two

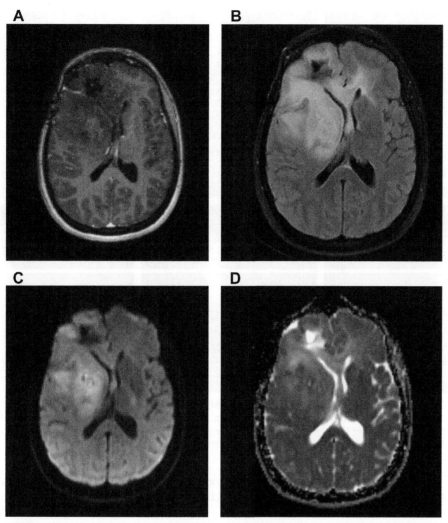

Fig. 3. Brain MRI in a patient who underwent right frontal craniotomy for the subtotal resection of right frontal anaplastic astrocytoma. Magnetization-prepared rapid gradient-echo (MPRAGE) image demonstrate ill-defined and heterogenous areas of enhancement in the right frontal lobe, basal ganglia, right anterior thalamus, and corpus callosum, which is concerning for tumor progression. TSE FLAIR image demonstrates hyperintensity throughout the right frontal lobe, subcortical structures, corpus callosum, and the left frontal lobe with associated worsening mass effect, right ventricular effacement, and leftward midline shift. Simultaneous multislice (SMS) accelerated DWI/ADC images demonstrate restricted diffusion with ADC hyperintensity in the right basal ganglia corresponding to the region of ill-defined enhancement, furthering concern for tumor progression. There are surrounding areas of DWI and ADC hyperintensity in the right frontal lobe that reflects T2 shine through. There is no evidence of acute infarction.

phase-encoded directions (commonly in the y and z planes) to reduce acquisition time. While better than putting all the acceleration into a single direction, large total acceleration factors can still result in a high SNR penalty, often prohibitive above a total acceleration factor of approximately 3 to 4.[34]

A limitation of parallel imaging is that the modern coil array is relatively poor in discerning elements in untangling aliasing in the z-direction, thus, in the SMS method, the excitation of the multiple slices must be spaced widely apart. CAIPI assists the role of the coil sensitivity in the z-direction by using the phase of the RF pulse to shift the position of adjacent slices in a controlled fashion making the aliasing easier to undo.[35] CAIPI spreads voxel aliasing more uniformly and allows for more efficient disentanglement of adjacent slices.

Wave-CAIPI builds on CAIPI by using sinusoidal G_y and G_z gradients applied during readout of each k-space line.[36] The characteristic corkscrew

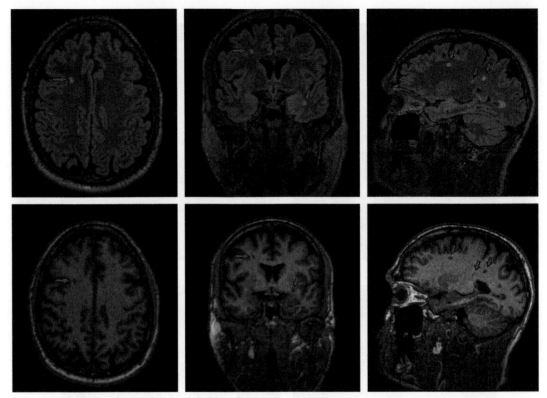

Fig. 4. WAVE-CAIPI SPACE-FLAIR (*top row*) and WAVE-CAIPI MPRAGE (*bottom row*) images demonstrate scattered foci of T2/FLAIR hyperintensity with corresponding T1 hypointensity in the periventricular, subcortical, and juxtacortical white matter throughout the supratentorial brain (arrow). This is consistent with a reported history of multiple sclerosis. There was no parenchymal enhancement to suggest active demyelination.

trajectory leads to the optimal synergy between aliasing and coil sensitivity profiles, allowing for highly accelerated volumetric imaging with low artifact and negligible g-factor penalty.[36] Wave-CAIPI has been used to accelerate 3D sequences such as MPRAGE (**Fig. 4**), SPACE-FLAIR (see **Fig. 4**), and SWI (**Fig. 5**).

Compressed Sensing

Compressed sensing (CS) is founded on the basis of reconstructing an image from incomplete k-space sampling by exploiting the existence of a sparse representation of the image (ie, a representation that will be represented with only a few variables), which is mathematically related to the ability to compress an image such as the well-known jpeg compression scheme.[37–39] Indeed, the inspiration for CS partly came from attempts to solve medical image compression. One of the solutions to medical image compression was lossy compression, whereby certain data elements are discarded.[40] Several research groups then applied this approach in reverse for MR imaging—if medical image data can be compressed by discarding certain

information, the initial image data acquisition can be limited to this compressed (under sampled) data-set which can be acquired much faster. Compression is simply a more efficient way of describing the image data; a general property of "naturalistic" images, whether photographs of scenes or medical images, is that they can be stored in this compressed representation and then reverted back with relatively little image degradation. The "compressed" data contain enough information to reconstruct images of similar quality as those that would arise from a fully sampled set.[37–39]

Application of CS in MR imaging is possible because of redundant image data and transform sparsity, meaning the object or image we are trying to recover has a sparse representation in a constrained transform domain.[39] Sparse representation means that essential information is contained in a few high-valued coefficients and most of the other coefficients can be discarded with no or negligible loss of information.[41] The final MR image can thus be recovered from under-sampled data using iterative knowledge-based reconstruction to fill in the empty k-space lines. The reconstruction method is nonlinear and enforces 2 conditions: (1)

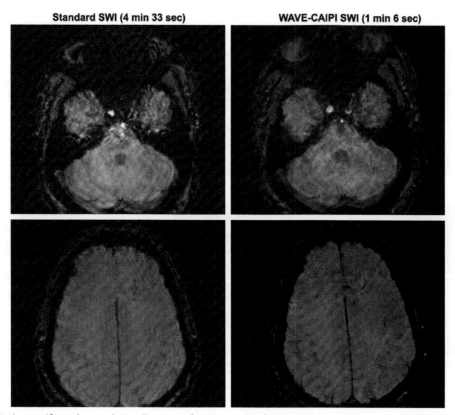

Standard SWI (4 min 33 sec)   **WAVE-CAIPI SWI (1 min 6 sec)**

Fig. 5. Motion artifact obscured visualization of supra- and infra-tentorial microhemorrhages on the standard SWI sequence due to the long acquisition time (4 min 33 sec). The presence of microhemorrhages is better seen on the WAVE-CAIPI SWI sequence, which is less affected by motion due to the shorter acquisition time.

the image data exhibit transform sparsity and (2) consistency of the reconstruction with the acquired data.[42] The first condition allows aliasing artifacts to be separated from the actual image signal and the second condition ensures that the actual image data are not replaced with arbitrary data. These 2 conditions balance the sparsity of the image and reconstruction of an image that is consistent with the collected image data. With CS, acquisition time can be reduced by half while maintaining high diagnostic quality. Because CS relies on image sparsity and not hardware, it is also not limited by the Nyquist limit like other techniques such as parallel imaging.[39] Compressed sensing has been applied to various 2D and 3D brain MR sequences such as T2-weighted imaging, FLAIR, 3D T1-echo-spoiled gradient echo (SPGR), and TOF MRA (**Fig. 6**).[18,43,44]

CLINICAL USE OF FAST MAGNETIC RESONANCE IMAGING
Pediatric Patients

MRI is preferred over CT as the imaging modality of choice for pediatric patients due to MRI's lack of ionizing radiation and excellent anatomic assessment of the brain. The same ionizing radiation dose from CT results in a 10-fold higher neoplastic potential for a child than an adult.[45] MRI is also superior to CT for evaluating the posterior fossa and ischemic stroke.[46] The long acquisition time, together with motion artifact associated with imaging young patients, can limit the diagnostic quality of MRI and may require sedation in some settings. Techniques to accelerate MRI acquisition have been used to overcome these limitations and studies have demonstrated clinical benefit for imaging pediatric patients in the emergency setting.[47]

Pediatric patients with ventricular shunt placement for hydrocephalus receive routine and emergency imaging to evaluate for shunt dysfunction. Single-shot fast spin-echo and ultrafast GRE T2-weighted imaging have been shown to be sufficient in most cases for catheter visualization and evaluation of shunt dysfunction.[48,49] Application of ultrafast brain MR imaging can also help avoid sedation and reduce motion artifact.[50]

Combining different acceleration techniques such as parallel imaging and EPI, a recent group

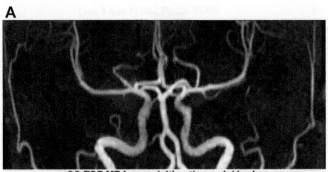

CS-TOF MRA: acquisition time = 1:11 min

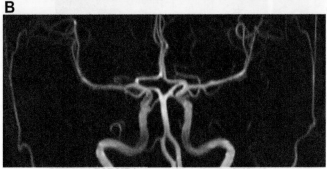

Standard TOF MRA: acquisition time = 6:43 min

Fig. 6. Example of CS-TOF MRA (*A*) and standard TOF MRA (*B*) MIP images in a healthy volunteer. Visualization of the proximal major intracranial vessels is similar between CS-TOF MRA and the standard TOF MRA images despite a 5-fold reduction in acquisition time for the CS sequence.

from Korea demonstrated that a 1-min ultrafast pediatric brain protocol consisting of T1-, T2-, and T2*-weighted imaging, FLAIR, and DWI sequences showed sufficient image quality for diagnostic use for a broad range of indications.[17] Accelerated MRI sequences have also been used for pediatric traumatic brain injury, including the use of single-shot fast spin-echo T1-and T2-weighted sequences, and accelerated EPI T1-weighted, FLAIR, and DWI sequences.[51] Kralik and colleagues reported similar sensitivity and specificity for the detection of trauma using accelerated EPI-DWI and EPI-T2*-weighted images when compared with their conventional counterparts.[52] Limitations of ultrafast brain MRI in pediatric patients include reduced sensitivity for certain pathology such as skull fractures and very small hemorrhages.[52–55]

Stroke Evaluation

Neuroimaging plays a critical role in the initial evaluation of acute ischemic stroke. MRI is superior to CT for the assessment of parenchymal integrity, tissue viability, and ischemic core.[56,57] DWI / FLAIR mismatch on MRI is suggestive of ischemic stroke less than 4.5 hours, which is a crucial patient selection criteria for IV-tPA, and is extremely helpful when the symptom of onset is unknown.[58,59] DWI also allows for the superior assessment of ischemic core volume than other techniques such as CT perfusion, and facilitates selection of patients likely to benefit from mechanical thrombectomy and late-window thrombolysis.

To reduce scan time and reduce motion degradation, fast brain MR protocols for acute stroke evaluation have been developed using ss-EPI and parallel imaging techniques.[60] A previously proposed protocol for comprehensive stroke evaluation included accelerated versions of DWI, FLAIR, GRE, DSC perfusion, and MRA.[60] The acquisition time of this protocol was 6-min long and demonstrated diagnostic image quality in greater than 90% of the cases. When the acceleration of ss-EPI and parallel imaging is pushed too far, however, image distortion and dropout artifacts can occur due to local field inhomogeneity and geometric distortion. Furthermore, SNR and sensitivity of detecting small areas of ischemia or hemorrhage are reduced.

Multi-shot echoplanar imaging (ms-EPI) is a high efficiency interleaved EPI imaging technique that uses multiple excitations, resulting in significantly reduced geometric distortion and higher SNR than ss-EPI.[61,62] Prototype ms-EPI brain MR protocol (T1-, T2-, T2*-weighted, FLAIR, and DWI) are being evaluated at our institution (**Fig. 7**).[63] The prototype fast brain ms-EPI-based protocol

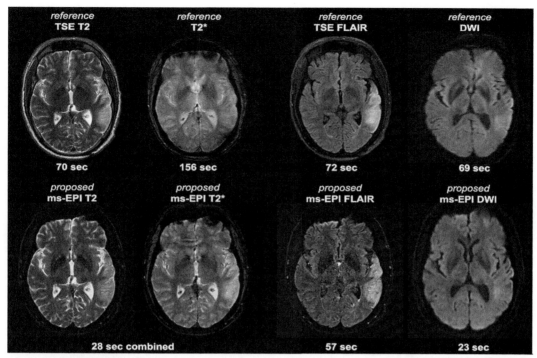

Fig. 7. ms-EPI MR sequences compared with standard brain MR sequences in a patient presenting with aphasia for 2 weeks. In both the ms-EPI and standard brain MR images, there was obvious T2/FLAIR hyperintensity in the left temporal lobe with subtle associated high DWI signal, suggestive of late subacute infarction. The overall diagnostic quality of the images was similar between the ms-EPI and the standard images. The acquisition times for the sequences are listed below each image in seconds.

totals approximately 2 minutes. Preliminary results demonstrated that while noise and artifact were increased on ms-EPI sequences compared with conventional sequences, the detection of image findings, including ischemic stroke evaluation, was not compromised.[63] Further efforts using machine-learning algorithms to improve image quality and to decrease image noise and artifact are currently ongoing.

Acute Nontraumatic Neurologic Presentation

Approximately 15% of emergency department visits are due to acute neurologic symptoms.[64] EPI and parallel imaging have been used in the emergency setting beyond ischemic stroke evaluation in these scenarios. Kazmierczak and colleagues and Prakkamakul and colleagues deployed ultrafast brain MRI protocols in the emergency and neurologic intensive care unit settings, respectively.[65,66] These studies included a broad range of acute neurologic symptoms such as vertigo, paresthesia, impaired vision, aphasia, motor deficits, memory impairment, tremor, and others. They found that the ultrafast brain MRI protocols were superior to CT for detecting acute intracranial pathologies. While the ultrafast protocol was noninferior to the standard brain MRI protocol and did

not impact clinical care, several pathologies were missed or were less conspicuous on the ultrafast MR images. Depending on the symptoms and suspected pathology of the patients, the protocols can be individualized by adding or replacing certain sequences (eg, a 3D SPACE FLAIR offers higher sensitivity for demyelinating lesions than conventional 2D FLAIR if this is an acute concern; susceptibility-weighted images offer greater sensitivity for small foci of intracranial hemorrhage, and so forth). Recently, an adaptable ultra-fast brain MRI protocol "Neuro-Mix" was proposed, whereby image quality can be dynamically adjusted by substituting different fast MRI sequences depending on the clinical indication and the patients' ability to tolerate MRI scanning.[67]

Operational Impact of Fast Magnetic Resonance Imaging

Reducing scan time is beneficial for improving patient care and access. For certain populations, including patients who are acutely ill, in pain, have claustrophobia, or altered in mental status, remaining still for prolonged periods of time for conventional brain MRI can be very difficult. Implementation of accelerated MR sequences can increase access for patients that would otherwise not tolerate

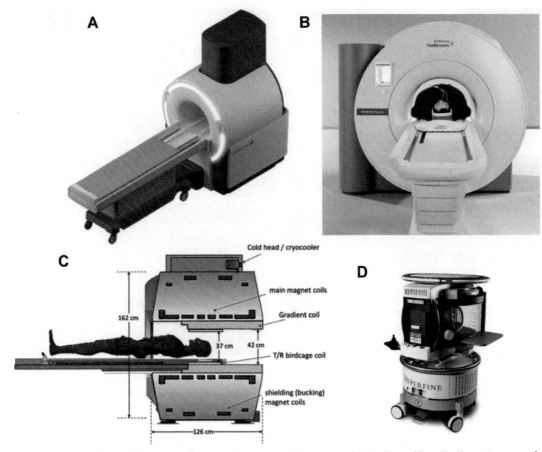

Fig. 8. Commercially available point-of-care and portable MRI systems. (*A*) Dedicated head-only MRI scanner for point-of-care imaging from Synaptive. (*B*) Siemens Healthineers moves into new clinical fields with its smallest and most lightweight 80 cm bore whole-body MRI. (*C*) Small-footprint, lightweight, high-performance 3T MRI scanner for advanced brain imaging with reduced installation costs. (*D*): Hyperfine Swoop® Portable MR Imaging SystemTM. (*From* [*A*] Panther et al (reference 88), Proc. ISMRM 2019 p. 3679, owner ISMRM; [*B*] Siemens Healthineers SHAPE 21 Imaging Press Conference, November 18, 2020. Available at: https://www.siemens-healthineers. com/press/releases/magnetom-free-max.html. [*C*] Foo TKF et al, Magn Reson Med. 2018 Nov;80(5):2232-2245. PMID: 29536587. [*D*] Proc. ISMRM 2020 abstract 555, owner ISMRM.)

the long scan times of standard MR protocols. Further advantages include a reduced number of repeat scans from motion degradation and improved patient satisfaction and comfort, all the while maintaining adequate diagnostic imaging quality.

The utilization of diagnostic imaging, including brain MRI, in the emergency setting has also been increasing.[68,69] This is partly due to increased MRI scanner availability, increased demand by clinicians and patients, and increased surveillance of patients with diseases such as cancer.[70–72] Strategies to meet the increasing imaging demand include acquiring more scanners, hiring of additional personnel, and acquisition of new space, but these are all associated with significant financial costs. Accelerated MRI protocols can improve scanner productivity without the additional financial

burden and mitigates downstream costs.[73] Implementation of accelerated brain MRI sequences at our institution was shown to reduce acquisition time by approximately 40% in the outpatient setting, suggesting that substantial improvement in operational efficiency can potentially be achieved in the emergency department as well.

POINT-OF-CARE AND PORTABLE MAGNETIC RESONANCE IMAGING
Expanding the Role of Magnetic Resonance Imaging in the Emergency Department with Small Foot-Print and Portable Scanners

The size, footprint, and siting needs of conventional high-field MRI scanners have traditionally prohibited their installation in specialized areas such as the emergency department (ED) or Intensive Care Unit

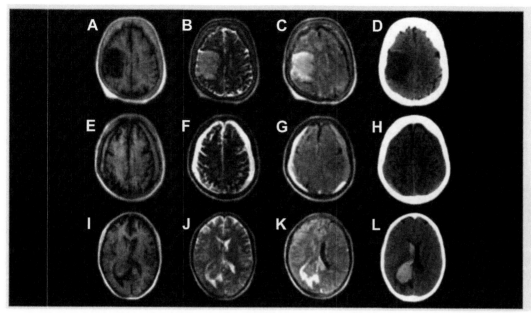

Fig. 9. Clinical examples of portable 0.063T MR images (axial T1, T2 and FLAIR) compared to non-contrast CT images respectively from left to right. Top row: Subacute right MCA ischemic infarct (a-d). Middle row: Bilateral subacute subdural hematomas (e-h). Bottom row: Suspected right splenial hemorrhagic mass (i-l) in a patient with metastatic Ewing's sarcoma.

(ICU). Recent technological work has focused on altering the system design to reduce the siting constraints and even produce truly portable MRI scanners that can be wheeled to the patient bedside. This has been primarily enabled by the design of scanners focusing on a particular body part, such as the brain, and by lowering the field strength of the magnet and compensating for the reduced image quality with computational filtering approaches (denoising) and utilization of state-of-the-art sequences and receive-coil technology. Other technical components that must be addressed to reduce system cost and siting needs include the magnet's magnetic footprint, power consumption, cooling of electrical components, cryogen use and venting, acoustic noise, and reduction of artifacts from electro-magnetic Interference (EMI) sources. The latter are typically eliminated through the use of a specialized shielded room, which must be eliminated in a truly portable scanner. When discussing portable and point-of-care MRI, it is important to keep in mind that the goal is not replacing conventional high-field scanners, but rather to supplement them by providing systems that expand the use of MRI in a new setting.

Rethinking System-Level Approaches for Portable Magnetic Resonance Imaging

To reimagine MRI as a portable device for use in the ED, a new system-level approach is needed.

The simplest approach is to continue the industrial effort into shortening the bore of conventional super-conducting magnet-based systems such as the current standard (the 1.5 T scanner). However, even after decades of effort, this system remains a multi-ton, nontransportable system with high power and cooling needs and a relatively large magnetic field footprint. Relaxing some of the features of this workhorse conventional scanner is required to make it truly easy to site in an ED (or portable). Reducing the focus from whole-body to brain-only yields the largest potential gains for increasing the range of siting locations. Other obvious departures include lowering the static magnetic field strength (at the expense of sensitivity) and/or the magnet's homogeneity, which alters the imaging pulse sequences that can be used.[74–76] The result is cheaper, smaller superconducting magnets or permanent magnets where the magnetic energy density can be stored without the use of cryogens. Other departures include nonswitched readout gradients built into the static magnet design (saving power, cooling, and reducing acoustic noise),[77] encoding by the rotation of a built-in gradient (further reducing encoding electronics),[78–83] and shrinking the imaging field of view (FOV) even further to a subset of the organ and perhaps not fully encoding all spatial dimensions.

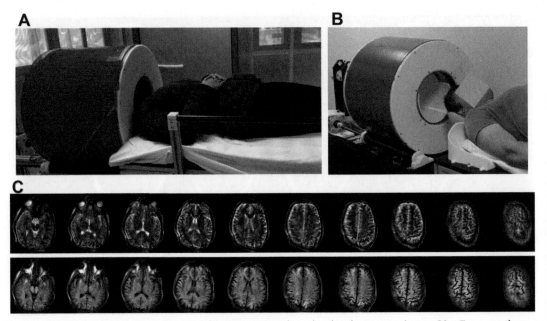

Fig. 10. The "Halbach Bulb," another portable MRI approach under development using an 80 mT rare earth magnet configuration with a magnet weight less than 100 kg. (*A*) A volunteer with head positioned inside the scanner (orange cylinder). The subject's shoulders remain outside the scanner allowing for a lightweight small bore design that fits the head only. (*B*) Another view of the scanner. (*C*) Representative T2 (*top row*) and T1 (*bottom row*) weighted images in a volunteer, obtained using this device. (*From* [*A*] Figure 1 of Cooley, C.Z., McDaniel, P.C., Stockmann, J.P. et al. A portable scanner for magnetic resonance imaging of the brain. Nat Biomed Eng 5, 229–239 (2021); [*B*] Original artwork; [*C*], Original artwork.)

Three Strategies for Portable Magnetic Resonance Imaging in the Emergency Department

We arbitrarily divide ED MRI use cases into 3 levels based on their degree of deviation from the standard 1.5 T scanner suite. The closest level uses modest deviations and attempts to improve siting (and perhaps cost) to facilitate siting within a tight ED space. This "easy-to-site suite" scanner could use a standard superconducting solenoid magnet architecture, perhaps at reduced field strength, but with modifications to decrease its cost, size, and stray-field footprint (**Fig. 8**). For example, the system might use a short-bore, conduction-cooled superconducting magnet to eliminate cryogens and the quench pipe. The footprint, size, and cost can be further reduced compared with conventional whole-body scanners if the magnet is sized for brain-only imaging and operated at mid-field (between 0.5 T and 1.0 T). This intermediate field strength is attractive because it can provide sensitivity and imaging contrasts similar to conventional 1.5 T scanners. This direction has been recently reviewed and put into historical perspective.[84] An additional technology that is on the near horizon is the addition of active Electro-Magnetic Interference (EMI) mitigation to eliminate

the standard RF shielded room. High-field (3T) superconducting head-only scanners can also be considered similarly "easy-to-site." These include the Siemens Allegra 3T clinical scanner[85] introduced in the early 2000s but no longer produced, and the more recent GE high-performance 3T head scanner using a conduction-cooled magnet with no cryogen vent pipe.[86] While the magnet and gradients of these high-field head-only systems are more compact, the focus of these 2 systems was on performance rather than siting alone.

Reduction of the magnet's B_0 field yields further siting benefits. A 0.5 T or 1.0 T superconducting magnet retains many aspects of conventional suites including high-power electrical hookups (for conventional gradients), maintenance-prone cryogenic equipment, water cooling, and a safety exclusion zone, but the potential siting benefits have motivated several commercial MRI manufacturers to initiate the development of this type of device (see **Fig. 8**). Two "mid-field" approaches (0.55 T[87] or 0.5 T[88–90]) have been introduced leveraging superconducting systems with cryogen-free refrigeration systems. Both use modern, high-performance gradient systems in standard architecture. Other efforts are underway with an even smaller head-focused 1.5 T high-temperature superconducting magnet.[91]

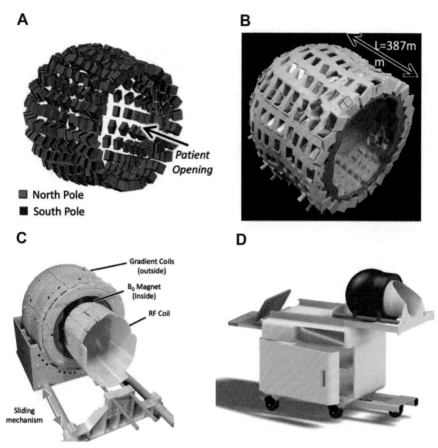

A

North Pole
South Pole

Patient Opening

B

L=387m
m

C

Gradient Coils (outside)
B₀ Magnet (Inside)
RF Coil
Sliding mechanism

D

Fig. 11. Illustration of the permanent low field magnet design used in the "Halbach Bulb" scanner. (*A*) Computer rendering of the rare earth metal array which creates a permanent magnetic field of 80 mT. (*B*) Photograph of the actual permanent magnet array used in the scanner. (*C*) Diagram of the scanner components, including the gradient coils, which are placed outside the permanent magnet array, and RF coil, which is placed inside the permanent magnet array. (*D*) Rendering of the scanner mounted on a portable frame that can be wheeled to the bedside for point-of-care imaging. (*From*: Original artwork.)

The second level would be a truly portable scanner that could be pushed from location to location within the ED. This device must operate using a standard electrical outlet or perhaps battery power. The mobile brain scanner would likely operate at low field (50 mT to 200 mT), need unconventional EMI mitigation, and must operate with substantially reduced electrical power compared with conventional systems and without water cooling or cryogenics. This class of POC devices is being actively pursued by several companies and academic groups. Notably, the first fully portable clinical MRI product scanner is now FDA approved for clinical care, the 64 mT Hyperfine scanner shown in **Fig 8**D.[92,93] **Fig. 9** shows some brain images taken with this system. **Figs. 10** and **11** show another approach under development, based on an 80 mT "Halbach-bulb" rare earth magnet configuration with a magnet weight less than 100 kg.[77,94,95]

Finally, the third class is a more speculative device that extends MRI to a near "hand-held" level, likely with greatly reduced imaging capabilities, but inexpensive and small enough to be considered an MR detector or monitoring device more than a diagnostic imaging device. Such a lightweight device could reach into the bed and monitors the brain, perhaps using 1D imaging or just the MR signal itself. This rethinks the role of MRI as a tomographic imager and, as such, is the most distant from conventional MRI scanner architectures. Nonetheless, examples of this more speculative device are starting to emerge in the literature, such as the 7 kg device shown in **Fig. 12**.[82] Even if detailed anatomy is not visualized, the MR data can be collected and monitored for changes that might accompany, for example, important intracranial pathology. This type of MRI is thus a patient monitoring device in the way a pulse-oximeter or ECG device is used at the

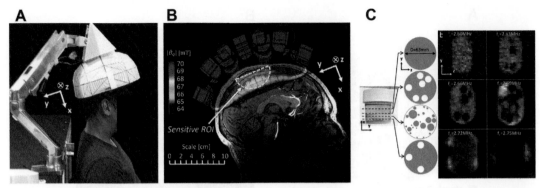

Fig. 12. (*A*) Concept drawing of the "MR Cap," a 7 kg device that can be positioned above the subject's head like a helmet. (*B*) Concept drawing illustrating the sensitive ROI of the scanner, superimposed on a sagittal T1-weighted image high-resolution image of the brain. (*C*) Images of a phantom were obtained using this scanner. Six images are shown on the right, at different depths of the phantom in the YZ (transverse) plane. (*From:* [*A, B*] from Figure 1 and C from Figure 9 of McDaniel, P.C., et al., *The MR Cap: A single-sided MRI system designed for potential point-of-care limited field-of-view brain imaging.* Magn Reson Med, 2019. **82**(5): p. 1946-1960. Owner: Wiley; [*C*], Original artwork.)

bedside in the ED or ICU. It is new territory for MRI and pushes the technology into a more radical configuration. As a monitoring device, the device must "reach" into the bed, operate adjacent to the patient (vs placing the anatomy inside the magnet), and be light and cheap enough for sustained operation as a monitoring device. An ED or ICU might benefit from such an MRI device to continuously image the brain watching for intracranial hemorrhage or changes in cerebral mass-effect through monitoring a ventricular/CSF left-right hemisphere asymmetry. An intracranial MR monitor could provide an early warning sign of impending herniation, particularly in patients whereby the clinical examination is difficult (eg, sedated patients). Single-sided spectrometers have also been introduced for assessing breast tissue[96,97] and muscle hydration.[98,99] Single-sided full imaging systems are less common, but have been demonstrated[100] and applied to burn depth.[101]

The above 3 visions for point-of-care portable MRI are not exhaustive, but we hope will stimulate emergency radiologists and emergency department clinicians to begin thinking of MRI as a tool that may soon be accessible at the bedside, and to understand and imagine how this emerging technology could benefit acute care in the near future.

SUMMARY

Challenges to MRI in the emergency setting include limited availability, limited throughput, siting constraints, costs, and motion artifacts. Fast brain MRI and portable MRI are emerging as promising technologies that can improve the efficiency of MR imaging in the emergency setting, and improve the availability of MRI in patient care settings whereby cost, siting, or scan-time considerations were previously prohibitive. MR acceleration techniques result in a substantial reduction in total acquisition times, while providing accurate diagnosis for the detection of major acute pathologies such as stroke, hemorrhage, mass effect, and hydrocephalus. Point-of-care and portable MRI systems can further expand the use of MRI by increasing the number of MRI departments able to afford and site and MRI scanner, by bringing the scanner to the bedside, and one day perhaps providing real-time monitoring of acute intracranial pathology. Though it remains to be seen, the ultimate goal of this technology development and clinical translation is to provide more timely, accurate, and available diagnostic information for acutely ill patients in emergency and acute care settings.

CLINICS CARE POINTS

- Use of fast MRI methods can be helpful in the evaluation of motion prone patients such as pediatric patients, critically ill patients and those with altered mental status.

- Decreasing the length of MR acquisitions can have beneficial impact on operational workflow and reduce the time required to obtain critical diagnostic information for acutely ill patients.

- Point-of-care and portable MRI technology is emerging as a promising tool to bring the diagnostic power of MRI to the bedside with reduced costs and relaxed siting constraints.

DISCLOSURE

J. Conklin: RSNA Research Seed Grant, research support from Siemens Healthineers. L.L. Wald: research support from Siemens Healthineers, Consulting and Equity from Neuro42 Inc. S. Huang: Research Support from the National Institutes of Health P41EB030006, and Siemens Healthineers

REFERENCES

1. The Joint Commission Stroke Certification Programs – Program Concept Comparison. Available at: https://www.jointcommission.org/-/media/tjc/documents/accred-and-cert/certification/certification-by-setting/stroke/dsc-stroke-grid-comparison-chart-42021.pdf, 2021. Accessed June 28, 2022.
2. Zaitsev M, Maclaren J, Herbst M. Motion artifacts in MRI: A complex problem with many partial solutions. J Magn Reson Imaging 2015;42:887–901.
3. Drose JA, Pritchard NL, Honce JM, et al. Utilizing Process Improvement Methodology to Improve Inpatient Access to MRI. Radiographics 2019;39:2103–10.
4. Tokur S, Lederle K, Terris DD, et al. Process analysis to reduce MRI access time at a German University Hospital. Int J Qual Health Care 2012;24:95–9.
5. Setsompop K, Feinberg DA, Polimeni JR. Rapid brain MRI acquisition techniques at ultra-high fields. NMR Biomed 2016;29:1198–221.
6. Goncalves Filho ALM, Conklin J, Longo MGF, et al. Accelerated Post-contrast Wave-CAIPI T1 SPACE Achieves Equivalent Diagnostic Performance Compared With Standard T1 SPACE for the Detection of Brain Metastases in Clinical 3T MRI. Front Neurol 2020;11:587327.
7. Hollingsworth KG. Reducing acquisition time in clinical MRI by data undersampling and compressed sensing reconstruction. Phys Med Biol 2015;60:R297–322.
8. Conklin J, Longo MGF, Cauley SF, et al. Validation of Highly Accelerated Wave-CAIPI SWI Compared with Conventional SWI and T2*-Weighted Gradient Recalled-Echo for Routine Clinical Brain MRI at 3T. AJNR Am J Neuroradiol 2019;40:2073–80.
9. Clifford B, et al. Clinical evaluation of an AI-accelerated two-minute multi-shot EPI protocol for comprehensive high-quality brain imaging. In: Proceedings of the International Society of Magnetic Resonance in Medicine. Intl Soc Magn Reson Med; 2021.
10. Lang M, Cartmell S, Tabari A, et al. Evaluation of the Aggregated Time Savings in Adopting Fast Brain MRI Techniques for Outpatient Brain MRI. Acad Radiol 2021. https://doi.org/10.1016/j.acra.2021.07.011.
11. Toga AW. Brain mapping: an encyclopedic reference, 2015. Elsevier Science. Available at: https://www.elsevier.com/books/brain-mapping/toga/978-0-12-397025-1.
12. Ogawa S, Lee TM, Kay AR, et al. Brain magnetic resonance imaging with contrast dependent on blood oxygenation. Proc Natl Acad Sci U S A 1990;87:9868–72.
13. Belliveau JW, Kennedy DN, McKinstry RC, et al. Functional mapping of the human visual cortex by magnetic resonance imaging. Science 1991;254(5032):716–9.
14. Kwong KK, Belliveau JW, Chesler DA, et al. Dynamic magnetic resonance imaging of human brain activity during primary sensory stimulation. Proc Natl Acad Sci U S A 1992;89:5675–9.
15. Delgado AF, Kits A, Bystam J, et al. Diagnostic performance of a new multicontrast one-minute full brain exam (EPIMix) in neuroradiology: A prospective study. J Magn Reson Imaging 2019;50:1824–33.
16. Skare S, Sprenger T, Norbeck O, et al. A 1-minute full brain MR exam using a multicontrast EPI sequence. Magn Reson Med 2018;79:3045–54.
17. Ha JY, Baek HJ, Ryu KH, et al. One-Minute Ultrafast Brain MRI With Full Basic Sequences: Can It Be a Promising Way Forward for Pediatric Neuroimaging? AJR Am J Roentgenol 2020;215:198–205.
18. Vranic JE, Cross NM, Wang Y, et al. Compressed Sensing-Sensitivity Encoding (CS-SENSE) Accelerated Brain Imaging: Reduced Scan Time without Reduced Image Quality. AJNR Am J Neuroradiol 2019;40:92–8.
19. Kozak BM, Jaimes C, Kirsch J, et al. MRI Techniques to Decrease Imaging Times in Children. Radiographics 2020;40:485–502.
20. Elster AD. Gradient-echo MR imaging: techniques and acronyms. Radiology 1993;186:1–8.
21. Winkler ML, Ortendahl DA, Mills TC, et al. Characteristics of partial flip angle and gradient reversal MR imaging. Radiology 1988;166:17–26.
22. Mugler JP 3rd, Brookeman JR. Three-dimensional magnetization-prepared rapid gradient-echo imaging (3D MP RAGE). Magn Reson Med 1990;15:152–7.
23.. Mansfield P. Multi-planar image formation using NMR spin echoes. J Phys C: Solid State Phys 1977;10:55–8.
24. Stehling MJ, Howseman AM, Ordidge RJ, et al. Whole-body echo-planar MR imaging at 0.5 T. Radiology 1989;170:257–63.
25. Poustchi-Amin M, Mirowitz SA, Brown JJ, et al. Principles and applications of echo-planar imaging: a review for the general radiologist. Radiographics 2001;21:767–79.

26. Feinberg DA, Oshio K. Phase errors in multi-shot echo planar imaging. Magn Reson Med 1994;32:535–9.

27. You S-H, Kim B, Kim BK, et al. Fast MRI in Acute Ischemic Stroke: Applications of MRI Acceleration Techniques for MR-Based Comprehensive Stroke Imaging. Investig Magn Reson Imaging 2021;25(2):81–92.

28. Deshmane A, Gulani V, Griswold MA, et al. Parallel MR imaging. J Magn Reson Imaging 2012;36:55–72.

29. Barth M, Breuer F, Koopmans PJ, et al. Simultaneous multislice (SMS) imaging techniques. Magn Reson Med 2016;75:63–81.

30. Todd N, Moeller S, Auerbach EJ, et al. Evaluation of 2D multiband EPI imaging for high-resolution, whole-brain, task-based fMRI studies at 3T: Sensitivity and slice leakage artifacts. Neuroimage 2016;124:32–42.

31. McNabb CB, Lindner M, Shen S, et al. Inter-slice leakage and intra-slice aliasing in simultaneous multi-slice echo-planar images. Brain Struct Funct 2020;225:1153–8.

32. Cauley SF, Polimeni JR, Bhat H, et al. Interslice leakage artifact reduction technique for simultaneous multislice acquisitions. Magn Reson Med 2014;72:93–102.

33. Mills SJ, Radon MR, Baird RD, et al. Utilization of volumetric magnetic resonance imaging for baseline and surveillance imaging in Neuro-oncology. Br J Radiol 2019;92:20190059.

34. Breuer FA, Blaimer M, Heidemann RM, et al. Controlled aliasing in parallel imaging results in higher acceleration (CAIPIRINHA) for multi-slice imaging. Magn Reson Med 2005;53:684–91.

35. Breuer FA, Blaimer M, Mueller MF, et al. Controlled aliasing in volumetric parallel imaging (2D CAIPIRINHA). Magn Reson Med 2006;55:549–56.

36. Bilgic B, Gagoski BA, Cauley SF, et al. Wave-CAIPI for highly accelerated 3D imaging. Magn Reson Med 2015;73:2152–62.

37. Candès EJ, Romberg J, Tao T. Robust Uncertainty Principles: Exact Signal Reconstruction From Highly Incomplete Frequency Information. IEEE Trans Inf Theory 2006;52:489–509.

38. Donoho DL. Compressed sensing. IEEE Trans Inf Theory 2006;52:289–1306.

39. Lustig M, Donoho D, Pauly JM. Sparse MRI: The application of compressed sensing for rapid MR imaging. Magn Reson Med 2007;58:1182–95.

40. Patidar, G., Kumar, .S. & Kumar, D. A review on medical image data compression techniques. 2nd International Conference on Data, Engineering and Applications (IDEA). Bhopal, India, February, 28-29, 2021.

41. Feng L, Benkert T, Block KT, et al. Compressed sensing for body MRI. J Magn Reson Imaging 2017;45:966–87.

42. Yang AC, Kretzler M, Sudarski S, et al. Sparse Reconstruction Techniques in Magnetic Resonance Imaging: Methods, Applications, and Challenges to Clinical Adoption. Invest Radiol 2016;51:349–64.

43. Sartoretti T, Reischauer C, Sartoretti E, et al. Common artefacts encountered on images acquired with combined compressed sensing and SENSE. Insights Imaging 2018;9:1107–15.

44. Jaspan ON, Fleysher R, Lipton ML. Compressed sensing MRI: a review of the clinical literature. Br J Radiol 2015;88:20150487.

45. Shah NB, Platt SL. ALARA: is there a cause for alarm? Reducing radiation risks from computed tomography scanning in children. Curr Opin Pediatr 2008;20:243–7.

46. Amlie-Lefond C, Sebire G, Fullerton HJ. Recent developments in childhood arterial ischaemic stroke. Lancet Neurol 2008;7:425–35.

47. Ramgopal S, Karim SA, Subramanian S, et al. Rapid brain MRI protocols reduce head computerized tomography use in the pediatric emergency department. BMC Pediatr 2020;20:14.

48. Miller JH, Walkiewicz T, Towbin RB, et al. Improved delineation of ventricular shunt catheters using fast steady-state gradient recalled-echo sequences in a rapid brain MR imaging protocol in nonsedated pediatric patients. AJNR Am J Neuroradiol 2010;31:430–5.

49. Boyle TP, Paldino MJ, Kimia AA, et al. Comparison of rapid cranial MRI to CT for ventricular shunt malfunction. Pediatrics 2014;134:e47–54.

50. Iskandar BJ, Sansone JM, Medow J, et al. The use of quick-brain magnetic resonance imaging in the evaluation of shunt-treated hydrocephalus. J Neurosurg 2004;101:147–51.

51. Kessler BA, Goh JL, Pajer HB, et al. Rapid-sequence MRI for evaluation of pediatric traumatic brain injury: a systematic review. J Neurosurg Pediatr 2021;1–9.

52. Kralik SF, Yasrebi M, Supakul N, et al. Diagnostic Performance of Ultrafast Brain MRI for Evaluation of Abusive Head Trauma. AJNR Am J Neuroradiol 2017;38:807–13.

53. Sheridan DC, Newgard CD, Selden NR, et al. QuickBrain MRI for the detection of acute pediatric traumatic brain injury. J Neurosurg Pediatr 2017;19:259–64.

54. Lindberg DM, Stence NV, Grubenhoff JA, et al. Feasibility and Accuracy of Fast MRI Versus CT for Traumatic Brain Injury in Young Children. Pediatrics 2019;144. https://doi.org/10.1542/peds.2019-0419.

55. Kabakus IM, Spampinato MV, Knipfing M, et al. Fast Brain Magnetic Resonance Imaging With Half-Fourier Acquisition With Single-Shot Turbo Spin Echo Sequence in Detection of Intracranial Hemorrhage and Skull Fracture in General Pediatric Patients: Preliminary Results. Pediatr Emerg Care 2021;37(12):e1168–72.

56. García-Bermejo P, Castano C, Davalos A. Multimodal CT versus MRI in Selecting Acute Stroke Patients for Endovascular Treatment. Interv Neurol 2013;1:65–76.

57. Chalela JA, Kidwell CS, Nentwich LM, et al. Magnetic resonance imaging and computed tomography in emergency assessment of patients with suspected acute stroke: a prospective comparison. Lancet 2007;369:293–8.

58. Emeriau S, Serre I, Toubas O, et al. Can diffusion-weighted imaging-fluid-attenuated inversion recovery mismatch (positive diffusion-weighted imaging/negative fluid-attenuated inversion recovery) at 3 Tesla identify patients with stroke at <4.5 hours? Stroke 2013;44:1647–51.

59. Gonzalez RG, Copen WA, Schaefer PW, et al. The Massachusetts General Hospital acute stroke imaging algorithm: an experience and evidence based approach. J Neurointerv Surg 2013;5 Suppl 1(Suppl 1):i7–12.

60. Nael K, Khan R, Choudhary G, et al. Six-minute magnetic resonance imaging protocol for evaluation of acute ischemic stroke: pushing the boundaries. Stroke 2014;45:1985–91.

61. van Pul C, Roos FG, Derksen OS, et al. A comparison study of multishot vs. single-shot DWI-EPI in the neonatal brain: reduced effects of ghosting compared to adults. Magn Reson Imaging 2004;22:1169–80.

62. Bilgic B, Chatnuntawech I, Manhard MK, et al. Highly accelerated multishot echo planar imaging through synergistic machine learning and joint reconstruction. Magn Reson Med 2019;82:1343–58.

63. Tabari A, Clifford B, Goncalves FALM, et al. Ultrafast Brain Imaging with Deep Learning Multi-Shot EPI: Preliminary Clinical Evaluation. Magnetom Flash 2021;79:66–70.

64. Moulin T, Sablot D, Vidry E, et al. Impact of emergency room neurologists on patient management and outcome. Eur Neurol 2003;50:207–14.

65. Kazmierczak PM, Dührsen M, Forbrig R, et al. Ultrafast Brain Magnetic Resonance Imaging in Acute Neurological Emergencies: Diagnostic Accuracy and Impact on Patient Management. Invest Radiol 2020;55:181–9.

66. Prakkamakul S, Witzel T, Huang S, et al. Ultrafast Brain MRI: Clinical Deployment and Comparison to Conventional Brain MRI at 3T. J Neuroimaging 2016;26:503–10.

67. Sprenger T, Kits A, Norbeck O, et al. NeuroMix-A single-scan brain exam. Magn Reson Med 2022;87(5):2178–93.

68. Redd V, Levin S, Toerper M, et al. Effects of fully accessible magnetic resonance imaging in the emergency department. Acad Emerg Med 2015;22:741–9.

69. Korley FK, Pham JC, Kirsch TD. Use of advanced radiology during visits to US emergency departments for injury-related conditions, 1998-2007, 1998-2007. JAMA 2010;304:1465–71.

70. Smith-Bindman R, Miglioretti DL, Larson EB. Rising use of diagnostic medical imaging in a large integrated health system. Health Aff (Millwood) 2008;27:1491–502.

71. Baker L, Birnbaum H, Geppert J, et al. The Relationship Between Technology Availability And Health Care Spending. Health Aff 2003;22(Suppl1):W3–537. https://doi.org/10.1377/hlthaff.w3.537.

72. McDonald RJ, Schwartz KM, Eckel LJ, et al. The effects of changes in utilization and technological advancements of cross-sectional imaging on radiologist workload. Acad Radiol 2015;22:1191–8.

73. Boland GW, Duszak R Jr. Modality Access: Strategies for Optimizing Throughput. J Am Coll Radiol 2015;12:1073–5.

74. Coffey AM, Truong ML, Chekmenev EY. Low-field MRI can be more sensitive than high-field MRI. J Magn Reson 2013;237:169–74.

75. Marques JP, Simonis FFJ, Webb AG. Low-field MRI: An MR physics perspective. J Magn Reson Imaging 2019;49:1528–42.

76. O'Reilly T, Webb A. Deconstructing and reconstructing MRI hardware. J Magn Reson 2019;306:134–8.

77. Cooley CZ, McDaniel PC, Stockmann JP, et al. A portable scanner for magnetic resonance imaging of the brain. Nat Biomed Eng 2021;5(3):229–39.

78. Cooley CZ, Stockmann JP, Armstrong BD, et al. Two-dimensional imaging in a lightweight portable MRI scanner without gradient coils. Magn Reson Med 2015;73:872–83.

79. Blumler P. Proposal for a permanent magnet system with a constant gradient mechanically adjustable in direction and strength. Concepts Magn Reson 2016;46(1):41–8.

80. Ren ZH, Maréchal L, Luo W, et al. Magnet array for a portable magnetic resonance imaging system. in IEEE International Microwave workshop series on RF and Wireless Technologies for Biomedical and Healthcare Applications (IMWSD-BIO). 2015. Taipei, Taiwan.

81. Ren ZH, Obruchkov S, Lu DW, et al. A low-field portable magnetic resonance imaging system for head imaging. in Progress in Electromagnetics

Research Symposium - Fall (PIERS - FALL). 2017. Singapore.

82. McDaniel PC, Cooley CZ, Stockmann JP, et al. The MR Cap: A single-sided MRI system designed for potential point-of-care limited field-of-view brain imaging. Magn Reson Med 2019;82:1946–60.

83. Vogel MW, Giorni A, Vegh V, et al. Rotatable Small Permanent Magnet Array for Ultra-Low Field Nuclear Magnetic Resonance Instrumentation: A Concept Study. PLoS One 2016;11:e0157040.

84. Runge, V.M. and J.T. Heverhagen, The Next Generation- Advanced Design Low-field MR Systems. Magnetom Flash, siemens.com/magnetom-world, 2020. special issue: Head-to-toe imaging: p. 11-19.

85. Mohr C. The Siemens Ultra High-field program MAGNETOM Allegra and Trio 3T MR The next dimension in clinical and research MR systems. Siemens Magnetom Flash 2002;1:21–2.

86. Foo T, et al. Dedicated High-Performance, Lightweight, Low-Cryogen Compact 3.0T MRI System for Advanced Brain Imaging. in Proc. of the ISMRM. Singapore. May 7-13, 2016.

87. Campbell-Washburn AE, Ramasawmy R, Restivo MC, et al. Opportunities in Interventional and Diagnostic Imaging by Using High-Performance Low-Field-Strength MRI. Radiology 2019;293:384–93.

88. Panther A, et al. A dedicated head-only MRI scanner for point-of-care imaging. in Proc. of the ISMRM. Montreal, May 11-16, 2019.

89. Stainsby J, et al. Imaging at 0.5T with high-performance system components, in Proc of the ISMRM. *Montreal, May*, 11-16, 2019

90. Stainsby J, et al. High-performance diffusion imaging on a 0,5T system. in Proc of the ISMRM. *Montreal, May*, 11-16, 2019

91. Vaughan J, et al. Progress toward a portable MRI system for human brain imaging. in Proc of the ISMRM. Singapore. May 7-13, 2016.

92. Welch EB, By S, Chen G, et al. Use environments and clinical feasibility of portable point-of-care bedside brain MRI. in Proc. of the ISMRM. 2020. virtual.

93. Sheth KN, Mazurek MH, Yuen MM, et al. Assessment of Brain Injury Using Portable, Low-Field Magnetic Resonance Imaging at the Bedside of Critically Ill Patients. JAMA Neurol 2021;78(1):41.

94. Cooley CZ, Haskell MW, Cauley SF, et al. Design of sparse Halbach magnet arrays for portable MRI using a genetic algorithm. IEEE Trans Magn 2018;54. https://doi.org/10.1109/TMAG.2017.2751001.

95. McDaniel P, Cooley C, Stockmann J, et al. Numerically optimized design for a low-cost, lightweight 86mT whole-brain magnet. in Proc of the ISMRM. 2019. Montreal Canada.

96. Ali TS, Tourell MC, Hugo HJ, et al. Transverse relaxation-based assessment of mammographic density and breast tissue composition by single-sided portable NMR. Magn Reson Med 2019;82:1199–213.

97. Tourell MC, Ali TS, Hugo HJ, et al. T1 -based sensing of mammographic density using single-sided portable NMR. Magn Reson Med 2018;80:1243–51.

98. Colucci LA, Corapi KM, Li M, et al. Fluid assessment in dialysis patients by point-of-care magnetic relaxometry. Sci Transl Med 2019;11. https://doi.org/10.1126/scitranslmed.aau1749.

99. Li M, Vassiliou CC, Colucci LA, et al. (1)H nuclear magnetic resonance (NMR) as a tool to measure dehydration in mice. NMR Biomed 2015;28:1031–9.

100. Perlo J, Casanova F, Blumich B. 3D imaging with a single-sided sensor: an open tomograph. J Magn Reson 2004;166:228–35.

101. He Z, He W, Wu J, et al. The Novel Design of a Single-Sided MRI Probe for Assessing Burn Depth. Sensors (Basel) 2017;17. https://doi.org/10.3390/s17030526.